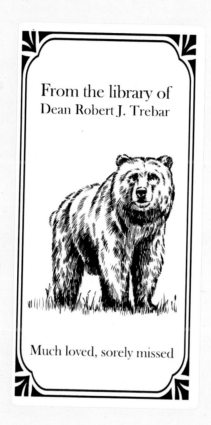

From the library of
Dean Robert J. Trebar

Much loved, sorely missed

ESSENTIALS OF ABDOMINAL WALL
HERNIAS

IN
MEMORY OF
THE FATHER OF INGUINAL HERNIA SURGERY

EDOARDO BASSINI
1844-1924

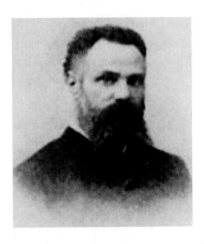

*"It will appear excess of daring to write at the present day
of the radical treatment of hernias"*

— Edoardo Bassini, 1890

*"The last chapter on the history of the groin anatomy and
operative repair of hernia defects has not yet been written"*

— Dr Lloyd Nyhus, decades after Edoardo Bassini

"The final word on hernia will probably never be written"

— Sir John Bruce, 1964

ESSENTIALS OF ABDOMINAL WALL
HERNIAS

VINOD KUMAR NIGAM
MS, FICS (USA), FIAGES
Consultant General & Laparoscopic Surgeon
The Apollo Clinic Gurgaon
Gurgaon, Haryana (INDIA)

SIDDHARTH NIGAM
MBBS, MS (General Surgery)
Consultant General Surgeon
The Apollo Clinic Gurgaon
Gurgaon, Haryana (INDIA)

I.K. International Publishing House Pvt. Ltd.
NEW DELHI • BANGALORE

DISCLAIMER

It is to confirm that the accuracy of the information presented in this book is based on generally accepted practices. However, authors and publisher are not responsible for any errors/omissions or any consequences arising due to the application of information provided in this book. Application of this information in a particular situation remains the responsibility of the professional using it.

The authors and publisher have checked the sources of materials, believed to be reliable and accord with acceptable practice and standard at the time of publication.

Published by

I.K. International Publishing House Pvt. Ltd.
S-25, Green Park Extension
Uphaar Cinema Market
New Delhi - 110 016 (India)
E-mail: ik_in@vsnl.net

ISBN 978-81-89866-93-8

Published by Krishan Makhijani for I.K. International Publishing House Pvt. Ltd., S-25, Green Park Extension, Uphaar Cinema Market, New Delhi - 110 016 and Printed by Rekha Printers Pvt. Ltd., Okhla Industrial Area, Phase II, New Delhi - 110 020.

Foreword

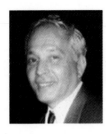 Those of us who know Dr Vinod Kumar Nigam are fully aware of his compulsive involvement and passion in the study of Abdominal Wall Hernias well for over a decade. Through this book his vast background and profound knowledge and understanding of this subject will be available to all surgeons interested in this subject, which in view of the overall prevalence of abdominal wall hernia, ipso facto includes every single surgeon.

Through historical background, detailed anatomy replete with explanatory line drawings, classification, clinical presentation of every variety of abdominal hernia and a lengthy discussion on operative treatment this book covers the complete gamut of hernia surgery. Dr Nigam's meticulous study is manifest in the minutiae of details, some of which may need correction. Seventeen procedures are described for tissue repair and fourteen for hernioplasty!

The language throughout is simple, sentences are brief and the coverage is in sequential point form, making the book both readable and educative. Particularly enjoyable are the quotations at the beginning of each chapter. There are numerous treatises on abdominal wall hernia, some of them very profound. This book is not profound – it is a book for the working surgeon. Dr Nigam's book on *Essentials of Abdominal Wall Hernias* will be a boon to the postgraduate student and is a credit to Indian surgical literature.

1st April 2008
Tehemton E. Udwadia
Emeritus Professor of Surgery, Grant Medical College and J.J. Hospital
Consultant Surgeon, Head, Department of M.A.S. Hinduja Hospital
Consultant Surgeon, Parsee General Hospital and Breach Candy Hospital, Mumbai

Foreword

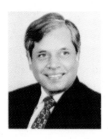

Hernia repair is one of the most commonly performed surgical procedures by a practising surgeon today. A hernia can be present at different ages, at different and sites at varying stages. Indeed, a surgeon practising hernia repairs has to necessarily possess a wide array of surgical repertoire and techniques. It is said that there are as many hernia repairs as there are surgeons. The gold standard in hernia repairs is not on the horizon yet. The numerous hernia repairs and techniques available can be bewildering and confusing to the busy practitioners.

We are witness to an era where hernia is represented by the Asia Pacific Hernia Society (APHS), American Hernia Society (AHS) and European Hernia Society (EHS). As President of APHS, it is a matter of great pride to write a foreword for an elegant textbook *Essentials of Abdominal Wall Hernias*.

I am aware that Dr V K Nigam has been a keen proponent of the art of hernia repair for several years. It is heartening to note that he has followed through with his passion to produce this textbook. An overview of the textbook reveals a well thought out plan and a lucid presentation of facts and details.

In the present era of specialization, we can envisage herniologists honing their skills to set up centers of excellence. I am certain that these surgeons would benefit from the insights and experience presented in the ensuing chapters. It is my desire that practising surgeons avail themselves of several suggestions and tips that have been presented in the book.

I congratulate the authors and publisher on a fine effort, which should go a long way in addressing many contentious issues with regard to hernia repair.

Dr Pradeep Chowbey
MS, MNAMS, FIMSA, FICS, FAIS, FACS
Padmashri Awarded by The President of India
Honorary Laparoscopic Surgeon to The President of India
Honorary Laparoscopic Surgeon to Armed Forces Medical Services (AFMS)
Doctor of Science (Honoris Causa)
Chairman - Minimal Access, Metabolic and Bariatric Surgery Centre,
Sir Ganga Ram Hospital, New Delhi (India)
President - Asia Pacific Hernia Society (APHS)
President - Obesity Surgery Society of India (OSSI)
Secretary General - Asia Pacific Bariatric Surgery Society(APBSS)

Foreword

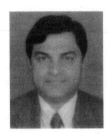

It is a pleasure to write about Dr V K Nigam and his most recent endeavour *Essentials of Abdominal Wall Hernias*. He is a very senior surgeon of National and International repute, well known for his innovative and original "Window Operation" for hydrocele which has been widely quoted and followed internationally and "Nigam's Reverse Curtain Hernioplasty", testimony of his keen interest and passionate involvement in the treatment of abdominal wall hernias.

Dr Nigam's decades of experience and knowledge about hernias are obvious in this book. The book has been written in an original and innovative style. He has made a commendable job in producing this book. Complex anatomy of the hernia has been simplified and made easy to understand by liberal use of diagrams, sketches and photographs in an exhaustive chapter. Other aspects of hernia have been comprehensively described in very well written chapters like aetiology, clinical features and contemporary management of abdominal wall hernias including the laparoscopic approach. The topic has been made so easy and interesting that even an undergraduate will find it a useful reading. On the other hand, the detailed and minute descriptions add to the knowledge of even a herniologist. The chapters on history, difficulties, important things, recent advances and arguments and controversies add extra flavor.

I congratulate Dr Nigam for producing such an excellent book and I am sure the monograph is going to be a landmark effort in the understanding and management of hernias and will be a valuable reading material for undergraduate, postgraduates students, practising surgeons and herniologists alike for years to come.

11th April 2008

Dr A.K. Kriplani
MS (Surgery)
Senior Consultant
Inderprastha Apollo Hospital, New Delhi
Laparoscopic, G. I. & Bariatric Surgeon
President, Indian Association of Gastrointestinal Endo Surgeons

Foreword

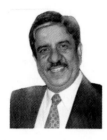

In the field of general surgery, hernia surgery remains the most common surgical procedure performed, with inguinal hernias leading the pack. While surgeons spent the early part of the twentieth century improving the technique of primary repair, the latter half was focused on developing techniques of mesh repair, minimizing incisions, and maximizing comfort –thanks to the controversy generated by laparoscopic repair! Despite many clinical trials, there is still no final consensus on timing of treatment, technique to be used, material, and mesh position.

Clinical advances of any significance cannot occur in isolation. As regards laparoscopic herniology, minimally invasive surgeons must join forces with their open surgical colleagues, so as to advance the field together. Free discussion and close collaboration are necessary to ensure that long-established surgical principles are adhered to, and outcomes are evaluated critically on an ongoing basis. Only by fulfilling its promise of being **"minimally invasive – maximally effective"**, will laparoscopy truly enter the mainstream.

Change must not be embraced just because it is different, or new. The tried and trusted must not be cast aside until its novel replacement has undergone an honest, duly diligent evaluation. Following this dictum, laparoscopy is being gradually incorporated into mainstream surgery, with appropriate caution and healthy, constructive critique.

Dr Vinod Kumar Nigam, with all his passion for perfection, has placed this monograph at an appropriate moment to bridge the gap. The essence of the book is the line diagrams which he has drawn with all the attention to detail. Dr Nigam has bundled his extensive experience with literature search for the ultimate benefit to the patient (through open as well as laparoscopic surgeons).

Essentials of Abdominal Wall Hernias is organised in a logical and readable way. The coverage is comprehensive; the teaching value behind it is priceless. I am particularly impressed by the choice and range of topics.

This book is directed to students (learners) of surgery at all levels from the surgical intern to the well established surgical practitioner. There are enough pearls of wisdom contained herein to enhance the readers' technical ability to treat and heal patients.

I look forward to the fruit that will continue to spring forth from the education and dissemination of this information.

11th April, 2008

Parveen Bhatia
Consultant Laparoscopic Surgeon & Medical Director
Global Hospital & Endosurgery Institute
New Delhi

Preface

Surgery (from greek *chirurgical*, and latin *chirurgial* meaning 'hand work') is the medical speciality that treats diseases or injuries by operative manual and instrumental treatment.

Hernia is one of the most important subjects in the field of general and laparoscopic surgeries.

This book is organized like a monograph using our patients to illustrate current surgical techniques that we use on a regular basis to treat various types of hernias. It strongly reflects the comprehensive, coordinated treatment plan used by us and various other excellent treatment centers. In putting together this material, we had several goals in mind. First was to educate health professionals about the new and rapidly growing field of Hernia Surgery. Second was to provide a reference for patients and their relatives, concerning treatments available and the type of results that might be expected. And finally, to reflect our own experience and philosophy as related to the treatment of this complex problem.

Laparoscopic surgery is a new technique of Hernia Surgery. It has many benefits over Open Hernia Surgery.

The book has been divided in five sections. **Section 1** presents the historical development, **Section 2** describes the anatomy of groin, **Section 3** provides clinical features of various types of hernias, **Section 4** explains various operative techniques and their complications, **Section 5** deals with allied subjects of hernia as well as clarifies all the doubts in the mind of surgeons and patients.

Due to its grounding in theory and research evidence, the book is well-designed for undergraduates, postgraduates, residents, general surgeons in training as well as trained surgeons, both general and laparoscopic. This book provides both theoretical and practical knowledge of hernia and its surgery.

Unfortunately, we could not stress on left-handed surgeons, as now some surgical instrument manufacturers are making instruments for left-handed surgeons also. On rough account, left-handed surgeons comprise 7%–9% of all surgeons worldwide.

We have purposely repeated some basic points which we feel are essential, as Moshe Schein also believes that "repetition of important points is critical in adult education".

VINOD KUMAR NIGAM
SIDDHARTH NIGAM

ALL INDIA INSTITUTE OF MEDICAL SCIENCES
Ansari Nagar, New Delhi-110029, India

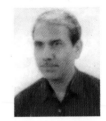

Dr. M.C. Misra MBBS, MS, FACS, FAMS, FRCS (Glasg.)
Professor & Head, DEPARTMENT OF SURGICAL DISCIPLINES
HEAD, MINIMAL ACCESS SURGERY UNIT,
ALL INDIA INSTITUTE OF MEDICAL SCIENCES
ANSARI NAGAR, NEW DELHI-110029
mcmisra@gmail.com

19th April 2008

Book review

At the outset the book "Essentials of Abdominal hernias" authored by Dr. Vinod Kumar Nigam and Sidharth Nigam and published by I.K. International Publishing House Pvt. Ltd. is likely to find space in personal library of any general surgeon practicing surgery of hernia.

Dr. Nigam has put in tremendous efforts to review embryology and anatomy of groin hernia extensively. He has not left any stone unturned when it came to give due recognition to those who have made scientific contribution in the understanding of this common surgical disease. He has been working on the manuscript and format of the book for number of years. He has been participating in different meetings on hernia both national and international and obtaining views of many specialists in the field of hernia.

Dr. Nigam has put in extra efforts to create his own artwork simplifying understanding of anatomy of groin hernia extensively. He has created himself over 350 line drawings depicting various facets of groinhernia anatomy and pathobiology. This book also has over 300 other pictures on groin and other abdominal wall hernia.

Of particular interest is the detailed description of various hernia classifications by renowned herniologists. These classifications have been explained on the basis of anatomy and Dr. Nigam has simplified the understanding for both undergraduate and postgraduate students through his original line drawings (artwork). Authors have tried to incorporate all-important aspects of anatomy, pathobiology and management of different abdominal wall hernias. The authors have ensured recent information being incorporated in the book by extensively reviewing published literature and quoting all relevant references.

I feel that the book is much different then the available texts in the market and libraries and offers simplified version of understanding the complexities of herniology for the readers. The book "Essentials of abdominal Hernias" must find place in the collection of average general surgeon dealing with this surgical disease in his or her clinical practice. Dr. Nigam's original artwork (line drawing) makes it more interesting and attractive for the learner.

I congratulate authors and the publishers for their effort for creating this masterpiece and wish them good luck for the success of the book.

Residence : C-II/11, Ansari Nagar, New Delhi-110029, **Phone** Res. : 0091-11-26589655, 26594531
Office : 0091-11-26594776, **Mobile** : 0091-9811896246, 9868397701, **Fax** : 0091-11-26588663, 26588641
E-mail : mcmisra@gmail.com, misramahesh@hotmail.com, mcmisra@aiims.ac.in, kkcorporation@mac.com

A Word from a Herniologist

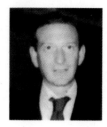

In the last few decades, the world of Hernia has been revolutionised by the advancement of technologies and shift in medical and surgical practice towards a minimally invasive approach. The surgical repair has reached the gold standard in the 90's with the tension-free repair and in the last years also the hectic and challenging cure of incisional and ventral hernia has switched toward a minimal invasive approach by using laparoscopic repair. Initial experience seems very attractive and clinical results in selected cases showed excellent clinical outcome.

The reason of the adoption of these new approaches has been favoured by the motto that overall "Patient safety is paramount" in term of surgical technique but also in terms of low complications and recurrence rate. Soon after the use of the mesh for hernia repair, new and different surgical approach appear in the operating theatre from open anterior technique to posterior repair from endoscopic preperitoneal repair to the laparoscopic technique, all with good results and low complications rate if performed by surgeon with great skill and experience. Laparoscopic approach since the starting is lagging behind because of the different anatomy and difficult to teach and apparently to learn. I am really glad, my good friend Dr Vinod has written a comprehensive book on hernia that ranges from the anatomy (thanks to make it easy to learn) to the classification from the treatment to managing complications.

I believe that this book is dedicated to hernia, it will be a must and a reference point for junior and trained surgeons who want to deepen in the hernia field. It represents a concise and complete approach to hernia with excellent description, diagrams, drawings and collection of pictures.

I welcome and greatly recommend this book to all practising surgeons.

2nd April, 2008

Davide Lomanto
MD, PhD, FAMS (Surg.)
Secretary General of the Asia Pacific Hernia Society (APHS)
Director, Minimally Invasive Surgical Centre (MISC)
Director, Khoo Teck Puat Advanced Surgery Training Centre (ASTC)
Senior Consultant Surgeon
Department of Surgery
Yong Loo Lin School of Medicine
National University of Singapore
Singapore 119074

A Word from a Herniologist

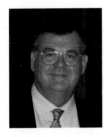 Last year I've met Dr Vinod Nigam at an International Meeting in Singapore where he was introducing his personal hernia repair procedure to audience in a very enthusiastic way. I appreciated a lot Dr Nigam's enthusiasm to do it. He was proud to show to colleagues the fruit of his work. He believe on it. Now with this textbook Dr Nigam not only introduce himself as new hernia repair supporter, but also as passionate, keen and clear-minded lover of the abdominal wall hernia surgery.

I appreciated in this textbook the scientific exactness in describing both anatomy and surgical steps, always in a precise, synthetic and didactic way. Very simple and clear are drawings and schemes that help to better understand anatomy and surgical techniques.

It's a book that doesn't waste one's time on useless and unnecessary descriptions, but sometimes enriches the reader with an historical information, a learned quotation or a gossip news, like that ones on Madonna or Harrison Ford.

The hernia rate is the same around the world and its distribution is absolutely democratic because it doesn't spare anybody.

Many congratulations again to Dr Nigam for his big passion for hernia repair and for his wide learning that has come off in this book *Essentials of Abdominal Wall Hernias*. It is a text that could be read very easily and that is very useful both for experts and for beginners in this so much involving field of the surgery.

From Italy I wish to Dr Nigam and to his textbook all the best in your wonderful country and all around the world.

13th March, 2008

Andrea Coda, MD
"The Hernia Centre of Turin", Director
Clinica Cellini
Via Cellini 5, 10125 Turin, Italy

Acknowledgements

Though, dreamt over a decade by us to write a book on hernia, it has materialized now. The foundation of the book is our experience in clinical and surgery in India, Yemen Arab Republic, USA and UK.

When we were students of surgery, we strongly felt the deficiency of a "complete book" on abdominal wall hernias. This inspired us to write this book.

We would like to remember our teachers Late Prof. Tara Chand, former Professor and Head of the Department of Surgery, GSVM Medical College, Kanpur; and Dr Hari P Gautam, renowed Cadiothoracic Surgeon, former UGC Chairman, former Vice-Chancellor, Banaras Hindu University and Dr B-C Roy Awardee, for their constant persuasion to write a book on hernia.

We owe a lot to Dr Parveen Bhatia, Medical Director and Laparoscopic Surgeon, Bhatia Global Hospital and Endosurgery Institute, New Delhi, and Honorary Secretary, IAGES for his valuable advises and for providing laparoscopic picture to be put on in this book.

We are indebted to Dr Pradeep Chowbey, Chairman, Department of Minimal Access Surgery, Sir Ganga Ram Hospital, New Delhi, for providing pictures of operative proceedings of his patients to be used in this book.

Our heartfelt thanks for Dr Asok Kumar Bose, former Professor and Head of the Department of Anatomy, MKCG Medical College, Berhampur, Orissa for helping us during preparation of chapter on anatomy.

We also wish to thank Kunal Nigam for helping us in preparation of parts pertaining to anatomy.

We are indebted to Mr Mukul Sharma, Consultant Editor, Times of India, and Science Writer, for enabling us to write "epilogue" and for his words of encouragement and inspiration to embark upon this book.

Words of encouragement, friendship and good wishes of our colleagues is greatly acknowledged.

We are greatly indebted to our family members for giving us everything to realise our potential.

And special thanks to Mr. Krishan Makhijani, the publisher and his entire editorial and production team.

VINOD KUMAR NIGAM
SIDDHARTH NIGAM

Contents

Abbreviations

ACS	=	Abdominal Compartment Syndrome
ASIS	=	Anterior Superior Iliac Spine
AWH	=	Abdominal Wall Hernia
BPH	=	Benign Prostatic Hyperplasia
CAPD	=	Continuous Ambulatory Peritoneal Dialysis
CBD	=	Common Bile Duct
CE	=	Clinical Examination
CF	=	Cremasteric Fascia
CL	=	Cooper's Ligament
CM	=	Cremaster Muscle
COPA	=	Cuffed Oro-Pharyngeal Airway
CT	=	Conjoint Tendon
CVS	=	Cardio Vascular System
DD	=	Direct Defect
DIH	=	Direct Inguinal Hernia
DIR	=	Deep Inguinal Ring
DRE	=	Digital Rectal Examination
DS	=	Direct Sac
DVT	=	Deep Vein Thrombosis
EH	=	Epigastric Hernia
E.I.V.	=	External Iliac Vessels
EOA	=	External Oblique Aponeurosis
ESF	=	External Spermatic Fascia
e-PTFE	=	Expanded Poly Tetra Fluoro Ethylene
FA	=	Femoral Artery
FBGFN	=	Femoral Branch of GFN
FC	=	Femoral Canal
FH	=	Femoral Hernia
FN	=	Femoral Nerve
FR	=	Femoral Ring
FT	=	Fascia Transversalis
FV	=	Femoral Vein
GA	=	General Anaesthesia
GBGFN	=	Genital Branch of GFN
GFN	=	Genito Femoral Nerve
GH	=	Gluteal Hernia
GPRVS	=	Giant Prosthesis for Reinforcement of Visceral Sac
GSV	=	Great Saphenous Vein
ICF	=	Internal Spermatic Fascia
IEV	=	Inferior Epigastric Vessels
IH	=	Incisional Hernia
IHN	=	Ilio Hypogastric Nerve
IIH	=	Indirect Inguinal Hernia
IIN	=	Ilio Inguinal Nerve
IL	=	Inguinal Ligament
ILH	=	Inferior Lumbar Hernia
IOM	=	Internal Oblique Muscle

IPOM	=	Intra Peritoneal Onlay Mesh
IPT	=	Iliopubic Tract
IS	=	Indirect Sac
IUL	=	Intra Uterine Life
IVC	=	Inferior Vena Cava
LA	=	Local Anaesthesia
LCNT	=	Lateral Cutaneous Nerve of Thigh
LFCT	=	Lateral Femoral Cutaneous Nerve
LH	=	Littre's Hernia
LL	=	Lacunar Ligament
LMA	=	Laryngeal Mask Airway
LS	=	Linea Semilunaris
LSCS	=	Lower Segment Caesarian Section
MAL	=	Mid Axillary Line
MAS	=	Minimal Access Surgery
OP	=	Operation Theatre
OH	=	Obstructed Hernia
OR	=	Operating Room
PB	=	Pubic Bone
PC	=	Pubic Crest
PDPH	=	Post Dural Puncture Headache
PH	=	Perineal Hernia
PONV	=	Post Operative Nausea and Vomiting
PS	=	Pubic Symphysis
PT	=	Pubic Tubercle
PUD	=	Peptic Ulcer Disease
PV	=	Portal Vein
RM	=	Rectus Muscle
RS	=	Rectus Sheath
QOL	=	Quality Of Life
SC	=	Spermatic Cord
SF	=	Scarpa's Fascia
SH	=	Spigelian Hernia
SIR	=	Superficial Inguinal Ring
SLH	=	Superior Lumbar hernia
SO	=	Saphenous Opening
SVC	=	Superior Vena Cava
SVH	=	Supravesical Hernia
TA	=	Testicular Artery
TAA	=	Transverse Abdominis Aponeurosis
TAAA	=	Transverse Abdominal Aponeurotic Arch
TAM	=	Transverse Abdominis Muscle
TAPP	=	Trans Abdominal Pre Peritoneal
TEP	=	Total Extra Peritoneal
TNS	=	Transient Neurological Syndrome
TV	=	Testicular Vessels
UH	=	Umbilical Hernia
VD	=	Vas Deferens
XP	=	Xiphisternum

Section 1
HISTORY

"O God
Great and Noble are those scientific
judgements that serve the purpose of
preserving health & lives of thy
creatures"
- Moses Bin Mirmon

1 Introduction

*"Arguably the most commonly performed general surgery procedure, ----
unfortunately, the attention given to this problem by the average general
surgeon has not always been consistent with the frequency with which it is
encountered"*
— Robert D Kugel (2007, Mastery of Surgery)

"All types of groin hernias are at risks of incarceration and strangulation"
— Patric J. Javid & David Brooks

*"To avoid recurrence,
A hernia should be operated when it is small, reducible and painless and not
when it becomes large, irreducible and painful*
— Author

HERNIA

"It is an abnormal protrusion of a viscus or a part of a viscus through an opening or weakness in the wall of the cavity that contains it."

Hernia is a Latin word which means a "tear or rupture", in Greek it means either an "offshoot" or "a budding" or "a bulge".

Although, hernia can occur at various sites of body, it is most commonly observed in the abdominal wall, particularly the inguinal region[1] (Figs. 1.1 & 1.2). Inguinal hernia is so common that when one talks about hernia it is generally taken as an inguinal hernia. Hernia occurs only in humans and does not occur in any other mammal. It is the penalty we pay for being given erect posture. Hernia may be

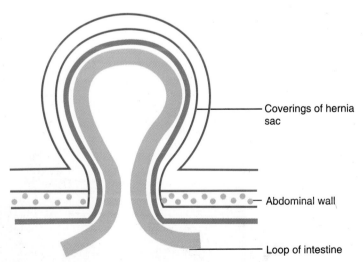

Fig. 1.1. A hernia, protrusion of loop of intestine through a weak area of abdominal wall.

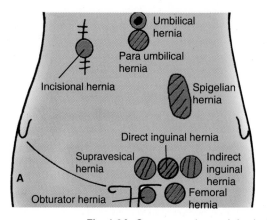

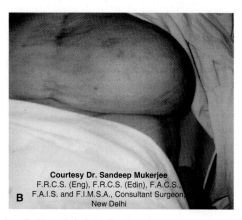

Courtesy Dr. Sandeep Mukerjee
F.R.C.S. (Eng), F.R.C.S. (Edin), F.A.C.S.,
F.A.I.S. and F.I.M.S.A., Consultant Surgeon,
New Delhi

Fig. 1.2A. Common and rare abdominal wall hernias, **B.** Huge left Spigelian hernia.

a protrusion of brain through foramen magnum or herniation of a muscle through a weak part of its covering fascia.

A lot of progress has been made in understanding the anatomy of hernia-prone regions of anterior abdominal wall and their treatment. Herniology is still developing and new methods of hernia treatment are being invented to reduce recurrence, post-operative complications and discomfort to the patient. Search is on for a "*Zero Recurrence*" hernia repair procedure.

The surgical treatment of a hernia was brutal in earlier days but the treatment changed in the last century and has developed at a fast pace in the last 20 years. Though the references to the surgical treatment of inguinal hernia date back to the first century; however, formal descriptions of hernia repair did not appear until the 15th century.[2]

Collectively, inguinal, femoral, umbilical and epigastric hernias represent the most common group of major operations performed by general surgeons.[3] Abdominal wall hernia can be either small or very big (Figs. 1.3 & 1.4).

Inguinal hernia is the commonest hernia, 73% of all abdominal wall hernias.

Femoral hernia is about 17% of all abdominal wall hernias.

Umbilical and paraumbilical hernias are 8.5% of all abdominal wall hernias.

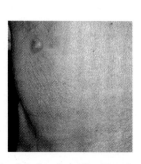

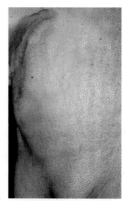

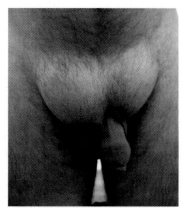

Fig. 1.3. Small umbilical hernia.   **Fig. 1.4.** Big incisional hernia.   **Fig. 1.5.** Big bilateral inguinal hernias.

Rare hernias are 1.5% of all abdominal wall hernias (Figs. 1.2A & B). Occurrence of incisional hernia is next to inguinal hernia.

It is important to know the detailed anatomy of anterior abdominal wall to avoid complications while placing ports and doing laparoscopic dissection or open tension-free repair.

> Laparoscopic hernia repair has just 5-15% market share, which is low as compared to laparoscopic cholecystectomy which has more than 93% share. It is due to the new developments in open hernia repair techniques which still have 85-95% share of the hernia market.[4]

Hernia represents the commonest surgical ailment and has a wide spectrum of study.[5]

As the surgical repair of the inguinal hernia is the most common general surgical procedure performed today[6], so every general surgeon should know about various aspects of it.

NOTE

"Surgeons not only must be masters of their crafts but also are responsible for identifying and learning new techniques, that are being introduced at an ever-increasing rate. They must overcome the instinctual mistrust of the new and, at the same time, avoid overenthusiastic, uncritical adoption of unproven procedures. Today's surgeons must also carefully assess and select the procedures and technologies that they will have time to learn and that will complement their practices and interests. More new things are coming along than any single individual can learn and practise with expertise, which makes general surgery a specialty with relative, as opposed to specifically, defined boundaries."[7]

KEY POINT

Surgery i s the only cure for hernia, as it is due to loss of structural integrity at musculo-tendinous layer.[8]

REFERENCES

1. **Townsend B** *et al.,* (2004). Sabiston textbook of surgery, 17th edition, **2**, p. 1199.
2. **Robert J, Fitzgibbons** *et al.,* (2005). Schwartz's principles of surgery, 8th edition, p. 1353.
3. **Rutkow IM.,** (1997). Surgical operations in the United States, then (1983) and now (1994): *Arch Surg.* 132: 983–90.
4. **Rodrique Z, Cuellar E, Villeta R, Ruiz P, Alcalde J.,** *et al.,* (2005). National project for management of clinical processes. Surgical treatment of inguinal hernia. *Cir. Esp.* 77: 194-202.
5. **Udwadia TE.,** (2006). Editorial, Surgery for hernia; Quo vadis? *Journal of Minimal Access Surgery,* **2 & 3,** p. 104.
6. **Rutkow I, Robbins AW.,** (1993). Demographic, classificatory, and socioeconomic aspects of hernia repair in the United States, *Surg. Clin. North Am.* 73: 413.
7. **Swanstrom LL.,** (2000). Laparoscopic hernia repairs: The importance of cost as an outcome measurement at the Century's end, *Surg. Clin. North Am.,* **80,** 4: L. 1341–1348.
8. **Franz MG.,** (2008). The biology of hernia formation, *Surg. Clin. N. Am.,* **88,** 1-15.

Historical Background

Hernia was mentioned in the Egyptian papyrus of Ebers in 1552 BC.

- Hernia surgery is being performed in India from ancient days. Hindus were known to use an abdominal or a preperitoneal approach for cases of strangulated hernia.[2]
- Hippocrates (460-375 BC) described umbilical hernia.
- Aulus Cornelius Celsus (25 BC- AD 50) was a Roman encyclopedist and possibly, although probably not, a physician. His work, the "De Medicina" is still remembered. Celsus is credited with recording the cardinal signs of inflammation: calor (warmth), dolor (pain), tumor (swelling) and rubor (redness and hyperaemia). He described the reduction and closure of umbilical hernia. He also treated and described inguinal hernia.

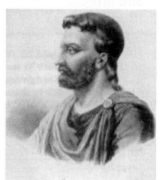

"Performed first surgical repair of umbilical hernia"
Aulus Cornelius Celsus, Roman Physician

- Heliodorus was the one who operated cases of inguinal hernia for the first time by properly dissecting the hernia sac from the spermatic cord structures.

- It was only in the late 18th century that articles started coming about anatomy, clinical features and operative procedures of hernia. It is known as the *"Age of Dissection"*.[3]

- Galen (131-201 AD), a Greek physician is second only to Hippocrates of Cos in importance to the development of medicine. He gave the concept that hernia occurs due to rupture of peritoneum and it should be treated with surgical repair.
- In 7th century, Paulus of Aegina described the operation and reduction of hernia.
- Guy de Chauliac, in 1363, differentiated femoral hernia from inguinal hernia.
- Franco, in 1556, described the use of "grooved hernia dissector" to cut the neck of hernia sac in strangulated hernia.

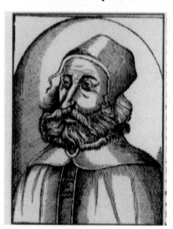

"Surgery is the ready motion of steady and experienced hands"
-Galen, Greek Physician

- Kaspar Stromayr in 1559 wrote how to differentiate direct inguinal hernia from indirect inguinal hernia.
- During 15th century and even later the treatment of hernia was very crude and brutal, as castration and cauterization were in practice. It was due to the total ignorance of the anatomy of the groin.

- Galilio suffered from hernia for long time.
- Michaelangelo was also suffering from hernia.
- Lord Nelson of United Kingdom suffered from a hernia after he was hit in abdomen in Battle of Cape St. Vincent in 1797.
- Sir Astley Cooper, himself a master of anatomy and surgery of hernia suffered from inguinal hernia.
- Sir Winston Churchill, the hero of World War-II suffered from inguinal hernia for long. He used a truss for a very long time. He was operated for hernia by Dr. Thomas P. Dunhill.

- Ambroise Pare (1510-1590) was a French surgeon. He was the official royal surgeon for Henry II, Francis II, Charles IX and Henry III. He is regarded as the Father of Surgery by some. He was also a leader in surgical techniques, especially, the treatment of wounds. He used the hernia truss for the first time.
He was the one who stopped the practice of doing castration while performing herniotomy.

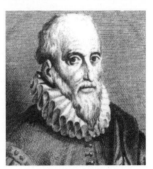

"I dressed him, and God healed him"
**- Ambroise Pare',
French Surgeon**

- In 1709, Jean Louis Petit (1674-1750), a French surgeon operated a case of strangulated hernia for the first time. He also described the inferior lumbar triangle, now called Petit's triangle. Inferior lumbar hernia comes out through Petit's triangle. His name is linked to an *external herniotomy'* which is done without incision into the sac.[2] *"What use is it to open the sac? The only purposes, that I know of, are to expose the intestine and omentum to remedy morbid changes ...."*   **- J. Louis Petit**
- Sir Percivall Pott (1714-1788), a surgeon in London, wrote "Treatise on Rupture" in 1756, about hernias. He was the first who described congenital hernia. His name is linked with Pott's disease (tubercular spondylitis), Pott's fracture (fracture of lower part of fibula and tibia with outward displacement of foot) and Pott's puffy tumour (Osteitis of skull).[2]
"All that can be done by surgery towards the cure of hernia, is to replace the prolapse body or bodies in the cavity belly and to prevent them from flipping out again"   **- Sir Percivall Pott**
- Pieter Camper (1722-1789) has born in the Netherlands. He was a great anatomist, anthropologist, artist, physician and surgeon. He described Camper's fascia and processus vaginalis for the first time. His illustrated work *"Icones herniarum"*, is a masterpiece of hernia anatomy. He was a doctor of philosophy as well as a doctor of medicine.
- Don Antonio de Gimbernat (1734-1816) was born in Terragona, Spain. He was sent to study surgery to Paris and London, by Charles III, King of Spain. He demonstrated to John Hunter, how to incise the lacunar ligament to facilitate the reduction of strangulated femoral hernia. Since then John Hunter started calling lacunar ligament as Gimbernat's ligament.[3]
"Why the treatment of it (hernia) remained in the hands of persons without education and without the smallest acquaintance either with human body or with the disorders they attempt to remedy"   **- Gimbernat,** He was opposed to quacks.

- August Gottlieb Richter (1742-1812) was born in Halle, Germany. He wrote a book on hernia *"Abhandlung Von den Brüchen"*. It was the best book on hernia at that time.[3] His name is linked with:
  - Richter's hernia
  - Richter's suture (interrupted silver sutures for wounds of intestine)
  - Monro-Richter line (a line passing from umbilicus to left ASIS)

  He thought that inflammation was a way to cure a reducible hernia.

  "A truss with a hard pad should be employed for this purpose, drawn sufficiently tight to cause pain"
  - Richter

- Antonio Scarpa, an Italian surgeon and anatomist (1747-1832), described the following structures:
  - Sliding hernia
  - Scarpa's fascia (deeper or membranous layer of superficial fascia)
  - Scarpa's triangle (femoral triangle)
  - Scarpa's sheath (cremasteric fascia)
  - Scarpa's ganglion (ganglion of eighth nerve in internal auditory meatus)
- Many of surgical successes can be traced back to the anatomical knowledge gained from 1750 to 1800.[4]

- Sir Astley Paston Cooper (1768-1841), first Baronet, an English surgeon and anatomist, made historical contributions to otology, vascular surgery, the anatomy and pathology of the mammary glands and testicles, and to the pathology and surgery of hernia.[5] He described:
  - Cooper's fascia
  - Cooper's ligament
  - Cooper's testis
  - Cooper's hernia
  - Fascia transversalis

  In 1804, he performed a successful herniotomy.

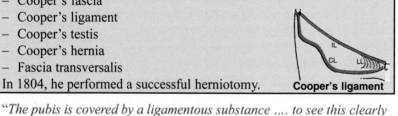

Cooper's ligament

"The danger is in the delay, not in the operation"
- Sir Astley Paston Cooper
English Surgeon & Anatomist

"The pubis is covered by a ligamentous substance .... to see this clearly in dissection, the fascia covering the pectineus muscle, together with the muscle itself, must be cut away."
(His own description of Cooper's ligament)

- Annet Jean Bogros (1786-1823), described "Space of Bogros" in the groin region of anterior abdominal wall.
- Jules Germain Cloquet (1790-1883), a Paris surgeon and anatomist described:
  - Iliopubic tract
  - Femoral septum
  - Haller habenula (a persistent remnant of foetal canal that once connected the tunica vaginalis with the peritoneal sac)
  - Cloquet's lymph node in femoral canal

  Edoardo Bassini was born in 1844 in Pavia, the son of a farmer, he changed the history and course of hernia surgery. He studied medicine at the University of Pavia, graduated in1866, at the age of only 22 years. During the Prussian-Austrian war, he joined the unification movement under Giuseppe Garibaldi as a foot soldier and in 1867 sustained a bayonet wound in the groin and was taken prisoner. For several months he was under treatment for faecal fistula which was successfully treated by Luigi Porta (1800-1875).[15]

After his release, Bassini returned to Pavia and became the assistant of the Chief of Surgery, Luigi Porta. At the suggestion of his mentor, he went abroad for further training. He worked at Christian Theodor Billroth's Centre in Vienna. He then went to Berlin to work with Bernhard Rudolph Konrad von Langenbeck (1810-1887), and learned the basics of plastic surgery and the design of surgical instruments. From Berlin, he travelled to London where he visited Thomas Spencer Wells and Joseph Lister and learned techniques of antiseptic surgery.

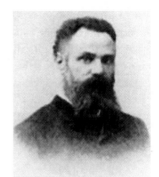

"It reconstructs inguinal canal as it is physiological"
Edoardo Bassini,
Father of modern herniorrhaphy

At the age of 30, he returned to Pavia as second assistant to Porta, who died one year later. Bassini lost the struggle for the appointment as Surgeon in Chief, and disappointed, he quit and returned to London to continue his studies. After returning to Italy, he became Head of the Department of Surgery at the La Spezia Hospital. In 1878, he was appointed a lecturer of Surgery at Parma.

In 1882, he moved to the University of Padua as head of surgical pathology, and in 1888, he succeeded Tito Vanzetti (1809-1888) in the chair of Clinical Surgery, a position he held until 1919.

Bassini carried out his method of inguinal hernia operation for the first time in 1884. In 1887, he presented his paper before the Italian Association of Surgery. In 1890, he published an article in *"Archiv Fur Klinische Chirurgie"* and it was only then that his method became known outside Italy.

- Bassini was considered a meticulous and careful operator, and an interesting and able teacher.
- Bassini introduced herniorrhaphy, ligation and resection of hernia sac with reconstruction of posterior wall of inguinal canal in inguinal hernia repair. He is now known as the *"Father of modern herniorrhaphy"*.
- Bassini was not limited only to herniology but also contributed in the development of other procedures such as suprapubic cystostomy, incision of thyroid operation, femoral hernia repair, ileocoloplasty, nephropexy, subtotal hysterectomy and hip disarticulation.[14]

BASSINI'S OPERATION

In standard surgical procedure for inguinal hernia, the hernia sac is removed and conjoint tendon is approximated to inguinal ligament.

"In order to achieve a radical cure of inguinal hernia, it is absolutely essential to restore those conditions in the area of hernial orifice which exist under normal circumstances"   **– Edoardo Bassini**

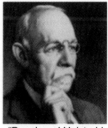

"Developed Halsted I, Halsted II operations for inguinal hernia and complete Halsted, a technique of mastectomy"
William Stewart Halsted

Bassini-Kirschner Technique

This technique is based on suturing of the inguinal ligament with non-absorbent material.

- William Stewart Halsted (1852-1922) is known as the "Father of American surgery". Born in New York City, he was the founder of the American residency training system. William S. Halsted was named the first chief of the Department of Surgery at Johns Hopkins Hospital. He modified herniorrhaphy for inguinal hernia. He also introduced the use of surgical gloves during operation. He was the first who used silk in hernia repair. He gave modified mastectomy technique for carcinoma of breast.

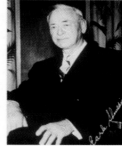

- Edward Earl Shouldice developed a new method of herniorrhaphy. Shouldice' operation for inguinal hernia is based on Bassini's repair. He started his technique in 1945, in which the posterior wall of inguinal canal is repaired by a double layer repair of fascia transversalis and double layer approximation of conjoint tendon and inguinal ligament.

"Walking early and often is key to postoperative recovery"
Edward Earl Shouldice

- Mair used skin strips taken from incision edge.
- In 1894, Philips used *"Silver coil"* for inguinal hernia repair.
- In 1952, Babcock Wayne Babcock (1872-1963), an American surgeon used stainless steel wire mesh to repair inguinal hernia.
- Various organic synthetic prosthetic materials were also used for mesh in hernioplasty, e.g., cloth, nylon, teflon, polyethylene and polyvinyl sponge but none could be accepted universally due to intense inflammatory reaction.
- Mc. Arthur used strips of external oblique aponeurosis in Bassini's repair.
- William Edward Gallie (1882-1959), a Canadian surgeon, used strips of fascia lata in inguinal hernia repair. This technique is called Gallie transplant.
- Handly used silk in darning of hernia in 1918 for the first time.
- In 1948, Maloney described *"darn"* using nylon suture.
- Haxton was the first who used nylon monofilament in herniorrhaphy.
- Melick was the first who used braided nylon herniorrhaphy.

- **It was the introduction of mesh by FC Usher *et al.* in 1958 that opened a new era for hernia surgery.**[6] Usher[7] introduced Marlex-50 (polyethylene plastic mesh) which gradually modified to polypropylene mesh. Usher called it "tension eliminating technique"[8] Marlex or prolene is used universally and is the most commonly used prosthetic material.

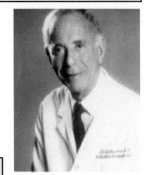

- Rene F. Stoppa, in 1975, used GPRVS (Giant Prosthetic Reinforcement of the Visceral Sac) for the first time. He used a giant-sized prosthesis covering the lower part of abdomen and pelvis in preperitoneal space.
- In 1983, Goretex (e-PTFE) was used for the first time in hernia repair.
- Newman of New Jersey developed tension-free technique for inguinal hernia using a polypropylene mesh onlay patch that he sutured over the posterior wall. Lichtenstein and Amid popularized Newman's technique.[9]

- Irving L. Lichtenstein in 1984 used the term *"tension-free hernioplasty"* with use of polypropylene mesh and established a milestone. He changed the course of hernia treatment. Lichtenstein's technique became Gold standard for hernia repair.
  Lichtenstein died in 2000.

"This factor of tension is eliminated and recurrence becomes less likely"
Irving L. Lichtenstein
Creator of tension-free hernioplasty

- Macewan, in 1888, attempted to block the internal inguinal ring by reefing the peritoneal sac and transfixing it. Gilbert originated the process of using the mesh with the internal inguinal ring[10].
- In 1989, Bogojavalenski did laparosocopic plugging of the hernia defect with prolene mesh.

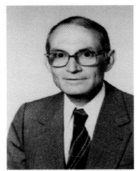

"introduced the term GPRVS, where giant prosthesis replaces endopelvic fascia"
Rene F. Stoppa

- In 1990, E.H. Phillips and J.B. Mc. Kernan introduced TEP (Total extraperitoneal) technique of laparoscopic inguinal hernioplasty.
- In 1991, Arregui introduced TAPP (Transabdominal preperitoneal) laparoscopic repair for inguinal hernia.

- Arthur I. Gilbert used sutureless hernioplasty in 1992 by placing the mesh without sutures.
- In 1992, IPOM (Intraperitoneal onlay mesh) repair for groin hernia was developed by Franklin, Rosenthal and Fitzgibbons.
- In 1992, LeBlanc and Booth used e-PTFE.
- Polyglycolic acid (Dixon) and polyglactin (Vicryl) are used as slowly absorbable meshes.
- Development of prosthetic mesh has reached a new height. Nowadays, partially absorbable meshes are used which are found to be more body friendly with less complications.
- Light weight, self-gripping dual meshes are expensive but avoid adhesion formation from abdominal organs and intestine, composite mesh causes less adhesions and visceral erosion.[26]
- Use of Fibrin glue is replacing the mesh fixation devices.
- It is only few years that proper studies started to understand wound healing and its relation to hernia development. Abnormal collagen metabolism studied and immature collagen isoforms measured, altered fibroblasts functioning and abnormal population found leading to increased incidence of recurrent incisional hernia in each attempt to repair it.[16-20]
- Role of growth factors and nutrition in wound healing in incisional hernias in under study.[21-25]

NOTE

- *As the use of mesh has become more widespread, recurrence rate in the future is likely to be lower than past.[11]*
- *Technical approach to hernia surgery continues to change significantly and so is the behaviour of patients and surgeons to ambulatory operations and earlier return to activity.[12]*

KEY POINT

It can be argued that more progress has been made in hernia surgery in the last 15 years than had been made in the previous 1500 years.[13]   *- Robert D. Kugel*

REFERENCES

1. **Udwadia TE.,** (2006). Inguinal hernia repair: The total picture, *Journal of Minimal Access Surgery*, **2,** 144.
2. **Chowbey P.,** (2004). Endoscopic repair of abdominal wall hernias, p. 1.
3. **Rutkow IM:** A selective history of hernia surgery in the late 18th century: The treatise of Percivall Pott, Jean Louis Petit, D August Gottlieb Richter, Don Antonio de Gimbernat and Pieter Camper., (2003). *Surg. Clin. North Am.*, 1021.

4. **Rutkow IM.**, (1997). Surgical operations in the United States, then (1983) and now (1994): *Arch. Surg.*, 132: 1021.

5. **Cooper A.**, (1804). The anatomy and surgical treatment of abdominal hernia, Philadelphia, Lee and Blanchard, p. 26.

6. **Read RC.**, (2004). Milestones in the history of hernia surgery: Prosthetic repair. Hernia, 8: 8–14.

7. **Usher F, Ochsner J, Tuttle LL Jr.**, (1958). Use of marlex mesh in the repair of incisional hernias. *Am. Surg.* 24: 969–974.

8. **Usher FC.**, (1962). *Arch Surg.*, 84: 325.

9. **Gilbert AI.**, (2007). Generations of the plug and patch repair. Its development and lessons from history, Mastery of surgery, 5th edition, Lippincott Williams & Wilkins, p. 1941.

10. **Gilbert AI.**, (2007). Generations of the plug and patch repair: Its development and lessons from history, Mastery of surgery, 5th edition, Lippincott Williams & Wilkins, p. 1940.

11. **Voyles CR, Hamilton BJ, Johnsan BD,** *et al.,* (2002). Meta-analysis of laparoscopic inguinal hernia trials favours open hernia repair with preperitoneal mesh prosthesis; *Am. J. Surg.*, 184: 6–10.

12. **Voyles CR.**, (2003). Outcomes analysis for groin hernia repairs, *Surg. Clin. North Am.*, 83: 1279.

13. **Kugel RD.**, (2003). The Kugel repair for groin hernias, *Surg. Clin. North Am.*, 83: 1119.

14. **Terranova O, Santis LD, Frigo F.**, The Bassini operation, http://www.masteryofsurgery.com/pt/re/fischer/book.

15. **Zimmerman and Heller.**, (1937). *Surg. Gynaecol. Obstet.*, 64: 971.

16. **Read RC.** (2006). Introduction. *Hernia*; 10(6): 454–5.

17. **Junge K., Klinge U.,** *et al.* (2004). Decreased collagen type I/III ratio in patients with recurring hernia after implantation of alloplastic prostheses. Langenbecks *Arch Surg,* 389(1): 17–22.

18. **Flum D.R., Horvath K., Koepsell T.** (2003). Have outcomes of incisional hernia repair improved with time? A population based analysis. *Ann Surg,* 237(1): 129–35.

19. **Katsumi A., Naoe T., Matsushita T.** *et al.* (2005). Integrin activation and matrix binding mediate cellular responses to mechanical stretch. *J. Biol. Chem.* 280(17): 16546–9.

20. **Dubay D.A.,** *et al.* (2005). Progressive fascial wound failure impairs subsequent abdominal wall repairs: a new animal model of incisional hernia formation. Surg. 137(4): 463–71.

21. **Roberts A.B.** (1995). Transforming growth factor beta: activity and efficacy in animalmodels of wound healing. *Wound Repair Regen* 3(4): 408–18.

22. **Best W.R., Khuri S.F.,** *et al.* (2002). Identifying patient preoperative risk factors and post-operative adverse events in administrative databases: results from the department of veterans affairs national surgical quality improvement program. *J. Am. Coll. Surg.* 194(3): 257–66.

23. **Williams J.G., Barbul A.** (2003). Nutrition and wound healing. *Surg. Clin. North Am.* 83: 571–96.

24. **Korenkov M., Beckers A., Koebke J.,** *et al.* (2001). Biomechanical and morphological types of the linea alba and its possible role in the pathogenesis of midline incisional hernia. *Eur. J. Surg.* 167(12): 909–14.

25. **Dubay D.A., Choi W., Urbanchek M.G.,** *et al.* (2007). Incisional herniation induces decreased abdominal wall compliance via oblique muscle atrophy and fibrosis. *Ann. Surg.* 245(1): 140–6.

26. **Gray SH.,** *et al.* (2008). Surgical progress in inguinal and ventral incisional hernia repair. *Surg. Clin. N. Am.*; 88, 17–26.

Section 2
ANATOMY

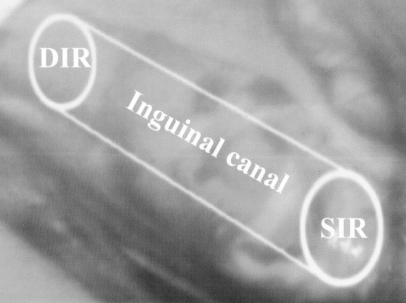

DIR

Inguinal canal

SIR

"Anatomy is Destiny" -*Sigmund Freud*

Embryology

*"Where have I come from", baby asked mother, "you were hidden in my
heart as its desire, my darling".*
— **Rabindranath Tagore**
Nobel Laureate, Literature

Inguinal canal is the passage of gubernaculum (Latin = a guiding structure) through anterior abdominal wall. The gubernaculum is attached from the base of gonad to labioscrotal swelling.

The inguinal canal is very small in early life and later increases in length due to gradual development and widening of pelvis. With the growth of pelvis, superficial inguinal ring remains at the same place but deep inguinal ring shifts laterally, that is why, in infants the superficial inguinal ring is superimposed on deep inguinal ring and there is almost no inguinal canal.

DESCENT OF TESTES

Testes develop on the posterior abdominal wall from the genital ridge. These are situated in lumbar region in front of kidneys (Fig. 3.1). The testes descend in scrotum to reside in optimum temperature environment required for normal spermatogenesis and hormones production. The scrotum is a

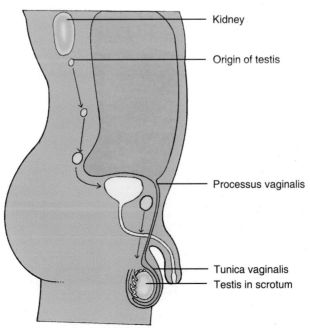

Fig. 3.1. Path of descent of testes.

thermoregulator to the testes, and keeps the temperature at least 2°F lower than that of inguinal canal.[5] The actual mechanism of descent of testes remains uncertain.[1]

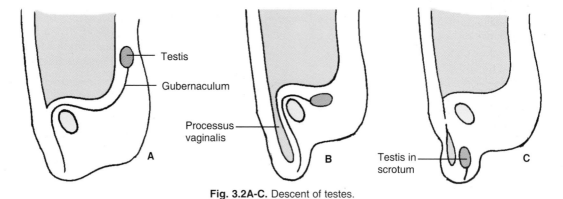

Fig. 3.2A-C. Descent of testes.

An epithelial diverticulum follows the path of gurbernaculum and pierces the anterior abdominal wall. The coelomic diverticulum is called "*Processus vaginalis*" and its path in anterior abdominal wall forms "Inguinal canal" (Figs. 3.2A-C). Gubernaculum was first described by John Hunter (1727-1793), Surgeon, St George's Hospital, London.

The final descent of testes through inguinal canal to scrotum is controlled by the following factors (Fig. 3.3):

• Testosterone
• Maternal gonadotrophins
• Differential growth of the body wall
• Gubernaculum (by shortening and active contraction of gubernaculum)
• Intraabdominal temperature
• Intraabdominal pressure
• Active contraction of lower fibres of internal oblique muscle which squeezes the testis through the inguinal canal to the scrotum

The testis descends through the processus vaginalis due to propulsive force generated by muscle derived from the gubernaculum. The descent of testis through the muscles of anterior abdominal wall forms inguinal canal traversing through the three abdominal wall muscles from deep inguinal

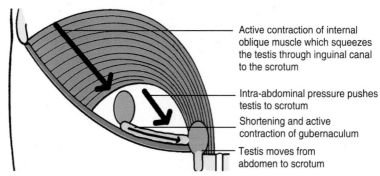

Fig. 3.3. Factors responsible for descent of testis.

ring in fascia transversalis to superficial inguinal ring in external oblique aponeurosis. (Fig. 3.4 A and B).

After propelling the testis, these muscles undergo programmed cell death (atrophy) for obliteration of processus vaginalis. The programmed cell death depends upon sympathetic activity, which is androgen dependent. It occurs during third trimester of pregnancy. Decrease in sympathetic activity produces hernia.[8]

This hypothesis supports the view that adult indirect inguinal hernia is congenital.

Genitofemoral nerve supplies cremaster muscle which develops in gubernaculum. It has been experimentally proved that if genitofemoral nerve is divided in fetus, the descent of testis is prevented.

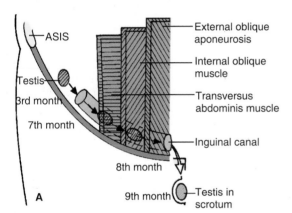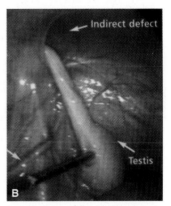

Fig. 3.4A. Descent of testis through abdominal wall muscles and development of inguinal canal, **B.** Right inguinal hernia defect with undescended testis, seen laparoscopically. Courtesy: Dr Parveen Bhatia, Global Hospital, New Delhi.

FATE OF PROCESSUS VAGINALIS

The processus vaginalis initially remains patent and then gets blocked at two sites before or after the birth:
• At internal inguinal ring.
• At the level just above the testis.
• The lower part of processus vaginalis becomes tunica vaginalis.
• The processus vaginalis between two obstructed sites is called funicular process. It gets blocked and becomes a fibrous cord, a rudiment of the processus vaginalis.
• The processus vaginalis closes earlier on left side than on right side and thus, hernia incidence is more on right side as it remains open for a longer period of time.
• The processus vaginalis usually closes few months before the birth or near the birth. It leads to a high incidence of inguinal hernias in premature infants.[2]
• The processus vaginalis obliterates earlier in girls than boys, in the 7th month of gestation.
• In females, the ovary descends into pelvis following the gubernaculum. The gubernaculum gets attached to either side of the developing uterus and the ovary does not descend further. The part of gubernaculum, extending from the uterus into the developing labium majus, persists as round ligament of uterus.

Almost all groin hernias in children are indirect inguinal hernias.[6]

A high prevalence of inguinal hernia is well known among patients suffering from certain congenital connective tissue disorders[3] such as **Ehlers-Danlos syndrome** and **Hurler-Hunter syndrome**.
Familial predisposition plays an important role[4] in the aetiology of hernia.

Indirect inguinal hernias in children are basically an arrest of embyronic development rather than an acquired weakness which explains the increased incidence of it in premature infants.[6]

- The incidence is much higher in premature infants, inguinal hernias develop in 13% of infants born before 32 weeks gestation and in 30% infants less than 1000 g.[7]
- Siblings of patients with inguinal hernia have a genetic risk of getting hernia. Sisters of affected girls have highest risk 17.8[9] brothers of a sibling have risk 4-5.[10,11]

KEY POINT

Adult indirect inguinal hernia is a congenital condition due to patent processus vaginalis. The development of processus vaginalis, its migration into the scrotum, and its final obliteration are intimately linked to the descent of the testis from the abdomen into the scrotum.

REFERENCES

1. **Peter William** *et al.,* (1993). Gray's anatomy, ELBS editions, p. 257.
2. **Brunicardi FC** *et al.,* (2005). Schwartz's principles of surgery, McGraw-Hill, 8th edition, p. 1505.
3. **Wirtschafter ZT, Bentley JP.**, (1964). Hernias as a collagen maturation defect. *Ann. Surg.,* 160: 852.
4. **Abramson JH, Gofin J, Hopp C**, *et al.,* (1978). The epidemiology of inguinal hernia: A survey in Western Jerusalem, *J. Epidemiol Community Health,* 32: 59.
5. **Rains JH.,** *et al.,* (1971). Bailey and Loves short practice of surgery, 15th edition, p. 1240.
6. **Brandt ML.**, (2008). Paediatric hernias, *Surg. Clin. N. Am.*; 88, 27–43.
7. **Kurkchubasche A, Tracy T.** (2008). Unique features of groin hernia repair in infants and children. In: Fitzgibbons R, Greenburg A, editors. Nyhus and Condon's hernia. Philadelphia: Lippincott Williams & Wilkins; 2002. p. 435–51.
8. **Tanyel FC, Okur HD.** (2004). Autonomic nervous system appears to play a role in obliteration of processus vaginalis. *Hernia*; 8(2): 149–54.
9. **Jones ME, Swerdlow AJ, Griffith M,** *et al.* (1998). Risk of congenital inguinal hernia in siblings: a record linkage study. Paediatr Perinat Epidemiol; 12(3): 288–96.
10. **Gong Y, Shao C, Sun Q,** *et al.* (1994). Genetic study of indirect inguinal hernia. *J. Med. Genet.*; 31(3): 187–92.
11. **Czeizel A, Gardonyi J.** (1979). A family study of congenital inguinal hernia. *Am. J. Med Genet*; 4(3): 247–54.

4

Anatomy of Anterior Abdominal Wall

"No disease of the human body belonging to the provision of the surgeon requires in its treatment a better combination of accurate anatomy knowledge with surgical skill than Hernia in all varieties"
— **Sir Astley Paston Cooper (1768-1841)**

"The anatomy of the groin is, by no means, the easiest to understand, incorporate or retain!"
— **R Bendavid (2007)**

"If anatomy, born as a purely descriptive and macroscopic science, had only studied the arrangement, the structure and the special relationships of the various organs of the body, it would have been of little use to medicine and to general science"
— **Dr Giovanni Lazzetti, Dr Enrico Rigutti, Atlas of Anatomy**

Groin is one of the weakest areas in the anterior abdominal wall and the commonest site for hernia.

(I) SURFACE ANATOMY OF GROIN

"The anatomy of groin is probably the most used, most studied and most confusing region of the body"

- **Harold Ellis, Emeritus Professor of Surgery, University of London**

Groin

Groin (Fig. 4.1) is the junctional region between the abdomen and the thigh. Groin is also called *region-inguinalis* or iliac or inguinal region (Latin – *Inguen*, plural – *inguinal*).

The term *"Groin Hernias"* includes following hernias:
- Indirect inguinal hernia
- Direct inguinal hernia
- Femoral hernia

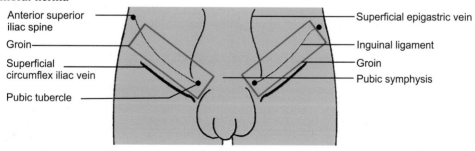

Fig. 4.1. Surface anatomy of groin.

Skin Creases

In the lower abdomen, two skin creases (Fig. 4.2) are visible:
- Abdominal crease
- Groin crease

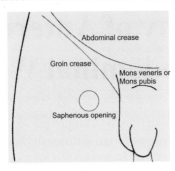

Fig. 4.2. Skin creases of groin.

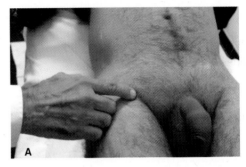

Fig. 4.3A. Demonstrating creases of groin (adult).

The upper crease is called the "abdominal crease" and the lower crease the "groin crease". Abdominal crease runs from one ASIS to another whereas the groin crease runs on each side, from near ASIS to the medial part of upper thigh. Abdominal crease separates a triangular area of fleshy prominence over pubic symphysis from abdomen which is called "Mons veneris[1]" or "Mons pubis". Mons pubis is situated anterior to pubic symphysis and is formed by subcutaneous adipose tissue (Fig. 4.2).

NOTE

The groin crease is used for incisions in groin hernia repair in girls for aesthetic purposes.

Inguinal Ligament

Inguinal ligament runs from ASIS to pubic tubercle. It is represented by a line connecting ASIS and pubic tubercle. It lies beneath the skin fold in groin and can be felt along its full length.

ASIS (Anterior Superior Iliac Spine)

ASIS lies at the level of sacral promontory. ASIS is easy to be seen and felt, but pubic tubercle is sometimes difficult to feel.

Inguinal Canal

Inguinal canal is an oblique passage through the lower abdominal wall. It can be marked by two parallel lines, 1 cm apart and 1.25 cm above the medial half of inguinal ligament.

Deep Inguinal Ring

The deep inguinal ring is the entrance to the inguinal canal. It is marked as an oval opening 1.25 cm above the mid inguinal point.

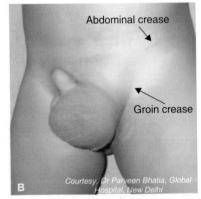

Fig. 4.3B. Demonstrating skin creases of groin (infant).

Superficial Inguinal Ring

Superficial inguinal ring is a triangular opening just above the pubic turbercle with its centre 1 cm above and lateral to pubic turbercle, and its apex faces upwards.

Superficial Epigastric Vein and Superficial Circumflex Iliac Vein (Fig. 4.1)

These two veins can be seen individually in anterior abdominal wall and upper part of thighs respectively.

Linea Alba (Fig. 4.4)

It is a vertical groove in the centre of abdomen dividing the anterior abdominal wall into two halves.

Linea Semilunaris (Figs. 4.5A & B)

It is a vertical curved groove running from cartilage of ninth costal cartilage to pubic tubercle. It corresponds to lateral margin of rectus abdominis muscle[2].

Arcuate Line of Douglas (Figs. 4.5A & B)

It is named after James Douglas (1675-1742), Scottish anatomist. It is a semilunar line, convex up and 2.5 cm below umbilicus from linea alba to linea semilunaris.

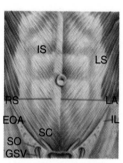

Fig. 4.4. Anatomical landmarks.

Monro's Line

It is a line from umbilicus to right anterior superior iliac spine.

Monro-Richter's Line (Fig. 4.5A)

It is a line from umbilicus to left anterior superior iliac spine.

Importance of Monro's Lines

The two Monro's lines and a line joining the two ASIS form a triangle. The "Spigelian belt" (hernia prone area) is an area that lies between the Monro's line and the interspinous line in Spigelian aponeurosis.

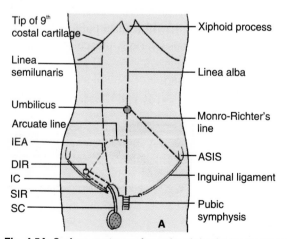

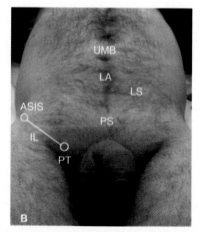

Fig. 4.5A. Surface anatomy of anterior abdominal wall and groin, **B.** Surface anatomy of anterior abdominal wall and groin in patient.

Mid Inguinal Point (Fig 4.6A)

It is a point at the centre of line between ASIS and pubic symphysis.

Middle Point of Inguinal Ligament (Fig. 4.6A)

It is a point at the centre of line between ASIS and pubic tubercle.

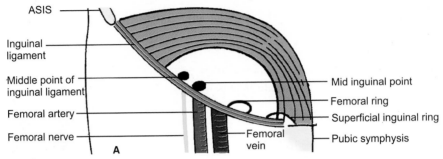

Fig. 4.6A. Surface landmarks of groin.

Pubic Turbercle (Figs. 4.6B & C)

It is a rounded bony prominence situated at the lateral end of pubic crest.

Pubic tubercle is a medial attachment of the inguinal ligament in the floor of the superficial inguinal ring and is crossed by the spermatic cord; ascending loops of cremaster are also attached to it[3]. It lies beneath the skin crease of lower abdomen, at a distance of 2-3 cm away from midline.

Methods of palpation of pubic tubercle

- Put your finger on the center of the abdominal crease, push deep until you feel pubic crest then move your finger sideways until you reach the tubercle (Fig 4.7A).
- You can also feel the pubic tubercle by invaginating the scrotum with examining finger.
- Another method of finding pubic tubercle is to follow inguinal ligament medially. The medial end of the inguinal ligament is attached to pubic tubercle. The first bony prominence felt at the medial end is pubic tubercle.
- In obese persons, follow the adductor longus tendon upwards. It will lead to pubic tubercle.
- Pubic tubercle and ASIS are important to hernia surgeon because various musculoaponeurotic and ligamentous structures are attached to them.
- Pubic tubercle can be palpated in a female through the lateral margin of labium majus.

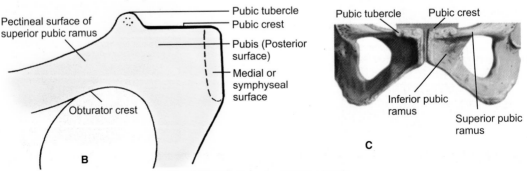

Fig. 4.6B & C. Bony landmarks of groin.

Structures attached to pubic tubercle (Fig. 4.7B)

- Inguinal ligament
- Conjoint tendon
- Ascending loops of cremaster muscle
- Lateral head of rectus abdominis muscle

Pubic Symphysis

It is a cartilaginous joint that unites the superior rami of the left and right pubic bones. Upper margin of pubic symphysis and pubic bones can be felt through the lower part of anterior abdominal wall, just above the root of penis or at mons veneris.

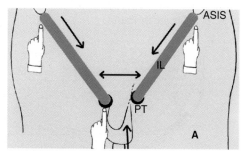

Fig. 4.7A. Examination of pubic tubercle.

Inferior Epigastric Vessels

If a line drawn from mid inguinal point to umbilicus, the lower two-thirds of this line represent inferior epigastric vessels.

Femoral Artery

It enters the thigh behind the inguinal ligament at the mid inguinal point. It is represented by the upper two-thirds of a line joining the mid inguinal point to adductor tubercle.

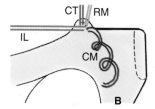

Femoral Vein

It leaves the thigh by passing under the inguinal ligament medial to femoral artery. Some as femoral artery except that the upper point is taken 1 cm medial to mid ixguinal point andlower point 1 cm lateral to adductor tubercle.

Fig. 4.7B. Structures attached to pubic tubercle.

Femoral Canal

Lower opening of femoral canal lies approximately 4 cm below and lateral to pubic tubercle.

Femoral Ring

It is represented by a horizontal line, 1.2 cmlong over the inguinal ligament and 1.2 cm medial to mid-inguinal point.

Femoral Nerve

It enters the thigh behind the point of the inguinal ligament. It is lateral to femoral artery and outside the femoral sheath.

> **KEY POINT**
>
> *Surface anatomy is important from the surgical point of view. Proper incision in relation to surface anatomy of the organ gives good exposure and easy dissection.*

(II) INGUINAL CANAL (FIGS. 4.8A-D)

Inguinal canal is a passage in the lower part of anterior abdominal wall, above the medial half of inguinal ligament. It extends from deep inguinal ring to superficial inguinal ring, formed due to migration of testis out of the abdominal cavity to scrotum for normal spermatogenesis. Weakening of this area of anterior abdominal wall makes it prone to hernia. Inguinal canal is present in both the sexes. It is larger in males.

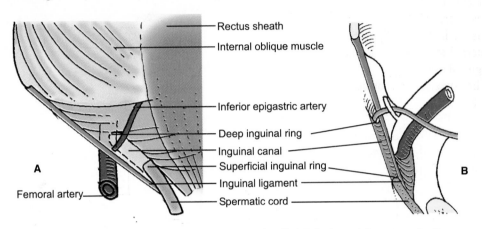

Fig. 4.8A. Inguinal canal, diagrammatic representation, **B.** Inguinal canal, laparoscopic view.

Length

It is 3.75 cm to 4 cm in an adult extending from deep inguinal ring to superficial inguinal ring.

In a newborn, it is very short, as superficial and deep inguinal rings are superimposed.

In many West African adults, it remains short with the two rings widened and almost on top of one another.[45]

Direction

The inguinal canal extends from deep inguinal ring to superficial inguinal ring in the following direction:

- Downwards
- Forward
- Medially

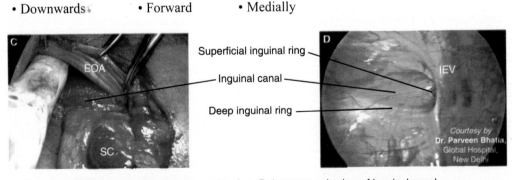

Fig. 4.8C. Inguinal canal, anterior view, **D.** Laparoscopic view of inguinal canal.

In 23 per cent people, the inguinal canal area is weak and easily predisposed to inguinal hernia.

Deep or Internal Inguinal Ring (Figs. 4.9A-G)

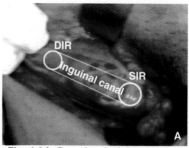

Fig. 4.9A. Deep inguinal ring, inguinal canal and superficial inguinal ring.

- It is a 'U'-shaped opening in fascia transversalis, which forms the posterior wall of inguinal canal. It is situated 1.25 cm above the mid inguinal point.
- It is lateral to inferior epigastric artery.
- It is the internal end of inguinal canal.
- Internal spermatic fascia arises from the margins of deep inguinal ring.
- It has two margins or crura:
  - Superior margin or crus.
    It is formed by transverse abdominal arch. It is the longer crus.
  - Inferior margin or crus.
    It is shorter crus and is made by following structures:
    a) Iliopubic tract
    b) Inferior epigastric vessels
    c) Interfoveolar ligament (Hesselbach's ligament)

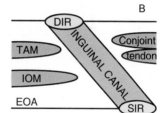

Fig. 4.9B. Inguinal canal, its relations.

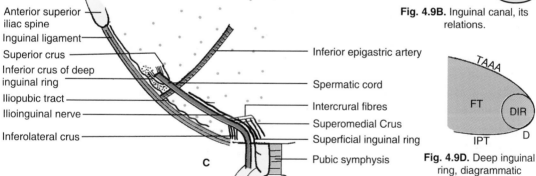

Anterior superior iliac spine
Inguinal ligament
Superior crus
Inferior crus of deep inguinal ring
Iliopubic tract
Ilioinguinal nerve
Inferolateral crus

Inferior epigastric artery
Spermatic cord
Intercrural fibres
Superomedial Crus
Superficial inguinal ring
Pubic symphysis

Fig. 4.9C. Anterior view of deep inguinal canal.

Fig. 4.9D. Deep inguinal ring, diagrammatic representation.

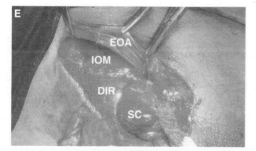

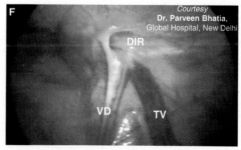

Fig. 4.9E & F. Deep inguinal ring, exploration and laparoscopic view.

- It has a long vertical axis.
- It is larger in males than in females.
- Its size varies in different individuals.
- It transmits spermatic cord in males and round ligament in females.

Superficial or External Inguinal Ring (Figs. 4.10A & B)

It is a triangular defect in external oblique aponeurosis. The base of the triangle is formed by pubic crest. It is pointing obliquely, medially and down. It is situated 1.25 cm above the pubic tubercle.

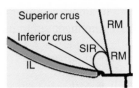

Fig. 4.9G. Superficial inguinal ring diagrammatic representation.

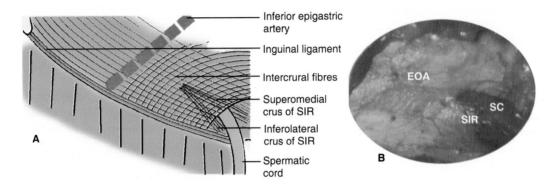

Fig. 4.10A. Superficial inguinal ring, diagrammatic representation, **B.** Laparoscopic view of superficial inguinal ring.

The two margins of superficial inguinal ring are called crura. There are two crura:

- Superomedial crus
- Inferolateral crus
  - Superior crus is formed by aponeurosis of the external oblique muscle and is attached to lateral border of the rectus sheath.
  - Inferior crus is formed by inguinal ligament and is attached to pubic tubercle.
  - The inferolateral crus is stronger.
  - The crura at apex are united by intercrural fibres.
    a) The superficial inguinal ring is 2.5 cm long and 1.2 cm wide at base.
    b) It has a long oblique axis in direction of external oblique aponeurosis.
    c) It is smaller in females than males.

- Superficial inguinal ring passes through the following structures in males:
  - Spermatic cord
  - Ilioinguinal nerve
- Superficial inguinal ring passes through the following structures in females:
  - Round ligament of uterus
  - Ilioinguinal nerve

In a normal adult, the superficial inguinal ring does not allow a finger to pass, except the tip of the little finger. In an indirect inguinal hernia, which comes through the superficial inguinal ring, the superficial inguinal ring permits a finger or two, as it gets dilated.

The margins of superficial inguinal ring are attached to external spermatic fascia.

> - In females, the term spermatic fascia should not be used but coverings of round ligament of uterus should be used.
> - Due to the attachment of internal spermatic fascia to the margins of deep inguinal ring and external spermatic fascia to the margins of superficial inguinal ring, these two rings cannot be observed externally.

Boundaries of Inguinal Canal (Figs. 4.11A-E)

Anterior wall of inguinal canal

- Along the whole length of the canal
  - Skin
  - Superficial fascia
  - External oblique aponeurosis
- Along the lateral one-third of the canal
  - The fleshy fibres of the internal oblique muscle are also present deep to the external oblique aponeurosis.

    The anterior wall of inguinal canal is formed in the whole length by the aponeurosis of external oblique muscle. It is reinforced by the fibres of internal oblique muscle at the weakest part of the posterior wall of inguinal canal medially over deep inguinal ring.

Posterior wall of the inguinal canal

- Along the whole length of the canal
  - Fascia transversalis
  - Extraperitoneal tissue
  - Parietal peritoneum
  - Inferior epigastric vessels (in lateral part)
- Along the medial two-thirds of the canal (Fig. 4.11C)
  - Conjoint tendon
  - Reflected part of inguinal ligament
  - Interfoveolar ligament in the lateral one-third

  The posterior wall of inguinal canal is mainly formed by conjoint tendon on medial side, which is formed by fibres of:
  - Internal oblique muscle
  - Transversus abdominis muscle

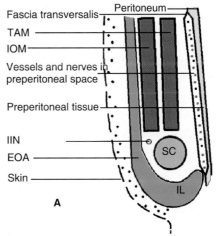

Fig. 4.11A. Boundaries and contents of inguinal canal.

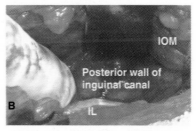

Fig. 4.11B. Posterior wall of inguinal canal.

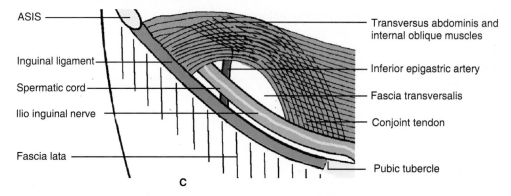

Fig. 4.11C. Anterior and posterior walls of inguinal canal.

The posterior wall of inguinal canal is formed by fascia transversalis along its entire length. It is strenghened by conjoint tendon where it lies opposite the weakest part of anterior wall of inguinal canal, i.e., superficial inguinal ring (Figs. 4.11 D & E).

> **NOTE**
>
> *The true posterior wall of inguinal canal is formed by the aponeurosis of the transversus abdominis. What constitutes the true defect leading to a direct inguinal hernia is the weakness of a layer of connective tissue between the transversus aponeurosis and tranversalis facia that Fruchaud has described as the vascular lamina...... It is a connective tissue layer that degenerates as a result of the metabolic defects that leads to hernia.*[38]

- **Roof of inguinal canal is formed by:**
  - Internal oblique muscle
  - Transversus abdominis muscle
- **Floor of inguinal canal is formed by:**
  - Grooved upper surface of inguinal ligament and its union with fascia transversalis.
  - Lacunar ligament (Gimbernat's ligament) at its medial end.

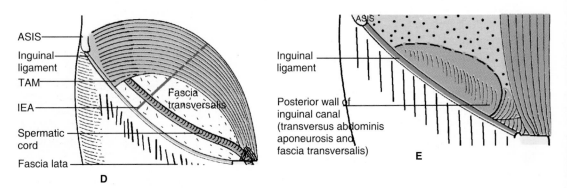

Fig. 4.11 D & E. Posterior wall of inguinal canal.

- The presence of inguinal canal weakens the lower part of anterior abdominal wall.
- The obliquity of the inguinal canal somewhat compensates for this weakness.
- The rise in intraabdominal pressure approximates the posterior and the anterior walls of inguinal canal and closes the inguinal canal.
- The conjoint tendon and reflected part of inguinal ligament are behind the superficial inguinal ring and strengthen the posterior wall of inguinal canal, on medial side.
- The fleshy fibres of internal oblique muscle are anterior to the deep inguinal ring and strengthen the anterior wall of inguinal canal.

Functions of Inguinal Canal

It allows the passage of spermatic cord in males and round ligament in females. Normal spermatogenesis takes place only if testis leaves the abdominal cavity and reaches the cooler environment of the scrotum.

Structures Passing Through Inguinal Canal

- Spermatic cord and its coverings in males and round ligament of uterus in females.
- Ilioinguinal nerve that enters the inguinal canal midway and comes out through superficial inguinal ring.
- Vestigial remnant of processus vaginalis is the prolongation of peritoneum which accompanies the descent of testis in the scrotum.
- Genital branch of genitofemoral nerve that enters the deep inguinal ring and becomes part of spermatic cord and supplies cremaster muscle and skin of scrotum.

Constituents of Spermatic Cord (Figs. 4.12A-D)

- Vas deferens
- Arteries
  - Cremasteric artery
  - Artery to vas deferens
  - Testicular artery
- Pampiniform plexus of veins
- Nerves
  - Genital branch of genitofemoral nerve
  - Sympathetic plexus around artery to ductus deferens

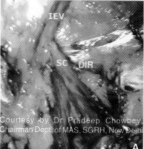

Fig. 4.12A. Spermatic cord structures, laparoscopic view.

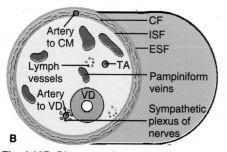

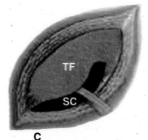

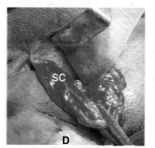

Fig. 4.12B. Diagrammatic representation of constituents of spermatic cord, **C.** and **D.** Anterior view of constituents of spermatic cord.

- Lymph vessels from testis
- Remnant of processus vaginalis

Coverings of Spermatic Cord (Figs. 4.13 A-C)

- Internal spermatic fascia is derived from fascia transversalis at deep inguinal ring.
- Cremasteric fascia is derived from internal oblique and transversus abdominis muscles.
- External spermatic fascia is derived from external oblique aponeurosis at superficial inguinal ring.

The testis descends into the scrotum through the abdominal wall along with nerves, vessels of testis and ductus deferens. These structures meet at deep inguinal ring and form spermatic cord, which extends from deep inguinal ring to posterior border of testis.

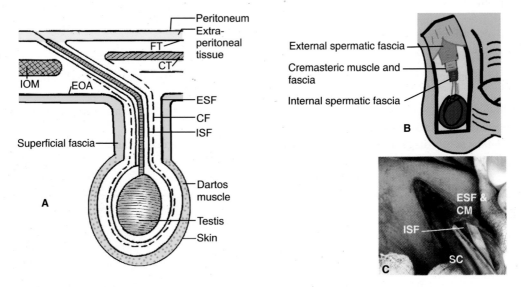

Fig. 4.13A. Coverings of spermatic cord, diagrammatic representation, **B.** and **C.** Anterior view of coverings of spermatic cord.

KEY POINT

Most of the external abdominal wall hernias occur in the groin."

(III) FEMORAL CANAL

"The body says what words cannot"   **- Martha Graham**

The **pelvicrural interval** (Fig. 4.14) is a space which connects the pelvic and abdominal cavities to thigh. It is situated under inguinal ligament.

The **pelvicrural interval** is divided into two spaces (Fig. 4.15):

- **Lateral space (Lacuna musculorum)**
  Iliopsoas muscle passes through this space.
- **Medial space (Lacuna vasculorum)**
  Femoral vessels and the canal pass[4] through this space (Fig. 4.16).
- Femoral canal extends from femoral ring to the saphenous ring or opening.
- Femoral canal is the medial compartment of femoral sheath.
- It is conical in shape.
- It is wide above and narrow below.
- It is closed above by septum crurale at femoral ring.

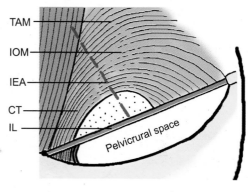

Fig. 4.14. Pelvicrural interval.

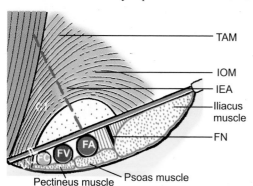

Fig. 4.15. Lacuna vasculorum and lacuna musculorum.

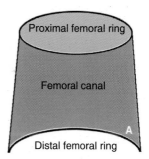

Fig. 4.16A. Femoral canal.

- It is closed below by cribriform fascia at saphenous opening which is present 3.75 - 4 cm below and lateral to pubic tubercle.

Size of Femoral Canal

Femoral canal is 1.25 cm long and 1.25 cm wide.

Femoral Rings

The base of femoral canal is called femoral ring (Figs. 4.16A & B). It is a weak area in anterior abdominal wall. Normally, the femoral ring admits the tip of little finger. Femoral rings are of two types: (i) Proximal or inner femoral ring; (ii) Distal or outer femoral ring.

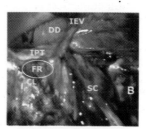

Fig. 4.16B. Femoral ring (FR), laparoscopic view.

Courtesy by Dr Pradeep Chowbey, Chairman Dept. of MAS, SGRH, New Delhi

Proximal or inner femoral ring

It is an oval opening of 1.25 cm diameter and is the entrance of peritoneal cavity to femoral canal. It is larger in females than in males.

> Femoral ring is a kind of safety valve for the expansion of the femoral vein in the upright position.[5] The inner femoral ring is bounded as described below[6, 7]:
> - Anteriorly by iliopubic tract.
> - Posteriorly by Cooper's ligament (Fig. 4.17).
> - Laterally by medial inter-compartmental septum edge.
> - Medially by transversus aponeurosis or lacunar ligament or both.

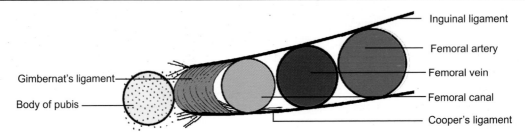

Fig. 4.17. Proximal femoral ring and its relations.

Distal or outer femoral ring (Fig. 4.18)

It is the exit of femoral canal to fossa ovalis[39].

The distal femoral ring is bounded as described below:
- Anteriorly by fascia lata and cribriform fascia.
- Posteriorly by fascia of pectineus muscle.
- Medially by iliopubic tract or lacunar ligament.
- Laterally by edge of medial inter-compartmental septum.

Boundaries of Femoral Canal

Anterior wall

- Iliopubic tract or inguinal ligament or both

Posterior wall

- Astley Cooper's ligament (iliopectineal ligament)
- Fascia iliaca

Medial wall

- The aponeurotic insertion of the transversus abdominis muscle
- Fascia transversalis
- Lacunar ligament (rarely)

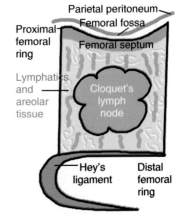

Fig. 4.18. Contents of femoral sheath, femoral septum and fossa.

> **NOTE**
>
> *McVay demonstrated that the medial boundary of femoral ring is the lateral edge of the aponeurosis of the insertion of the transversus abdominis muscle with transversalis fascia onto the pecten of the pubis but not the lacunar ligament.*

Lateral wall

- Inter-compartmental septum, which separates femoral canal from the central compartment containing femoral vein.

Relations of Femoral Canal

Femoral canal starts at the junction of abdomen and thigh and lies medial to the femoral vein in femoral sheath. It is related to following structures:
- **Inferior epigastric vessels**
  - These are related to the junction of lateral and anterior walls of the femoral ring, and should be taken care of during cutting the femoral ring.
- **Femoral septum (Fig. 4.18)**
  - It is a part of extraperitoneal connective tissue. It is pierced by lymphatics. It closes the femoral ring opening by plugging it. It is also called "Septum crurale".
- **Femoral fossa (Fig. 4.18)**
  - It is a depression in parietal peritoneum, covering the opening of femoral canal and femoral septum from above.

Femoral Sheath (Figs. 4.19A-C)

It is a funnel-shaped fascial sheath enclosing upper 3-4 cm of femoral vessels. It envelops femoral vessels. The sheath rests upon pectineus and adductor longus muscles medially and psoas major and iliacus muscles laterally. Femoral canal lies in front of the pectineus muscle.

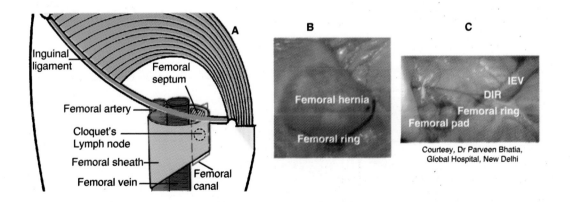

Fig. 4.19A-C. Femoral sheath, contents and ring.

Walls of Femoral Sheath (Figs. 4.20 & 4.21)

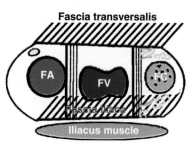

Fascia transversalis

Anterior wall

- It is formed by fascia transversalis.

Posterior wall

- It is formed by fascia iliaca which covers iliacus muscle.

Fig. 4.20. Walls of femoral sheath.

Lateral wall

- It is vertical.

Medial wall

- It is oblique.

Inferiorly the fascia joins the connective tissue around femoral vessels.

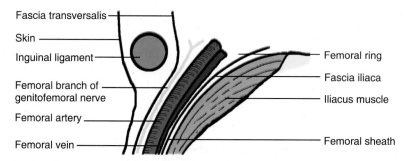

Fig. 4.21. Formation of femoral sheath.

Compartments of Femoral Sheath (Fig. 4.22)

Lateral or arterial compartment

It contains:
- Femoral artery
- Femoral branch of genitofemoral nerve.

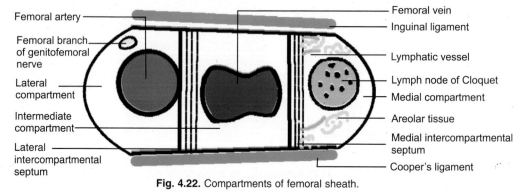

Fig. 4.22. Compartments of femoral sheath.

Intermediate or central or venous compartment

It contains:
• Femoral vein

Medial or lymphatic compartment

It is also called femoral canal. It is the smallest of all compartments. It contains:
• Lymph node of Cloquet

Contents of Femoral Canal (Fig. 4.22)

• Lymph node of Cloquet or Rosenmullar's lymph node. It is named after Jules Germain Cloquet, 1790-1883, Professor of Anatomy and Surgery, St. Louis Hospital, Paris, France. It drains
  – Glans penis in males
  – Clitoris in females
• Lymphatics
• Areolar tissue and fat
• Femoral artery and vein are inside femoral sheath but femoral nerve is outside the femoral sheath and is lateral to femoral artery.

The femoral canal contents collectively make "femoral pad", which acts in the following manner:
• Cushions the femoral vein to expand in valsalva maneuver.
• As a plug to avoid abdominal contents from entering the thigh.

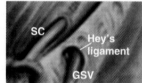
Fig. 4.23. Hey's ligament, left side.

Hey's Ligament (Figs. 4.18 & 4.23)

The lateral margin of saphenous opening is also called Hey's ligament. It is named after William Hey, English Surgeon (1736-1819) who described it. Hey's ligament helps the femoral hernia sac to divert upwards.

KEY POINT

All femoral hernias must be operated as there is high risk of strangulation. Strangulation is the initial presentation of 40% of femoral hernias.

(IV) VARIOUS LIGAMENTS IN RELATION TO GROIN HERNIA

"The surgical student's illustration is the living patient and his black board is the operation table."
                                                                    - Ian Aird

The various ligaments present in the groin hernia are described below:

Inguinal Ligament (Poupart's Ligament, Crural Arch, Fallopian Arch, Femoral Arch, Arcus Inguinalis, Fallopian Ligament, *Ligamentum Inguinale* or Superficial Crural Arch)

NOTE

The inguinal ligament is a band and not a ligament.[8]
It is named after Francoi's Poupart (1661-1708), Surgeon at Hotel Dieu, Paris, France. He wrote
"They are attached...... They perform the friction of bone in this region because they give the three great muscles of the abdomen, that is to say the external oblique, the internal oblique and the transverse".[9] The inguinal ligament was first described by Gabrielle Fallopio, Padua, Italy in 1561 and not by Poupart.

• It is a ligamentous thickened lower part of external oblique aponeurosis (Figs. 4.24 A & B), which at its lower end folds inwards.

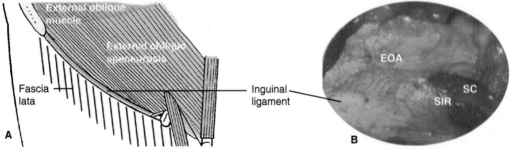

Fig. 4.24A. External oblique aponeurosis forming inguinal ligament, diagrammatic representation, **B.** Anterior view of external oblique aponeurosis forming inguinal ligament.

• It extends from ASIS to pubic tubercle, 12-14 cm in length.
• Its medial one-third has a free edge.
• Its lateral two-thirds is attached with ilio-psoas fascia.
• It has a grooved (deep or internal) abdominal surface which forms the floor of inguinal canal (Figs. 4.24 D & E).
• It is convex towards thigh and is continuous with fascia lata. The convexity is due to the pull of fascia lata.
• The lateral part of inguinal ligament is rounded and more oblique, the medial part is more horizontal and wide.
• It is situated at the junction of anterior abdominal wall and front of thigh, beneath the fold of groin.

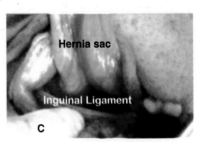

Fig. 4.24C. Inguinal ligament.

Attachments of inguinal ligament (Fig. 4.24F)

- Fascia lata is attached at its lower border. The ligament is convex downwards due to traction of fascia lata.
- Upper surface of inguinal ligament forms three muscles:
  - **Internal oblique muscle**
    It arises from the lateral two-thirds of inguinal ligament.
  - **Transversus abdominis muscle**
    It arises from lateral one-third of inguinal ligament.
  - **Cremasteric muscle**
    It arises from middle part of inguinal ligament.

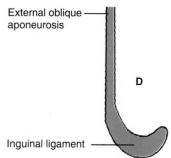

Fig. 4.24D. External oblique aponeurosis and Inguinal ligament.

Extensions of Inguinal Ligament (Fig. 4.25)

There are three extensions of inguinal ligament:
- Lacunar ligament
- Pectineal ligament
- Reflected part of inguinal ligament

Relations of inguinal ligament

Medial half of the upper grooved surface of inguinal ligament forms the floor of inguinal canal and contains spermatic cord or round ligament of uterus.

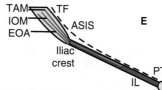

Fig. 4.24E. Iliac crest and inguinal ligament with attached muscles and fascia.

Lacunar Ligament (Gimbernat's Ligament or Pectineal part of Inguinal Ligament) (Fig. 4.25)

It is named after Manuel Louise Antonio Don Gimbernat (1734-1816), Professor of Anatomy, Barcelona, Spain . He attended lectures of William Hunter, brother of John Hunter in London. He became surgeon to King Carlos III. He demonstrated the lacunar ligament in 1768. In 1793, he wrote "A new method of operation on crural hernia". John Hunter started calling lacunar ligament "Gimbernat's ligament" after Gimbernat showed him how the incision of lacunar ligament facilitated reduction of strangulated femoral hernia.[10]

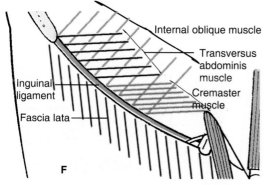

Fig. 4.24F. Attachments of inguinal ligament.

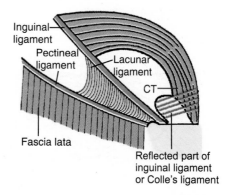

Fig. 4.25. Extensions of inguinal ligament.

- Lacunar ligament is the lower part of inguinal ligament. The fibres of lacunar ligament recurve down and are attached to pectinate ligament (Cooper's ligament). Sometimes, it forms the medial border of femoral canal.
- The deep part (abdominal) of lacunar ligament is called 'classical lacunar ligament' which extends from medial part of inguinal ligament to pecten pubis. It has the following features:
    - **Shape:** It is triangular in shape.
    - **Size:** It measures 2 cm from base to apex.
    - **Base:** It is laterally concave and forms medial rim of femoral ring.
    - **Apex:** It is attached to pubic tubercle.
    - **Anterior margin:** It is continuous with inguinal ligament.
    - **Posterior margin:** It is attached to pecten pubis and is continuous with pectineal fascia. Pectineal ligament or Sir Astley Paston Cooper's ligament extends laterally from its base.
    - It is horizontal in position.
    - It supports the spermatic cord.
    - It is strengthened by the pectineal fascia and by fibres from the linea alba.
- Fascial lacunar ligament is formed by fascia lata.

Iliopectineal or Pectineal Ligament (Sir Astley Paston Cooper's ligament) (Figs. 4.26 A-D)

It is named after Sir Astley Paston Cooper, a surgeon and anatomist, Guy's Hospital, London. He attended lectures of John Hunter as student. Perhaps the greatest English surgeon and anatomist. He called Cooper's ligament "ligament of pubis".

- It extends laterally from the base of lacunar ligament along pecten pubis. It is augmented by:
    - Pectineal fascia
    - Linea alba (adminiculum linea albae)
- It is formed by:
    - Fibres of lacunar (Gimbernat's) ligament
    - Periosteum and fascia along superior ramus of pubis
    - Aponeurotic fibres which are made up of three muscles:
        a) Internal oblique muscle
        b) Transversus abdominis muscle
        c) Pectineus muscle
    - Inguinal falx (Henle's ligament)

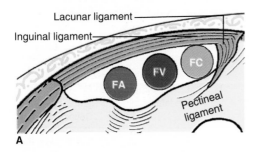 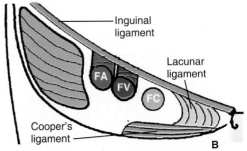

Fig. 4.26A. Inguinal, lacunar and pectineal ligaments, above or superior view, **B.** Front or anterior view of inguinal, lacunar and pectineal ligaments.

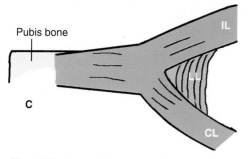

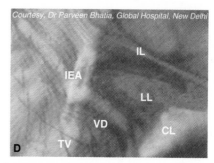

Fig. 4.26C. Inguinal, lacunar and Cooper's ligaments, diagrammatic representation, **D.** Laparoscopic view of inguinal, lacunar and Cooper's ligaments.

- It is fixed medially to superior pubic ramus and laterally to ileum.
- It is an extension of lacunar ligament from the posterior part of its base.
- It is regarded as thickening in the upper part of pectineal fascia.
- It forms the posterior border of femoral ring.

> **NOTE**
>
> *If a surgeon incises the inguinal ligament in a tightly incarcerated femoral hernia, then he will find that hernia cannot be reduced. It is because of the deeply placed Cooper's ligament. Laparoscopic hernioplasty dissection with grasper can cause injury to pudendal veins over Cooper's ligament and to obturator vessels below Cooper's ligament.*

Reflected Part of Inguinal Ligament (Colles' Ligament) (Figs. 4.27 A & B)

It is named after Abraham Colles (1773-1843), Professor of Anatomy and Surgery, Dublin, Ireland. He worked with Sir Astley Paston Cooper. His name is linked with the following:
- Colles' fracture of radius
- Colles' fascia
- Colles' ligament
- These fibres run from inferior crus of superficial inguinal ring to linea alba.
- It is an expansion of inferiolateral crus of superficial inguinal ring.
- It lies in front of falx inguinalis and behind the external oblique aponeurosis and superficial to inguinal ligament.
- Fibres of right and left ligaments decussate in linea alba.

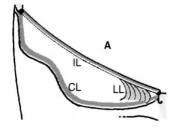

Fig. 4.27A. Course of Cooper's ligament.

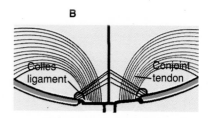

Fig. 4.27B. Colles' ligament.

Conjoint / Conjoined Tendon (Henle's Ligament or Inguinal Falx or *Falx Inguinalis,* L = Sickle, L = Inguinal) (Figs. 4.28A & B)

It is a conjoint tendon of:
- Internal oblique muscle
- Transversus abdominis muscle
- Transversus abdominis aponeurosis

It is attached to:
- Pubic crest
- Pecten pubis
  - It descends behind superficial inguinal ring.
  - It supports the weak area of anterior abdominal wall at superficial inguinal ring.
  - Medially, it fuses with anterior wall of rectus sheath.
  - Laterally, it may fuse with interfoveolar ligament.
  - It is mainly formed by the fusion of lowest aponeurotic fibres of internal oblique and fibres of transversus abdominis muscle.

"Some authors state that conjoint tendon is found in 5% cases only. They call it conjoint area"[49].

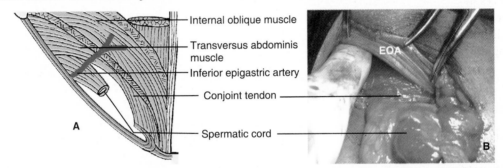

Fig. 4.28A. Conjoint tendon, diagrammatic representation, **B.** Open view of conjoint tendon..

> **NOTE**
>
> *Conjoint tendon insertion extends laterally 1-2 cm beyond pubic tubercle where it fuses with iliopectineal ligament of Astley Cooper. When this lateral extension is not present, the strength of the posterior wall is reduced and it predisposes to direct hernia (Figs. 4.29 A & B).[11]*

Interfoveolar Ligament (Hesselbach's Ligament) (Fig. 4.29A)

It is a false ligament and not a true ligament. It is a thickening of fascia transversalis at medial

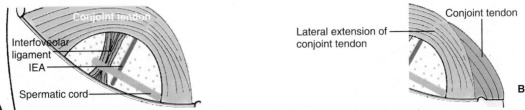

Fig. 4.29A. Interfoveolar ligament, **B.** Lateral extension of conjoint tendon.

border of deep inguinal ring, anterior to inferior epigastric vessels. It is attached above to transversus abdominis muscle and below to inguinal ligament.

Iliopubic Tract (Thomson's Ligament) (Figs. 4.30 A-D)

- In 1836, Alexander Thomson was the first who described the iliopubic tract.[47]
- The lower part of fascia transversalis is thickened to form the iliopubic tract.
- It is a band of aponeurotic fibres, which is a fascial condensation.
- It lies posterior to and adjacent to the inguinal ligament.
- If iliopubic tract is well-developed (in majority of cases), then it can be used in groin hernia repair.
- It is a member of "deep musculoaponeurotic layer of inguinal region".
  The deep musculoaponeurotic layer of inguinal region consists of:
  - Transversus abdominis muscle
  - Transversus abdominis aponeurosis
  - Fascia transversalis
  - Iliopubic tract
- It is a condensation of fascia transversalis.
- It is a lateral extension of fascia transversalis.
- It runs from iliopectineal arch and ASIS to superior pubic ramus. It normally inserts for a distance of 1-2 cm along the pectinate line and the mid portion of superior pubic ramus.
- It is anterior to Cooper's ligament and posterior to inguinal ligament.
- It separates deep inguinal ring from femoral canal.
- It is seen as a white fibrous tract.
- It forms the upper boundary of "Triangle of Pain".
- It forms the inferior crus of deep inguinal ring while transversalis fascia forms superior crus.
- Iliopubic tract ends medially in a fanning out manner by attaching to superior pubic ramus and Cooper's ligament.

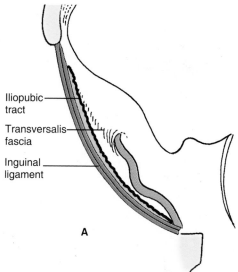

Fig. 4.30A. Course of Iliopubic tract.

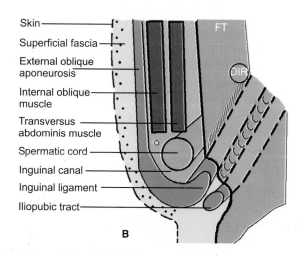

Fig. 4.30B. Iliopubic tract and its relations.

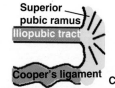

Fig. 4.30C. Iliopubic tract and Cooper's ligament.

> **NOTE**
>
> *The medial fibres of iliopubic tract are inserted in superior pubic ramus and Cooper's ligament. Fibres inserted on Cooper's ligament form medial border of femoral canal rather than lacunar ligament[46] (Fig. 4.30D).*

Course of iliopubic tract

It is a separate tract from inguinal ligament. It is attached laterally to iliac crest and ASIS. It runs medially crossing internal inguinal ring inferiorly then crosses femoral vessels and is attached medially to pubic ramus. It runs parallel to inguinal ligament. It is sometimes confused with inguinal ligament when underdeveloped (Fig. 4.30A).

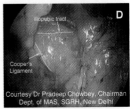

Courtesy Dr Pradeep Chowbey, Chairman
Dept. of MAS, SGRH, New Delhi

Fig. 4.30D. Iliopubic tract, laparoscopic view.

> **NOTE**
>
> *Iliopubic tract is an extremely important structure in repair of hernia in both the anterior and posterior approach.[12]*

Iliopectineal Arch (Fig. 4.31)

- It is the thickening of iliopsoas fascia and separates lacuna vasculorum from lacuna musculorum.
- It gives attachment to:
  - External oblique aponeurosis
  - Inguinal ligament
  - Internal oblique muscle fibres
  - Transversus abdominis muscle fibres
  - Iliopubic tract

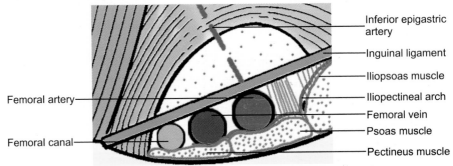

Fig. 4.31. Iliopectineal arch.

> **KEY POINT**
>
> *Knowledge of groin ligaments is important for both the open tension-free repair as well as the laparoscopic repair of inguinal hernia, and specially the knowledge of inguinal ligament, iliopubic tract, lacunar ligament and Cooper's ligament.*

(V) IMPORTANT STRUCTURES IN GROIN

"There is no more difficult art to acquire than the art of observation"

— Sir William Osler

Transversalis Fascia or Fascia Transversalis (Fascia of Gallaudet) (Figs. 4.32A-F)

> Fruchaud's view was that "the fundamental cause of all groin hernias is failure of the transversalis fascia to retain the peritoneum". Stoppa used prosthesis to replace fascia transversalis over Fruchaud's MPO.[13]

Transversalis fascia is perhaps the most commonly misunderstood structure in the literature devoted to groin hernia. It was first described by Cooper[14].

- It is a continuous sheet that covers the extraperitoneal space and that is why it is sometimes known as "wallpaper of abdominal cavity" or "Endoabdominal fascia".
- It lines the whole abdominal cavity. The part of fascia which lines the transversus abdominis muscle is called fascia transversalis.
- It is two-layered in inguinal region and envelops the inferior epigastric vessels.
- The fascia transversalis is attached anteriorly to linea alba and continues posteriorly with lumbar and renal fascia.
- It is continuous above as diaphragmatic fascia.

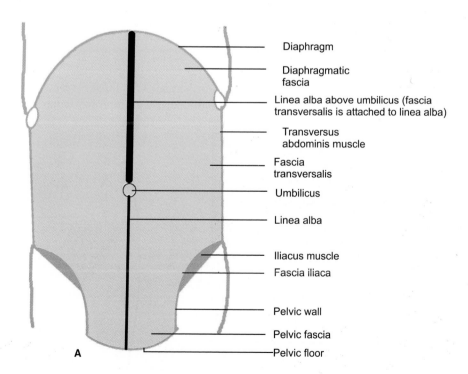

Fig. 4.32A. Transversalis fascia and its extent.

- Its lower part is attached to:
  - Iliac crest
  - Inguinal ligament
  - Pubic tubercle
  - Pubic crest
- A part of transversalis fascia extends below inguinal ligament as femoral sheath. Transversalis fascia is separated from peritoneum by a layer of preperitoneal adipose tissue called "Fascia propria", some call it Dulucq's fascia.

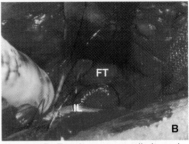

Fig. 4.32B. Fascia transversalis in groin, Achilles heel of groin.

- Transversalis fascia bridges the space between transversus arch above and inguinal ligament and iliopubic tract below. This area is a weak area in groin, known as "Achilles heel of groin". Direct inguinal hernia occurs here (Fig. 4.32B).
- It is of varying thickness and structure in different parts of abdominal cavity, according to the need of local part. Around kidneys, it contains plenty of fat and areolar tissue to give cushion effect to kidneys. In some regions, there occur aligned bundles of collagen, sometimes elastic fibres, particularly in the pelvis and bundles or sheets of non-striated muscle[15]. It gives strength to groin region and prevents hernia development.

- The fascia transversalis around deep inguinal ring forms superior and inferior crura. These two crura form a sling of fascia transversalis "Monk's Hood"-shaped structure around deep inguinal ring. It is also called "Sling of Keith" after Sir Arthur Keith, (1882-1931) Scottish anatomist (Fig. 4.32C). This fascial sling has a pulling effect outwards and above the deep inguinal ring and prevents indirect inguinal hernia formation.

- **Transversalis fascia and groin hernias**
  - Transversalis fascia plays an important role in preventing groin hernias.
  - Weakness of transversalis fascia leads to groin hernias so it must be repaired well and its anatomic integrity must be maintained to avoid recurrence. Improper repair of transversalis fascia is one of the causes of high recurrence.

Transversalis fascia analogous or derivatives:

- Iliopectineal arch
- Iliopubic tract
- Crura of deep inguinal ring
- Cooper's ligament
- Interfoveolar ligament
- Anterior femoral sheath

- **Thomson's fascia (Fig. 4.32D)**
  It covers femoral vein. It is not always present, but if present it is used in Cooper's ligament repair in femoral hernia operation.[15]

The anterior lamina of fascia transversus is adherent to rectus and transversus abdominis muscle and the posterior layer lies over

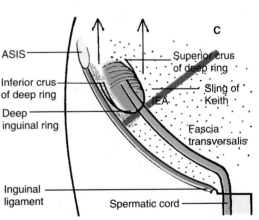

Fig. 4.32C. Fascia transversalis and sling of Keith.

peritoneum and divides the preperitoneal "Space of Nyhus" into the following two spaces:

- **Anterior space or vascular space (Fig. 4.32E)**
  - It is the space between anterior and posterior lamina of fascia transversalis.
- **Posterior space or space of Bogros (Fig. 4.32E)**
  - It is the space between posterior lamina of fascia transversalis and peritoneum.

    Both laminae of fascia transversalis are fused to Cooper's ligament inferiorly.

    Preperitoneal space is also called properitoneal space.

- The condensation of fascia transversalis forms three structures:
  - Interfoveolar ligament.
  - Iliopubic tract.
  - Iliopectineal arch.

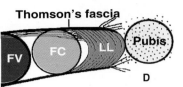

Fig. 4.32D. Thomson's fascia.

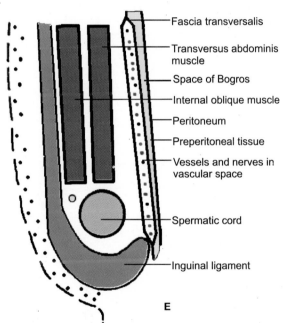

Fig. 4.32E. Vascular space and space of Bogros.

Boundaries of Fascia Transversalis

- **Anterior:** It is adherent to linea alba above the umbilicus.
- **Posterior:** It merges with thoracolumbar fascia and is continuous with renal fascia.
- **Superior:** It is continuous with diaphragmatic fascia.
- **Inferior:**
  - Laterally, it is attached to
    a) Inner lip of iliac crest
    b) Inguinal ligament

- Medially, it is attached to:
  - Pubic tubercle
  - Pubic crest
  - Pectineal line.

- It is also prolonged into thigh as anterior wall of femoral sheath.

Openings in fascia transversalis

- Deep inguinal ring

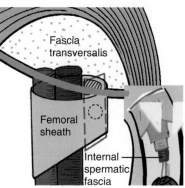

Fig. 4.33. Prolongations of fascia transversalis.

> **Prolongations of fascia transversalis (Fig. 4.33)**
>
> Fascia transversalis prolongs downwards in two directions:
> - Medially, propagates to internal spermatic fascia which is a tubular prolongation around spermatic cord.
> - Laterally, propagates to anterior wall of femoral sheath.

Relation to vessels and nerves

Femoral vessels lie inside the femoral sheath whereas femoral nerve lies outside the femoral sheath.

Preperitoneal Space of Nyhus (Fig. 4.34)

It is a space bounded anteriorly by anterior layer of fascia transversalis and posteriorly by peritoneum. It contains:
- Connective tissue
- Fat
- Vessels
- Nerves
- Lymph nodes and lymphatics

Arteries

- External iliac artery with its branches.
- Deep circumflex iliac artery.
- Suprapubic and retropubic arteries, accessory obturator artery, cremasteric artery.
- Inferior epigastric artery with its branches.

Veins

- External iliac vein.
- Deep circumflex iliac vein.
- Inferior epigastric vein:
  - Suprapubic and retropubic tributaries.

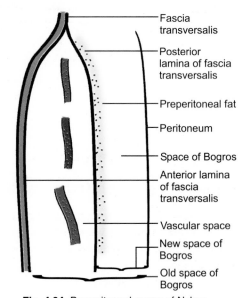

Fig. 4.34. Preperitoneal space of Nyhus.

– Rectusial tributaries from the rectus abdominis.
– Accessory obturator veins.
  All these veins form the "Bendavid circle".

Nerves

* Ilioinguinal nerve.
* Iliohypogastric nerve.
* Spermatic plexus of sympathetic and sensory nerves.
* Ventral rami of L1, L2, L3.
* Genitofemoral nerve. It has two branches:
  – Genital branch
  – Femoral branch
* Femoral nerve.
* Lateral femoral cutaneous nerve or lateral cutaneous nerve of thigh.

Space of Bogros (Fig. 4.35A-C)

This preperitoneal space was described by French anatomist Annet Jean Bogros (1786-1823) in 1823, the year he died.

The preperitoneal space was thought to be a single space but later on the space between anterior lamina of fascia transversalis and peritoneum was found to be divided by posterior lamina of fascia transversalis into two spaces:

* Anterior preperitoneal space or vascular space
* Posterior preperitoneal space or "space of Bogros"

Importance of space of Bogros (Fig. 4.35C)

Prosthetic mesh is placed in this space to cover hernia prone area completely.

> * The "Original Space of Bogros" was between peritoneum and anterior lamina of fascia transversalis.
> * "The New Space of Bogros" is a space between peritoneum and posterior lamina of fascia transversalis.
> * It is the lateral extension of retropubic space or cave of Retzius.

Space (Cave) of Retzius (Figs. 4.36 A-C)

It was described by Swedish anatomist, Anders Adolf Retzius (1796-1860) in 1858. It is a preperitoneal space in anterior abdominal wall lying behind supravesical fossa and medial umbilical fossa.

It contains:
* Normal and aberrant obturator vessels
* Accessory pudendal vessels in 10% persons

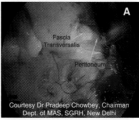

Fig. 4.35A. Space of Bogros, between fascia transversalis and peritoneum, laparoscopic view.

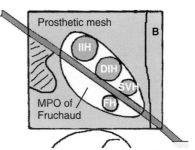

Fig. 4.35B. Mesh in space of Bogros, diagrammatic representation.

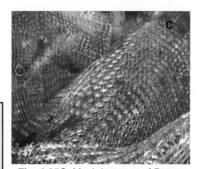

Fig. 4.35C. Mesh in space of Bogros.

- Loose connective tissue
- Fat
- Pubovesical ligaments

Boundaries of space of Retzius

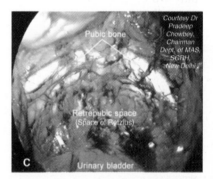

- **Anterior** – Posterior surface of pubis and rectus abdominis muscle.
- **Posterior** – Urinary bladder.
- **Superior** – Peritoneal reflection from urinary bladder to anterior abdominal wall.
- **Inferior** – Pubovesical ligaments.

Fig. 4.36A. Space of Retzius cross-section.

Importance of space of Retzius

Exploration of this space is important for proper fixation of mesh to cover whole hernia prone area in laparoscopic hernioplasty.

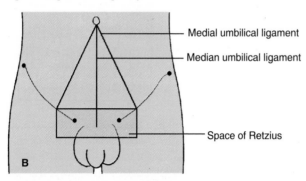

Fig. 4.36B. Space of Retzius, diagrammatic representation, **C.** Laparoscopic view of space of Retzius.

Hesselbach's Triangle (Figs. 4.37 A-C)

It was explained by Franz Caspar Hesselbach (1759-1816) in 1814.
- It is also called "Inguinal triangle".
- It is a weak area in anterior abdominal wall through which direct inguinal hernia occurs.
- It is bounded by:
  - **Superomedial boundary:** Lateral border of rectus muscle.
  - **Inferior boundary:** Inguinal ligament.
  - **Superolateral boundary**: Inferior epigastric vessels
  - **Fascia transversalis:** Forms the floor of the triangle.

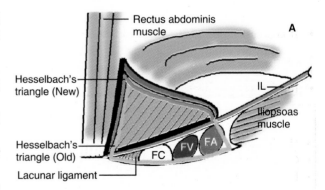

Fig. 4.37A. Hesselbach's triangle, new and old.

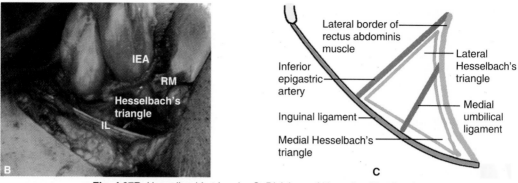

Fig. 4.37B. Hesselbach's triangle, **C.** Divisions of Hesselbach's triangle.

- The triangle is ressected by medial umbilical fold, which is formed by obliterated umbilical artery, into two compartments:
  - Medial compartment or supravescial fossa.
  - Lateral compartment or medial umbilical fossa.

NOTE

- *Direct inguinal hernia occurs through Hesselbach's triangle. It can occur in either of the two fossae, i.e., supravesical or medial umbilical fossa.*
- *Direct hernia occurs commonly through medial umbilical fossa, as in this area peritoneum is separated from external oblique aponeurosis by extraperitoneal tissue and fascia transversalis only, whereas in supravesical fossa conjoint tendon comes in the way and gives strength to the wall thus resisting the development of hernia. Therefore, supravesical hernia is less common.*

Today's Hesselbach's triangle is slightly smaller than the actual triangle described by Hesselbach in 1814. In the original triangle, the base was bounded by pubis pecten and pectineal ligament and not by inguinal ligament.

Hesselbach gave importance to the following two lower corners of triangle:

Medial corner

- It is between rectus muscle and pubis and is the site of direct inguinal hernia.

Lateral corner

- It is between pubic ramus and femoral vein and is the site of the neck of femoral hernia.

Hesselbach described the following structures:

- Hesselbach's triangle
- Corona mortis
- Hesselbach's hernia
- Hesselbach fascia (cribriform fascia)
- Hesselbach's ligament (interfoveolar ligament)

Lateral Triangle of Groin (Fig. 4.38)

MPO can be divided into three anatomic triangles, medial, lateral and femoral, also called triple triangles of groing which are the potential sites of groin hernia.

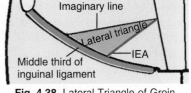

Fig. 4.38. Lateral Triangle of Groin.

Gilbert says that "failures following prior mesh repairs presented more commonly in the lateral triangle and became clinically evident within 2 years, following initial repair".[40]
The lateral triangle of groin has the following boundaries:

- **Base** – Middle one-third of inguinal ligament.
- **Medial boundary** – Deep epigastric vessels.
- **Lateral boundary** – A line from junctions of upper and middle one-third of the inguinal ligament to where the inferior epigastric vessels cross the lateral edge of rectus muscle.[41]

Myopectineal Orifice (MPO) of Fruchaud (Figs. 4.39 A-C)

It was described by H. Fruchaud, a French surgeon, in 1956. Fruchaud felt that this area in groin is the site of all common abdominal wall hernias.

Fruchaud hypothesis[42] is that "the fundamental cause of all groin hernias is failure of the fascia transversalis to retain the peritoneum". Stoppa used prolene mesh to reinforce fascia transversalis over MPO of Fruchaud. Fruchaud was Rene Stoppa's mentor. His influence on Stoppa led to the development of Stoppa's Giant Prosthetic Reinforcement of Visceral Sac (GPRVS).

It is an oval-shaped, funnel-like potential orifice.[48]

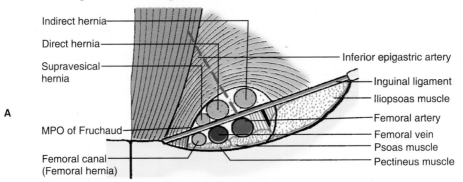

Fig. 4.39A. MPO of Fruchaud.

Boundaries of MPO of Fruchaud

- **Superior–** Arch of internal oblique and transversus abdominis muscles.
- **Lateral** – Iliopsoas muscle.
- **Medial** – Lateral border of rectus muscle.
- **Inferior** – Pubis pecten.

Iliopubic tract divides MPO into two parts:
- **Superior compartment:** It is further divided in two compartments by inferior epigastric vessels:
  - **Medial compartment or Hesselbach's triangle**
    It is the site of direct inguinal hernia.

– **Lateral compartment**
>   It contains deep inguinal ring—the site of indirect inguinal hernia.
- **Inferior compartment:** It is divided into two compartments:
  – **Lacuna vasculorum (Medial compartment)**
>   Through it, external iliac vessels pass into thigh and become femoral vessels. The medial compartment has femoral canal which lies medial to femoral vein and transmits femoral hernia.
  – **Lacuna musculorum (Lateral compartment)**
>   It is a neuromuscular compartment and allows femoral nerve and iliopsoas muscle to thigh.

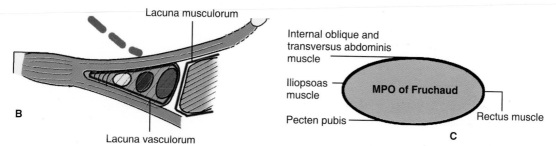

Fig. 4.39B. MPO of Fruchaud, inferior compartment.

Fig. 4.39C. MPO of Fruchaud.

Surgical Ellipse (Fig. 4.40)

All hernias develop from an elliptical area in groin, which is called "Surgical ellipse". Commonly, four hernias occur through this elliptical area:
- Indirect inguinal hernia
- Direct inguinal hernia
- External supravesical hernia
- Femoral hernia

This surgical ellipse has the following boundaries:
- **Floor** – Posterior wall, formed by transversus abdominis aponeurosis and fascia transversalis.
- **Superomedial edge**
  – Internal oblique muscle and aponeurosis
  – Transversus abdominis muscle and aponeurosis

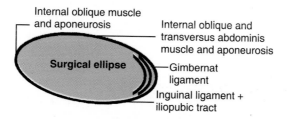

Fig. 4.40. Surgical ellipse.

- **Inferolateral edge**
  - Inguinal ligament
  - Iliopubic tract
  - Femoral sheath
  - Cooper's ligament
- **Medial apex** – Gimbernat's ligament
- **Lateral apex** – Arched fibres of internal oblique muscle and aponeurosis

Superficial Inguinal Pouch (Denis Browne)[16] (Figs. 4.41A & B)

It was described by Denis John Walker Browne (1892-1967), pioneer of British Pediatric Surgery, Hospital for Sick Children, Great Ormond Street, London, England.

It is a space occupied by loose areolar tissue. It is situated between following structures:
- External oblique aponeurosis
- Deep layer of superficial fascia (Scarpa's fascia)

Importance of inguinal pouch

- In children, retractile testis can retract in this pouch and mimic inguinal hernia.

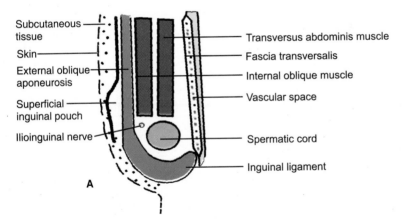

Fig. 4.41A. Superficial inguinal pouch.

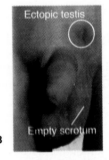

Fig. 4.41B. Retractile left testis in superficial inguinal pouch.

Pubis

It is the frontal part of pubic bone. It forms pubic symphysis by meeting the pubic bone of opposite side. It has three surfaces:
- Anterior surface
- Posterior surface
- Medial or symphyseal surface
- Anterior surface faces inferolaterally. It is attached to:
  - Medial femoral muscles
  - Pyramidalis muscle

- Posterior surface faces upwards and backwards. It is related to urinary bladder.
- Medial or symphyseal surface is united by a cartilage to the opposite pubis.

Pubic Crest (Fig. 4.42)

It is the upper border of pubis which hangs over the anterior surface. It is attached to:
- Rectus abdominis muscle
- Conjoint tendon

Superior Pubic Ramus

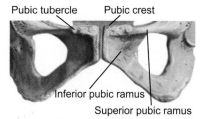

Fig. 4.42. Hernia landmarks in pelvis.

It extends from the body of pubis upward and laterally. It has three surfaces:

Anterior surface or pectineal surface (Fig. 4.43)

It is attached to pectineus muscle. Anteriorly, it is bounded by obturator crest and posteriorly by pecten pubis or pectineal line, which is a sharp line.

Dorsosuperior or pubic surface

It is bounded above by pecten pubis and below by a sharp inferior border.

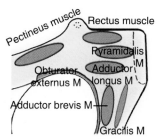

Fig. 4.43. Muscles attached to pubis.

Obturator surface

It is directed downwards and back. It is bounded posteriorly by a sharp inferior border and in front by obturator crest.

Pecten Pubis

It is also called "pectineal line". It is the sharp superior edge of the pectineal surface. It is attached to:
- Conjoint tendon
- Pectineal ligament or Cooper's ligament

KEY POINT

Transversus abdominis muscle, transversus abdominis aponeurosis and fascia transversalis are the most important layers in preventing inguinal herniation.

(VI) ANTERIOR ABDOMINAL WALL

"Ignorance is like knowledge, there is no end to it."

— **Albert Einstein**

"The anatomy of anterior abdominal wall has not changed but the understanding of it has changed due to introduction of laparoscopic hernia repair"

— **Author**

> *"The outline of the anterior abdominal wall is approximately hexagonal. It is bounded superiorly by the arched costal margin (with xiphisternal junction at the summit of the arch). The lateral boundary on either side is, arbitrarily, the mid-axillary line (between the lateral part of the costal margin and the summit of iliac crest). Inferiorly on each side, the anteriorly abdominal wall is bounded in continuity, by the anterior half of the iliac crest, inguinal ligament, pubic crest and pubic symphysis."*[17]
>
> - **Mahadevan V**

Anterior abdominal wall extends from subcostal margins above to inguinal ligaments and below to pubic symphysis. It is divided into two halves by a vertical groove. The linea alba lies underneath this groove. Normal abdominal wall is soft and moves inwards and outwards during respiration. The contour of abdomen depends upon muscle tone and fat. (Fig. 4.44).

McVay stresses that the terms anterolateral and posterolateral abdominal wall are more anatomically correct than anterior and posterior abdominal wall.[50]

Development of Anterior Abdominal Wall

The mesoderm of future abdominal wall divides and gives three flat muscles of abdominal wall, namely, external oblique, internal oblique and transversus abdominis muscles. By the third month of intrauterine life, abdominal wall closes except at umbilicus. Length of intestine increases faster than the abdominal cavity. So, intestines escape out of abdomen and

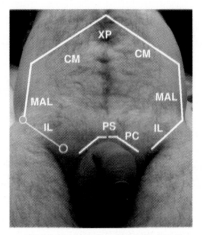

Fig. 4.44. Anterior abdominal wall.

enter the umbilical cord. When abdominal cavity develops sufficient space then intestines come back to abdominal cavity from umbilical cord and the umbilical ring closes. If any deviation happens in the development of anterior abdominal wall and the umbilicus does not close as scheduled, then umbilical hernia occurs.

Layers of Anterior Abdominal Wall (Fig. 4.45)

Abdomen has the following nine layers in its anterior abdominal wall:
- Skin
- Camper's fascia
- Scarpa's fascia
- External oblique muscle and aponeurosis
- Internal oblique muscle

- Transversus abdominis muscle
- Fascia transversalis
- Preperitoneal tissue
- Peritoneum

Most hernias are repaired through an anterior approach, therefore, it is essential to understand the anatomy of anterior abdominal wall—from skin to preperitoneal space.[18]

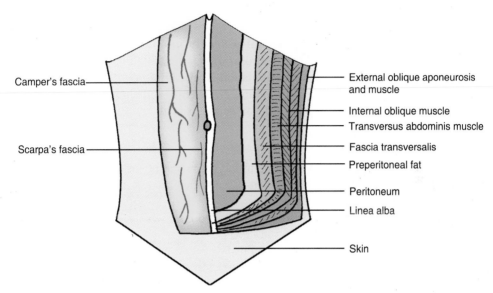

Fig. 4.45. Structure of anterior abdominal wall.

Skin

The skin is loosely attached to underlying structures except at umbilicus. At umbilicus, it is attached firmly with scar tissue.

The skin of anterior abdominal wall has great capacity to stretch so as to accommodate pregnancy, ascites and huge ventral hernias.

Langer's lines are the natural tension lines of strain due to pattern of collagen fibre bundles in the dermis. These are permanent lines and run in abdominal wall downwards and forwards, and almost horizontal in the middle of the trunk.

> **NOTE**
>
> *Incision should be made along Langer's lines to give a narrow scar as collagen fibres in dermis are in parallel rows. If the incision is across Langer's lines then the scar is puckered and heaped up.*

Linea Albicans

These are whitish lines or streaks on skin of lower part of anterior abdominal wall. These lines are formed due to the stretching of skin.

Linea Semilunaris

It is a visible curved vertical groove which extends from tip of the ninth costal cartilage in subcostal margin above and pubic tubercle below. It corresponds to the lateral margin of rectus abdominis muscle. It is clearly visible in thin persons with well developed muscles.

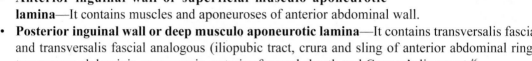

Fig. 4.46. Laminar structure of groin.

Laminar Structure of Groin (Fig. 4.46)

Groin wall is separated in two laminar structures by spermatic cord:
- **Anterior inguinal wall or superficial musculo aponeurotic lamina**—It contains muscles and aponeuroses of anterior abdominal wall.
- **Posterior inguinal wall or deep musculo aponeurotic lamina**—It contains transversalis fascia and transversalis fascial analogous (iliopubic tract, crura and sling of anterior abdominal ring, transversus abdominis aponeurosis, anterior femoral sheath and Cooper's ligament.[46]

Superficial Fascia (Figs. 4.47A & B)

It is a single-layered structure above umbilicus but below umbilicus it splits into two layers.

The structures found between two layers of superficial fascia are nerves, vessels, lymphatics and fat.

The superficial fascia of inguinal region is divided into two layers (Fig. 4.47):
- Camper's fascia – superficial part –a fatty layer
- Scarpa's fascia – deeper part –a membranous layer

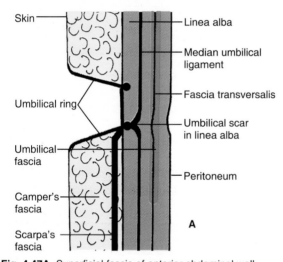

Fig. 4.47A. Superficial fascia of anterior abdominal wall.

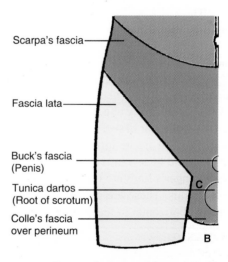

Fig. 4.47B. Extent of Scarpa's fascia

Camper's Fascia (Fig. 4.48)

It is named after Pieter Camper (1722-1789), Professor of Botany, Anatomy and Surgery, Groningen, the Netherlands. It extends upwards in anterior abdominal wall and down to perineum over thigh, buttocks and scrotum. It is continuous in other parts of body except:

- Penis–There is no fat in penis.
- Scrotum – It is replaced by dartos muscle.

Scarpa's Fascia (Fig. 4.48)

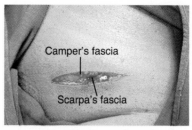

Camper's fascia

Scarpa's fascia

Fig. 4.48. Camper's and Scarpa's fascia.

It is named after Antonio Scarpa (1747-1832). He first studied in Bolagna, Italy and then became Professor of Surgery at Modena, Italy. Later on, he became Professor of Anatomy in Padua, Italy. Antonio Scarpa's name is associated with the following structures:
- Scarpa's triangle (femoral triangle).
- Scarpa's ganglion (ganglion in the eighth nerve in internal auditory meatus).

The subcutaneous fat contains Scarpa's fascia. It is a misnomer, since it is only a condensation of connective tissue.

Scarpa's fascia is of importance to hernia surgeon as it can hold the sutures.[19]

> Scarpa's fascia is a thin membranous layer. It extends from abdominal wall to penis, scrotum and perineum. It has different names at different positions:
> - **Scarpa's fascia** – in lower anterior abdominal wall
> - **Buck's fascia** – over penis
> - **Tunica dartos** – over scrotum
> - **Colle's fascia** – over perineum

The Scarpa's fascia and Colle's fascia are attached to deeper tissues in such a manner that they prevent the extravasation of urine after rupture of urethra, into ischiorectal fossa and thigh.

When Scarpa's fascia passes in front of thigh, it fuses with deep fascia of thigh, 1.5-2 cm below inguinal ligament. Posteriorly, it fuses with perineal body and posterior margin of perineal membrane.

The lines of attachment of this fascia are as follows:
- Holden's line (Line of attachment of Scarpa's fascia to thigh). It extends from just lateral to pubic tubercle to 8 cm laterally
- Pubic tubercle
- Body of pubis
- Pubic arch
- Perineal membrane

Extravasation of urine and Scarpa's fascia (Fig. 4.49)

Rupture of bulbar urethra can cause extravasation of urine in scrotum, perineum and penis and it can go deep into the lower part of anterior abdominal wall upto Scarpa's fascia. Urine does not extravasate in thigh because of attachment of Scarpa's fascia to fascia lata (Holden's line).

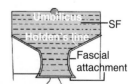

Umbilicus — SF

Holden's line

Fascial attachment

Fig. 4.49. Extravasation of urine and scarpa's fascia.

Importance of Scarpa's fascia

While closing abdominal wounds, the Scarpa's fascia must be sutured as it has the following advantages:
- It strengthens the wound.

- It strengthens the skin scar.
- Scar is better cosmetically.
- It can hold sutures.
- It prevents extravasation of urine in thigh.

Umbilicus (Figs. 4.50A-D)

Umbilicus is a scar in midline at the junction of third and fourth lumbar vertebrae.

Umbilicus is the site where the Veress needle is introduced to induce pneumoperitoneum in laparoscopic surgery, as the abdominal wall is thinnest and peritoneum is closer to the skin at umbilicus and is more densely adherent to the umbilicus than at any other site along the abdominal wall[20].

Umbilical hernia occurs through the umbilicus and paraumbilical hernia occurs above or below umbilicus in midline (Fig. 4.50).

Umbilical trocar site hernias occur in about 1% of the cases after laparoscopic herniorrhaphy[21].

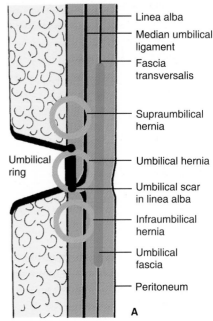

Fig. 4.50A. Umbilicus and umbilical fascia.

Umbilical ring (annulus umbilicalis) (Fig. 4.50)

It is the aperture in the abdominal wall through which the umbilical cord communicates with the foetus. After birth it is felt for sometime as a distinct fibrous ring surrounding the umbilicus. These fibres later shrink progressively.

Richet's Fascia (Fig. 4.50)

It was first described by Louis Alfred Richet (1816-1891), Professor of clinical surgery, Faculty of Paris, France. It is a fold of extraperitoneal fascia enveloping the obliterated umbilical vein.

- Umbilicus is the site of porto-caval anastomosis. These anastomoses open up in portal hypertension and form "caput medusae", which are dilated veins radiating from umbilicus.

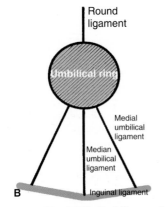

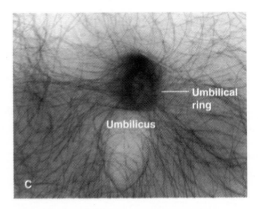

Fig. 4.50B. Umbilicus and ligaments, diagrammatic representation, **C.** External view.

- The venous blood flow and lymph flow of the anterior abdominal wall run upwards above and downwards below the plane of umbilicus. They do not cross umbilical plane.
- Umbilicus is supplied by T10 segment of spinal cord.
- Umbilicus is the meeting point of fourfolds (Fig. 4.50D) of embryonic planes:
  - Two lateral folds
  - One head fold
  - One tail fold
- Umbilicus is the meeting point of the following three systems:
  - Vitello-intestinal duct (digestive system)
  - Urachus (excretory system)
  - Umbilical vessels (vascular system)

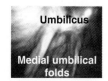

Fig. 4.50D. Umbilicus and medial umbilical folds.

- In early foetal life, loops of intestine escape from abdomen to umbilicus and later on gradually return back but sometimes this escape persists even at the time of birth and is called exomphalos.
- Weakness of umbilicus may lead to formation of umbilical hernia.

Cutaneous Nerves of Anterior Abdominal Wall (Figs. 4.51A & B)

- Anterior abdominal wall is supplied by:
  - Lower six thoracic nerves (T7-T12)
  - First lumbar nerve (L1)
- There are seven anterior cutaneous nerves. These are the branches of:
  - Lower five intercostal nerves
  - Subcostal nerve
  - Iliohypogastric nerve (T12, L1)
- Iliohypogastric nerve is situated 2.5 cm above superficial inguinal ring.
- Ilioinguinal nerve emerges through superficial inguinal ring and supplies external genitalia and medial side of thigh in upper part.

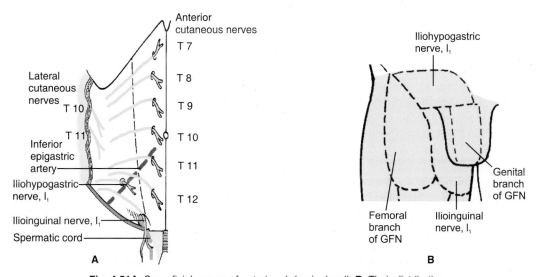

Fig. 4.51A. Superficial nerves of anterior abdominal wall, **B.** Their distribution.

- Two lateral cutaneous nerves supply side skin of the abdomen. They are derived from two lower intercostal nerves (T10, T11).
- Lateral cutaneous branches of subcostal nerve (T12) and iliohypogastric nerve (L1) supply anteriosuperior part of gluteal region.

Cutaneous Arteries of Anterior Abdominal Wall

Anterior cutaneous arteries (Fig. 4.52)

Anterior cutaneous arteries accompany anterior cutaneous nerves.
   These are the branches of:
- Superior epigastric artery
- Inferior epigastric artery

Lateral cutaneous arteries

These are branches of lower intercostal arteries and supply lateral side of anterior abdominal wall.
   Three superficial inguinal arteries are encountered in hernia surgery. These are:
- **Superficial epigastric artery**
  – It runs upwards and medially. It is encountered in medial part of incision for inguinal hernia. It is the branch of femoral artery.
- **Superficial external pudendal artery**
  – It runs upwards and medially. It passes in front of spermatic cord. It is a branch of femoral artery.
- **Superficial circumflex iliac artery**
  – It runs below the inguinal ligament and then it runs upwards and laterally. It is a branch of femoral artery.

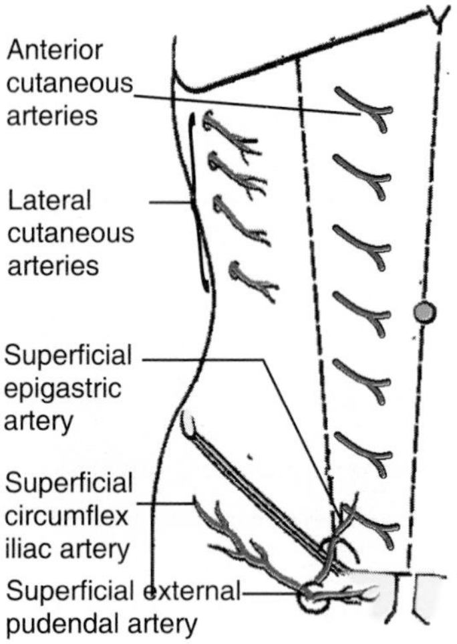

Fig. 4.52. Arteries of anterior abdominal wall.

Veins of Anterior Abdominal Wall (Fig. 4.53)

Veins of anterior abdominal wall accompany arteries. Superficial inguinal veins drain into great saphenous vein.
   In portal vein or superior venacava or inferior venacava obstruction, the superficial veins of anterior abdominal wall become dilated as they provide collateral circulation. So during the examination for anterior abdominal wall hernia if one finds dilated superficial veins, it could be due to PV/SVC/IVC obstruction, then investigate accordingly prior to surgery.
   In portal vein obstruction, blood flows upwards in superficial veins of abdomen above the umbilicus and downwards below the umbilicus. The dilated veins from the umbilicus are called 'caput medusae' (Fig. 4.54). The vein radiates from umbilicus in various directions.
- In SVC obstruction, the blood flows on the side of abdomen downwards.
- In IVC obstruction, the blood flows on the side of the abdomen upwards.

The superficial vessels in anterior abdominal wall form a network of vessels in subcutaneous tissue called "**panniculus adiposus**".

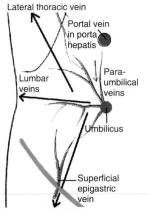

Fig. 4.53. Veins of anterior abdominal wall

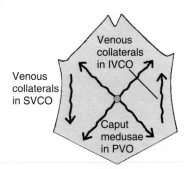

Fig. 4.54. Dilated veins of abdominal wall in IVCO, SVCO and PVO.

NOTE

Port site haematomas are formed due to injury to panniculus adiposus network in laparoscopic hernioplasty.

Deep Nerves of Anterior Abdominal Wall (Fig. 4.55)

Anterior abdominal wall is supplied by:
- Lower five intercostal nerves (T7- T11)
- Subcostal nerve (T12)
- Iliohypogastric nerve (L1)
- Ilioinguinal nerve (L1)

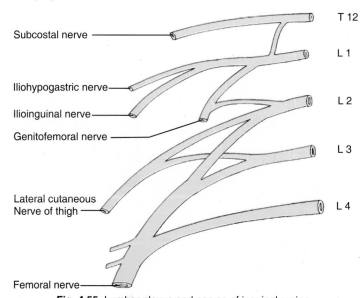

Fig. 4.55. Lumbar plexus and nerves of inguinal region.

NOTE

Following three nerves are most commonly injured during the open hernia operation.
* *Ilioinguinal nerve • Iliohypogastric nerve*
* *Genital branch of genito-femoral nerve*
Incision if applied without keeping anatomy of ilioinguinal nerve and iliohypogastric nerve in mind can inadvertently injure these nerves. The incision can be safely extended medially but lateral extension may cause injury to illioinguinal and illiohypogastric nerves (Fig. 4.56A). These nerves are usually not injured in laparoscopic surgery, but if excessive force is applied while applying staples or tacks, then they can get injured in laparoscopic surgery also.
Following three nerves are most commonly injured during the laparoscopic hernia operations. (Fig. 4.56B)
* *Lateral femoral cutaneous nerve • Femoral branch of genito femoral nerve • Intermediate cutaneous branch of the anterior branch of femoral nerve*
 Nerve entrapment causes severe pain, nerve transection numbness.

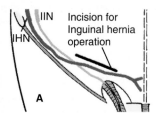

Fig. 4.56A. Incision for inguinal hernia causing injury to IIH and IIN

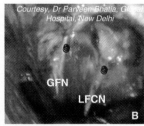

Fig. 4.56B. Common nerve injury in laparoscopic hernia repair.

Ilioinguinal Nerve (Figs. 4.57A-D)

It is a commonly damaged nerve during open hernia surgery and during mesh fixation in laparoscopic surgery. It can cause post-operative pain. Post-operative pain is now recognised as an important long term complication of inguinal hernia repair[22].

It pierces internal oblique muscle just below and medial to the iliohypogastric nerve, runs with

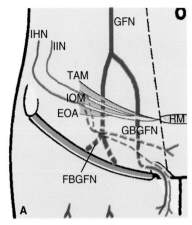

Fig. 4.57A. Ilioinguinal, iliohypogastric and genitofemoral nerves.

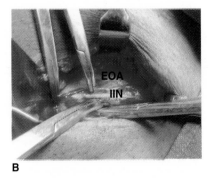

Fig. 4.57B. Ilioinguinal nerve exposed by incising external oblique aponeurosis.

the spermatic cord inside inguinal canal and becomes cutaneous by emerging through the superficial inguinal ring.

Pathway

It arises from L1, crosses quadratus lumborum muscle then crosses iliacus muscle, pierces transversus abdominis muscle near ASIS, then pierces internal oblique muscle, travels through inguinal canal then exits through external inguinal ring in front of spermatic cord (Fig. 4.57D).

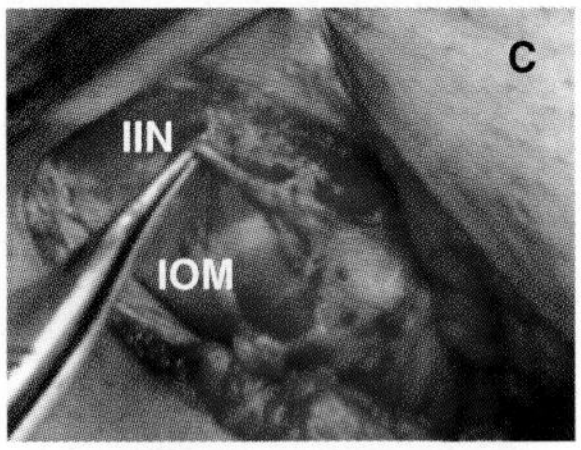

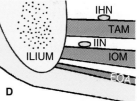

Fig. 4.57C. Isolation and preservation of ilioinguinal nerve.

Distribution

- Skin:
  - Root of penis
  - Anterior third of scrotum
  - Small area of thigh below medial part of inguinal ligament
  - Labia majora in females
- Abdominal musculature

Site of entrapment injury

- Medial to ASIS, during forceful fixation of mesh.

Clinical features of nerve injury

- Pain and burning (paraesthesia) in lower abdomen
- Hypoalgesia or hyperalgesia
- Tenderness medial to ASIS
- Limitation of internal rotation of hip
- Extension of hip causes pain
- Abdominal muscle weakness

Fig. 4.57D. Cross section of inguinal region, relation of nerves with muscles.

NOTE

Ilioinguinal nerve is most commonly injured nerve in open inguinal hernia repair while incising the external oblique aponeurosis and dividing superficial inguinal ring.

Iliohypogastric Nerve (Figs. 4.58A & B)

It pierces the internal oblique muscle from deep to superficial surface at about 2.5 cm in front of ASIS. It becomes cutaneous by piercing external oblique aponeurosis 2.5 cm above the superficial inguinal ring.

Pathway

It arises from T12 and L1, crosses quadratus lumborum muscle, pierces transversus abdominis muscle above iliac crest and then pierces internal oblique muscle just above and in front of ASIS, then it runs under external oblique muscle above inguinal canal, then pierces external oblique muscle above and medial to external inguinal ring.

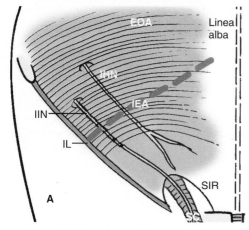

Fig. 4.58A. Ilioinguinal and iliohypogastric nerves.

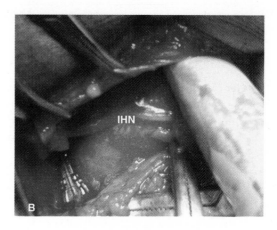

Fig. 4.58B. Iliohypogastric nerve.

Distribution

It supplies:
• Skin in suprapubic region.
• Posterolateral part of gluteal region with its lateral cutaneous branch.

Site of injury or entrapment

• It is more commonly injured in open hernia repair than in laparoscopic rapair while separating external oblique aponeurosis from internal oblique muscle.
• Medial to ASIS in forceful mesh fixation in laparoscopic repair.

Clinical features of nerve injury

• Pain and burning in the area of supply
• Hypoalgesia or hyperalgesia
• Tenderness medial to ASIS and suprapubic area
• Weakness of lower abdominal muscles

Genitofemoral Nerve (Figs. 4.59A-C)

Pathway

It originates from L1 and L2 crosses psoas muscle and divides into following two branches:
• Genital branch
• Femoral branch

• **Genital branch**
  The genital branch crosses the external iliac artery and enters the deep inguinal ring and travels through inguinal canal. It pierces the iliopubic tract lateral to internal inguinal ring and enters inguinal canal or pierces the transversalis fascia and travels with spermatic cord to scrotum.[53]
• **Femoral branch**
  It descends lateral to external iliac artery, crosses the deep circumflex iliac artery and passes behind the inguinal ligament to enter the thigh. It enters the femoral sheath lateral to femoral

artery then pierces the anterior layer of femoral sheath and fascia lata and supplies the skin of middle part of upper part of thigh.

Distribution (Fig. 4.59B)

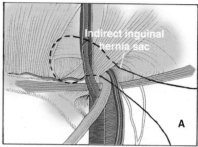

- **Genital branch**
  - It supplies to cremaster muscle, spermatic fascia and tunica vaginalis of testis.
  - It is the efferent branch for "cremasteric reflex".
  - In females, it is sensory to labia majora.
- **Femoral branch**
  - It supplies to skin over femoral triangle of thigh.
  - It is an afferent branch for "cremasteric reflex".

Fig. 4.59A. Reduction of indirect sac can cause injury to genital branch of genitofemoral nerve.

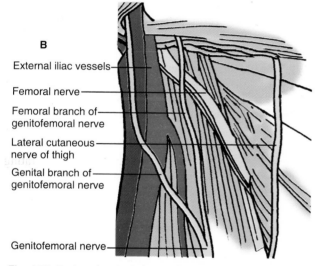

B

External iliac vessels

Femoral nerve

Femoral branch of genitofemoral nerve

Lateral cutaneous nerve of thigh

Genital branch of genitofemoral nerve

Genitofemoral nerve

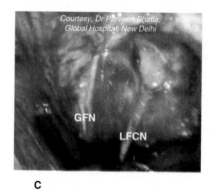

C

Fig. 4.59. B. Anterior view of genitofemoral, femoral and lateral femoral cutaneous nerves. **C.** Laparoscopic view of genitofemoral, femoral and lateral femoral, cutaneous nerves, Courtesy Dr. Parveen Bhatia, Global Hospital, New Delhi, India,

Sites of injury or entrapment

- It is usually injured or entrapped in inguinal or femoral area due to forceful fixation of mesh with staples or tacks.
- Genital branch can be damaged while reducing the sac in indirect inguinal hernia.
- Injury to genital branch is avoided by keeping the easily visible blue external spermatic vein (the blue line) with the spermatic cord while it is being lifted from the inguinal floor.[43,44]

Clinical features of nerve injury

- Pain in groin, scrotum and upper thigh
- Hyperalgesia or hypoalgesia
- Tenderness over inguinal canal area
- Walking or hyperextension of hip or external rotation of hip causes pain

- Loss of cresmasteric reflex
- Ejaculatory dysfunction

NOTE

There is evidence from a number of studies that upto 30% of patients will have some degree of discomfort or pain, one year or more after inguinal hernia repair[23]. This happens due to nerve injury.

Femoral Nerve (Fig. 4.60)

Origin

It arises from L2, L3 and L4.

Pathway

It emerges from lateral border of psoas muscle, travels under inguinal ligament lateral to the femoral artery outside the femoral sheath and divides into sensory and motor branches.

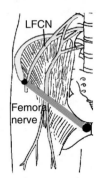

Fig. 4.60. Femoral and lateral femoral cutaneous nerves.

Distribution

- Sensory to medial and intermediate areas of thigh
- Motor to quadriceps muscles

Site of injury or entrapment

- Intermediate cutaneous branch of anterior branch of femoral nerve can be damaged during laparoscopic groin hernia repair.
- Femoral nerve can be damaged behind inguinal ligament.
    Femoral nerve although not routinely encountered during a preperitoneal dissection, but injuries have been reported [24] during groin hernia surgery.

Clinical features of femoral nerve injury

- Pain in groin, anterior and medial thigh
- Hyperalgesia or hypoalgesia
- Hip extension increases pain
- Quadriceps muscle weakness and atrophy
- Loss of patellar reflex

NOTE

Genitofemoral and lateral femoral cutaneous nerves are readily identified lateral to the spermatic vessels while performing a preperitoneal herniorrhaphy. They usually enter the thigh below the iliopubic tract, but exceptions have been described[25].

Lateral Femoral Cutaneous Nerve (Lateral Cutaneous Nerve of Thigh) (Fig. 4.60)

It is the most commonly injured nerve in laparoscopic hernia surgery.
The placement of staples outside the permitted area result in nerve injury.[26]

Origin

It originates from L2 and L3.

Pathway

It emerges from the lateral border of psoas muscle, crosses the iliac fossa over posterior wall, travels down lateral to iliac vessels and then emerges to thigh either through or below inguinal ligament 1 cm medial to ASIS.

Distribution

Lateral aspect of upper thigh.

Site of injury and entrapment

Above iliopubic tract.

Clinical features of nerve injury

- "Meralgia Paraesthetica" – Pain or numbness or severe burning sensation along its course.[54]

Deep Arteries of Anterior Abdominal Wall (Figs. 4.61- 4.64)

Anterior abdominal wall is supplied by two large arteries from above:
- Superior epigastric artery
- Musculo-phrenic artery
    Both of these arteries are two terminal branches of internal thoracic artery.
It is also supplied by two large arteries from below:
- Inferior epigastric artery
- Deep circumflex iliac artery
    These two arteries are branches of external iliac artery.

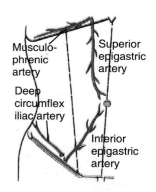

Fig. 4.61. Deep arteries of anterior abdominal wall.

Inferior Epigastric Artery (Figs. 4.61 & 4.62)

It is the branch of external iliac artery from the medial side of its lower end just above the inguinal ligament.

    Injury to the inferior epigastric vessels (during TAPP and TEP) may be treated by intracorporeal clipping.[27]

    It runs upwards and medially to deep inguinal ring and pierces transversalis fascia at lateral border of rectus muscle and enters posterior rectus sheath by passing in front of the arcuate line. It supplies rectus muscle and anastomoses with superior epigastric artery.

It has the following branches (Fig. 4.63):

- Cremasteric branch to spermatic cord. It runs laterally and upwards and penetrates the transversalis fascia and enters internal inguinal ring with spermatic cord.
- Pubic branch anastomoses, with pubic branch of oburator artery. Sometimes, it replaces obturator artery and then it is called abnormal obturator artery or aberrant obturator artery.
- Muscular branches to rectus abdominis muscle.
- Cutaneous branches to overlying skin.

Deep circumflex artery (Fig. 4.63)

It is the lateral branch of external iliac artery. It arises from the lateral side, opposite to the origin of inferior epigastric artery. It goes laterally and upwards behind inguinal ligament. It pierces transversus abdominis muscle and runs between it and internal oblique muscle.

Course

It has an ascending branch which originates near anterior superior iliac spine. It runs upwards between internal oblique and transversus abdominis muscles.

Muscles of Anterior Abdominal Wall (Figs. 4.64 A & B)

The following muscles form anterior abdomen wall:

- Large muscles
- Small muscles

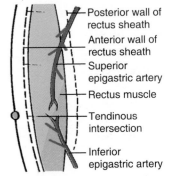

Fig. 4.62. Deep arteries of anterior abdominal wall.

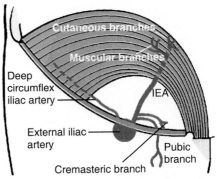

Fig. 4.63. Branches of inferior epigastric artery and deep circumflex iliac artery.

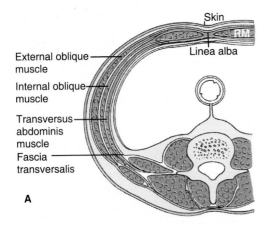

Fig. 4.64A. Muscles of anterior abdominal wall.

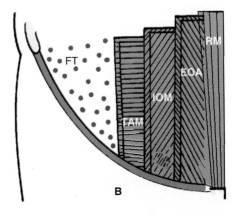

Fig. 4.64B. Directions of fibres of muscles of anterior abdominal wall.

Large muscles

These are four muscles on either side of midline:
- External oblique muscle
- Transversus abdominis muscle
- Internal oblique muscle
- Rectus abdominis muscle

The large muscles form anterior and lateral part of abdominal wall. Medially, these muscles except rectus abdominis end in strong sheets called aponeurosis. The aponeurosis on both sides of muscles meet in midline and decussate to form linea alba, a band in midline (Fig. 4.64A).

Small muscles

These are two muscles on either side of midline:
- Cremaster muscle
- Pyramidalis muscle

Fascia and aponeurosis (Fig. 4.65)

Fascia and aponeurosis are fibrous structures in muscles.
"Aponeurosis is a portion of muscle containing no muscle fibre, and is usually present at insertion points".
"Fascia is a fibrous tissue that lines or envelops a muscle."

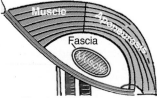

Fig. 4.65. Aponeurosis and fascia.

Large Muscles of Anterior Abdominal Wall

External oblique muscle (Fig. 4.66)

It is the most superficial muscle on the side of abdominal wall.

Origin

It arises from middle of the shaft of lower eighth ribs as eight muscle slips.

> Upper four slips interdigitate with those of serratus anterior muscle.
> Lower four slips interdigitate with those of latissimus dorsi muscle.
> The muscle fibres run in the following directions:

- Downward
- Medially
- Forward

Insertion

Muscle fibres end in aponeurosis which inserts in:
- Xiphoid process
- Linea alba
- Pubic symphysis
- Pubic crest
- Pectineal line of the pubis
- Lower fibres of muscle are inserted on outer lip of iliac crest on its anterior two-third

It is supplied by T7-T12 nerves.

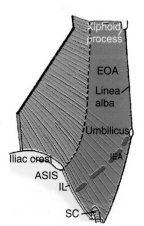

Fig. 4.66. External oblique muscle and aponeurosis.

External oblique fascia (Fig. 4.67)

It is a fascial sheet covering the external oblique muscle and aponeurosis over whole of the anterior abdominal wall. It is a weak layer of connective tissue.

External oblique aponeurosis (Fig. 4.68)

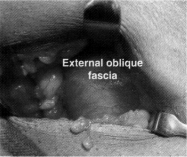

Fig. 4.67. External oblique fascia.

- The muscle is converted to a dense tendinous sheet called external oblique aponeurosis.
- The junction of muscle fibres and aponeurosis is represented by a line drawn from the ninth corsal cartilage down to the level of umbilicus, then this line curves laterally and meets ASIS.
- The aponeurosis of external oblique has a free inferior border which is folded inside and forms inguinal ligament. The external oblique aponeurosis has a free posterior border also.
- The aponeurosis forms anterior rectus sheath between linea semilunaris and linea alba.
- There is a triangular aperture in the aponeurosis of external oblique above the pubic crest called superficial inguinal ring.
- Fibres of external oblique course inferomedially as "hands in pockets".

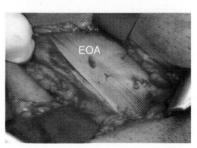

Fig. 4.68. External oblique aponeurosis.

- The external oblique aponeurosis divides in two layers at lateral border of rectus abdominis muscle above the arcuate line. One layer goes in front and another layer goes behind rectus abdominis muscle. Below arcuate line of Douglas, it goes in front of rectus abdominis muscle fusing with internal oblique and transversus abdominis aponeurosis and forms anterior rectus sheath.
- External oblique aponeurosis takes part in the formation of the following four ligaments:
  – Inguinal ligament (Poupart's ligament)
  – Lacunar ligament (Gimbernat's ligament)
  – Reflected inguinal ligament (Colles' ligament)
  – Pectineal ligament (Cooper's ligament)
- Rizk (1980)[28] found after extensive cadaveric study that external oblique aponeurosis is a bilaminar structure and not a unilaminar structure as thought previously.
  Two layers of aponeurosis are:
  – Superficial layer
  – Deep layer
  The fibres of both layers are at right angles to each other.

NOTE

Sometimes the infra-umbilical incision for laparotomy is closed by suturing the external oblique fascia and not the linea alba, which results in incisional hernia.

Internal oblique muscle (Figs. 4.69 & 4.70)

It lies deep to external oblique muscle and superficial to transversus abdominis muscle. Muscle and aponeurosis are covered with a fascia. It extends from iliopubic tract (iliopubic tract is a part of the iliopsoas fascia and lies behind the inguinal ligament which is a part of external oblique aponeurosis) to ribs.

Origin

It arises from:
- Inguinal ligament—It originates from lateral two-thirds part of inguinal ligament and is not attached to medial one-third part of inguinal ligament.
- Iliac crest—It is attached only to the intermediate strip of anterior two-thirds of iliac crest.
- Thoracolumbar fascia.

The fibres of internal oblique muscle run in the following directions:
- Upward
- Forward
- Medially

Muscle fibres of internal oblique cross the fibres of external oblique muscle at right angle.

Insertion

The muscle is inserted into the following structures:
- Lower three to four ribs and cartilages
- 7th, 8th and 9th costal cartilages
- Xiphoid process
- Linea alba
- Pubic crest
- Pectineal line of pubis

It is supplied by T7-L1 nerves.

> ### NOTE
>
> *Denervation of the internal oblique muscle by adjacent incisions (e.g., appendectomy) can also be associated with the eventual development of an indirect inguinal hernia.[29]*

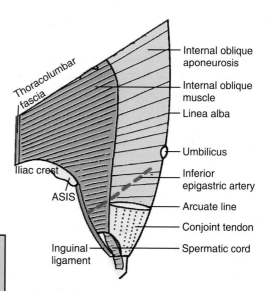

Fig. 4.69. Internal oblique muscle.

Aponeurosis of internal oblique (Fig. 4.69)

- The union of muscle fibres and aponeurosis is at the lateral border of rectus abdominis muscle.
- Aponeurosis takes part in the formation of rectus sheath as described below.

- **Below midway between umbilicus and pubic symphysis**
  It passes in front of rectus abdominis muscle forming anterior rectus sheath, as there is no posterior rectus sheath in this region.
- **Above midway between the umbilicus and pubic symphysis**
  Aponeurosis divides in two lamine at lateral border of rectus abdominis muscle. One lamina passes in front forming anterior rectus sheath and another passes behind rectus abdominis muscle forming posterior rectus sheath.

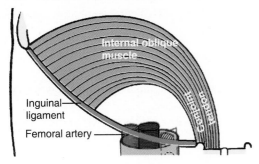

Fig. 4.70. Internal oblique muscle.

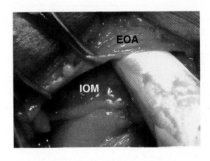

Fig. 4.71. Conjoint tendon.

The posterior rectus sheath is deficient below the level midway between umbilicus and pubic symphysis. This lower margin of posterior rectus sheath is downward concave in shape and is called "Arcuate line" or "Linea semicircularis" or "Fold of Douglas".

Lowest muscle fibres of internal oblique unite with lowest muscle fibres of transversus abdominis and form conjoint tendon.

Some fibres of internal oblique muscle wrap around spermatic cord and are called "cremasteric muscle".

Transversus abdominis muscle (Figs. 4.72 A & B & 4.73A-C)

Origin

It is the innermost muscle of abdominal wall. It originates from:

- Lateral one-third of the inguinal ligament.
- Anterior two-thirds of inner lip of iliac crest.
- Thoracolumbar fascia.
- Lower six costal cartilages.
- Iliopsoas fascia and inguinal region.

Muscle fibres of transversus abdominis run horizontally forward.

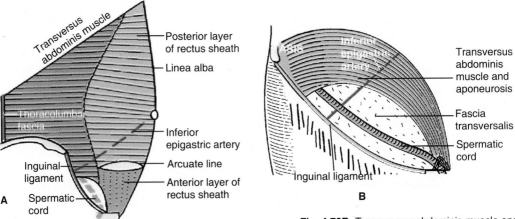

Fig. 4.72A. Transversus abdominis muscle and aponeurosis.

Fig. 4.72B. Transversus abdominis muscle and aponeurosis, in groin.

The muscle is inserted into the following structures:
- Xiphoid process
- Linea alba
- Pubic crest
- Pectineal line of pubis

It is supplied by T6-L1 nerves.

The neurovascular plane lies between internal oblique and transversus abdominis muscles. The neurovascular planes of anterior wall of abdomen and thoracic wall are continuous.

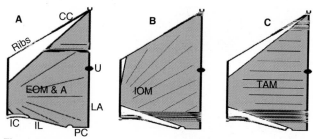

Fig. 4.73A-C. EOM covers groin better, IOM covers whole wall better and TAM covers middle part well. Jointly three muscles cover abdomen well and help trunk movement. CC = Costal Caritage   IC = Iliac Crest

Aponeurosis of transversus abdominis

- Above the level of arcuate line the aponeurosis transversus abdominis passes behind the rectus abdominis muscle along with posterior lamina of internal oblique muscle.
- Below the level of arcuate line the aponeurosis passes in front of rectus abdominis along with anterior rectus sheath.
- Aponeurosis of all abdominal muscles end in linea alba. Each aponeurosis splits into two laminae which interdigitate to give strength to anterior abdominal wall.

Transversus Abdominis Aponeurotic Arch (TAAA) (Fig. 4.74)

It is formed by the following structures:
- Transversus abdominis muscle
- Aponeurosis of transversus abdominis muscle
- Internal oblique muscle
- Aponeurosis of internal oblique muscle

Rectus abdominis muscle (Fig. 4.75)

Origin

Rectus abdominis is a long muscle, which runs vertically on either side of the midline of abdominal wall. It originates from two heads:
- **Lateral head:** It arises from lateral part of pubic crest.
- **Medial head:** It arises from anterior pubic ligament.

Insertion

It is inserted in the following structures:
- Xiphoid process
- 7th, 6th and 5th costal cartilages

It is supplied by T7-T12 nerves.

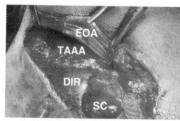

Fig. 4.74. Transversus abdominis aponeurotic arch.

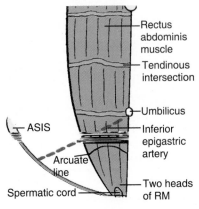

Fig. 4.75. Rectus abdominis muscle.

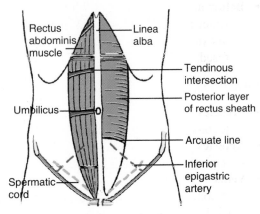

Fig. 4.76. Rectus sheath.

Rectus Sheath (Fig. 4.76)

Rectus abdominis muscle is enclosed in a sheath formed by aponeurosis of external oblique, internal oblique and transversus abdominis muscles.

This sheath is called rectus sheath. It has two walls:

- **Anterior wall**
  - It covers the rectus muscle completely.
  - It is firmly attached with tendinous intersections of muscle.
- **Posterior wall**
  - It is incomplete as it is absent above costal margins and below arcuate line.
  - It is free from rectus muscle and is not adherent to it.

Structure of rectus sheath (Fig. 4.77)

- **Above costal margin (Fig. 4.77a)**
  - Anterior wall: It is formed by external oblique aponeurosis.
  - Posterior wall: Deficient.
- **Between costal margin and arcuate line (Fig. 4.77b)**
  - Anterior wall: It is formed by external oblique aponeurosis and anterior lamina of internal oblique aponeurosis.
  - Posterior wall: It is formed by posterior lamina of internal oblique aponeurosis and aponeurosis of transversus abdominis.

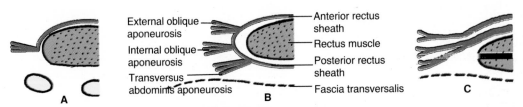

Fig. 4.77. Structure of rectus sheath.

- **Below arcuate line (Fig. 4.77c)**
  - Anterior wall: It is formed by aponeurosis of all three flat abdominal muscles. The aponeurosis of external oblique is separate but aponeurosis of both the internal oblique and transversus are fused.

Contents of rectus sheath

- **Muscles**
  - It contains two muscles: (i) Rectus abdominis muscle (ii) Pyramidalis muscle
- **Arteries**
  - It contains two arteries: (i) Superior epigastric artery (ii) Inferior epigastric artery
- **Veins**
  - It contains two veins: (i) Superior epigastric vein— It drains into internal thoracic vein. (ii) Inferior epigastric vein—It drains into external iliac vein.
- **Nerves**
  - It contains the following nerves: (i) Five lower intercostal nerves (ii) Subcostal nerve.

Functions of rectus sheath

- It increases the efficiency of rectus abdominis muscle during its contraction by checking the bowing of rectus muscle.
- It gives the strength to the anterior abdominal wall.

Tendinous intersections (Fig. 4.78A)

The rectus muscle is divided in four parts by three transverse fibrous bands called "tendinous intersections". These intersections:

- Explain the segmental origin of rectus abdominis muscle.
- Increases the power of rectus muscle by increasing the number of muscle fibres.

The three intersections found at three levels are as follows:

- Opposite free end of xiphoid process
- Opposite umbilicus
- Third intersection is in between the above two

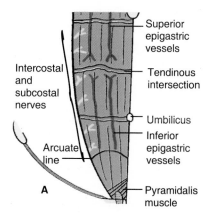

Fig. 4.78A. Tendinous intersections.

Linea Semilunaris

It is a curved line from tip of 9th costal cartilage to pubic tubercle. It corresponds to the lateral border of rectus abdominis muscle.

Arcuate Line (Linea Semicirularis or Semilunar Fold of Douglas) (Fig. 4.78A)

The posterior rectus sheath ends at a level midway between umbilicus and pubic symphysis. It is concave inferiorly and is also known as the fold or line of Douglas or linea semicircularis or arcuate line. It lies 2.5 cm below the umbilicus. The inferior epigastric artery enters the rectus sheath below the arcuate line. It is named after James Douglas (1675-1742), Anatomist and Obstetrician, London, England.

Linea Alba (Figs. 4.78B & C)

It is formed by decussating aponeurotic fibres of three flat muscles of anterior abdominal wall in the midline. It extends from pubic symphysis to xiphisternum. It is wide above the umbilicus and narrow below the umbilicus as the two rectus muscles touch each other below the umbilicus but these are separated above the umbilicus. It is avascular so the midline incisions are bloodless but healing is delayed and incisional hernia is common here.

Each lateral muscle of anterior abdominal wall has two laminae of aponeurosis, so six laminae from each side come in midline and decussate forming linea alba. Normally, it is a triple decussation. When there is single decussation, then it is in midline. When there is triple decussation, then one is in midline and two other decussations are on sides at the medial borders of two recti.

Sometimes it is difficult to recognize linea alba on exploration and midline incision goes to one side and exposes the rectus muscle which you do not want to see. Here is a solution "Lift the upper end of midline incision with introduction of index finger towards head and a ridge is raised". Incision on this ridge leads to linea alba.[51]

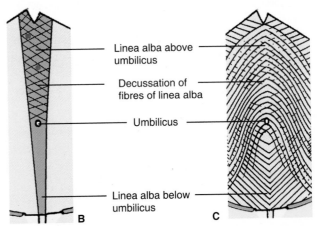

Fig. 4.78B. Single decussation, abnormal, **C.** Triple decussation, normal.

Functions of Anterior Abdominal Wall Muscles (Fig. 4.79)

- **Support to abdominal viscera**
  - It provides a support to abdominal organs against gravity by their muscle tone. **Internal oblique muscle** is the most important support of abdominal viscera.
- **Protection to abdominal organs**
  - Thick muscle sheets act as anchor sheets.
- **Assistance to expulsive acts**
They assist in all the expulsive acts like:
  - Micturition
  - Defaecation
  - Parturition
  - Vomiting
- **Support to muscles during respiration and during forceful expiratory acts**
  - The external oblique muscle helps during respiration

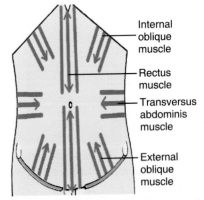

Fig. 4.79. Functions of anterior abdominal wall muscles.

by depressing and compressing the lower part of chest causing forceful expiratory acts such as coughing, sneezing, blowing and shouting.

- **Movements to trunk (Fig. 4.64A)**

Muscles of anterior abdominal wall are responsible for the following movements of body:
  - Flexion of trunk is helped by rectus abdominis muscle.
  - Lateral flexion is caused by oblique muscles.
  - Rotation of trunk is by the combined efforts of external oblique and internal oblique muscles.

Small Muscles of Anterior Abdominal Wall (Fig. 4.80)

Cremaster muscle (Fig. 4.80)

The cremaster muscle consists of muscle fasciculi embedded in cremasteric fascia. The muscle fasciculi form loops. These loops are attached on both ends with bone and muscles and thus facilitate in action of cremaster muscle.

The medial ends of loops are attached with:

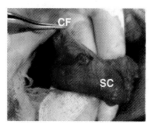

- Pubic tubercle
- Pubic crest
- Conjoint tendon

The lateral ends of loops are continuous with:

Fig. 4.80. Small muscles of anterior abdominal wall.

- Inguinal ligament
- Internal oblique muscle
- Transversus abdominis muscle

Cremasteric fascia (Fig. 4.81)

The cremasteric fascia actually is a collection of muscle loops with intervening connective tissue. It forms a layer around spermatic cord and testis. It is between internal spermatic fascia and external spermatic fascia.

Cremasteric muscle is fully developed in males. In females, it has only few fibres as there is no testis to be elevated.

It is supplied by genital branch of genitofemoral nerve (L1).

It suspends and elevates the testis. It tends to close the superficial inguinal ring when intra-abdominal pressure increases.

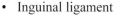

Fig. 4.81. Cremasteric fascia covering the spermatic cord.

Cremasteric reflex (Fig. 4.82)

If the skin of upper medial thigh is touched with hand, there is a reflex contraction of cremasteric muscle causing elevation of testis. The reflex is lost in L1 upper motor neuron lesion and is brisk in children.

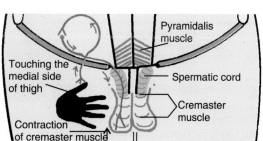

Fig. 4.82. Pathway of cremasteric reflex.

Pyramidalis muscle (Fig. 4.82)

It originates from anterior surface of body of pubis. It is inserted into linea alba. It is supplied by (T12) subcostal nerve.

It makes linea alba tense and stretched.

Functional Divisions of Anterior Abdominal Wall (Figs. 4.83 A - C)

The anterior abdominal wall is divided in two areas functionally as well as structurally:
- **Upper Zone – "Parachute area"**
  - It supports respiratory movements and gives support to the upper abdomen.
- **Lower Zone – "Belly Support area"**
  - It supports the lower abdomen.[30]

The functional failure in abdominal wall may lead to hernia formation in parachute area and belly support area.

- Functional failure in parachute area leads to:
  - Epigastric hernia.
  - Umbilical and paraumbilical hernia.

- Functional failure in belly support area leads to:
  - Inguinal hernia.
  - Femoral hernia.

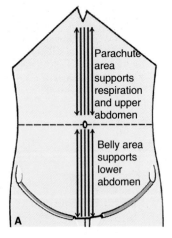
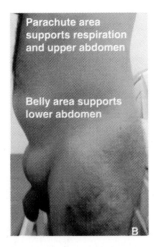
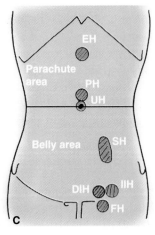

Fig. 4.83A. Functional divisions of anterior abdominal wall, diagrammatic view, **B.** Side view, **C.** Common hernias in front view.

Comparison between Supraumbilical and Infraumbilical Parts of Anterior Abdominal Wall (Fig. 4.84)

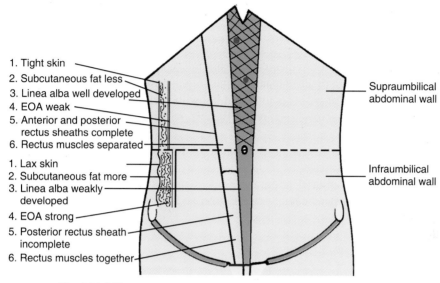

1. Tight skin
2. Subcutaneous fat less
3. Linea alba well developed
4. EOA weak
5. Anterior and posterior rectus sheaths complete
6. Rectus muscles separated

Supraumbilical abdominal wall

1. Lax skin
2. Subcutaneous fat more
3. Linea alba weakly developed
4. EOA strong
5. Posterior rectus sheath incomplete
6. Rectus muscles together

Infraumbilical abdominal wall

Fig. 4.84. Difference between supraumbilical and infraumbilical abdominal wall.

KEY POINT

In laparoscopic hernia surgery, you can see that the structures above iliopubic tract are the part of anterior abdominal wall and structures below iliopubic tract are the part of retroperitoneal area. Avoid dissection and fixation devices below iliopubic tract.

Lymphatic Drainage of Anterior Abdominal Wall (Fig. 4.85)

The lymphatic drainage of anterior abdominal wall above and below the umbilicus do not cross as there is a watershed line between them at the level of umbilicus.

The lymphatics of anterior abdominal wall above the umbilicus drain upwards towards axillary lymph nodes.

The lymphatics of anterior abdominal wall below the umbilicus drain downwards into superficial inguinal lymph nodes.

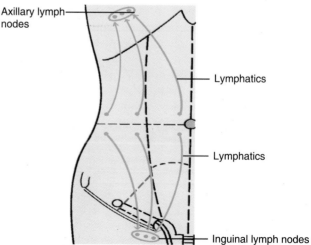

Axillary lymph nodes

Lymphatics

Lymphatics

Inguinal lymph nodes

Fig. 4.85. Lymphatic drainage of anterior abdominal wall.

(VII) LAPAROSCOPIC GROIN ANATOMY

"Remember that your patient is a human being like yourself, your knowledge of anatomy may save his or her life."

- Richard S. Snell

Before the beginning of laparoscopic hernia surgery, the familiarity with anatomy of posterior wall of inguinal canal was not much required and it was also not much understood. But now it is a must for every surgeon who wishes to practise laparoscopic groin hernia repair. Most of the surgeons are well versed with anterior view of groin anatomy but not with posterior view of groin anatomy.

During open hernia repair, some structures are visible, which are not seen during laparoscopic hernia repair and vice-versa.

It is essential to know the laparoscopic groin anatomy for the following purposes:
- Proper repair and fixation of mesh.
- To avoid complications and injuries to organs.

The posterior or inner or laparoscopic view of lower abdominal wall shows: (i) Five peritoneal folds and (ii) six fossae.

Five Peritoneal Folds (Fig. 4.86)

Five peritoneal folds are:
- **Median umbilical ligament or fold**
  - It is in the midline of anterior abdominal wall. It is the remnant of urachus.
- **Medial umbilical ligaments or folds**
  - These are two folds, one on either side of median umbilical ligament or fold. These are formed by peritoneal folds over obliterated umbilical arteries and are present upto internal iliac artery.

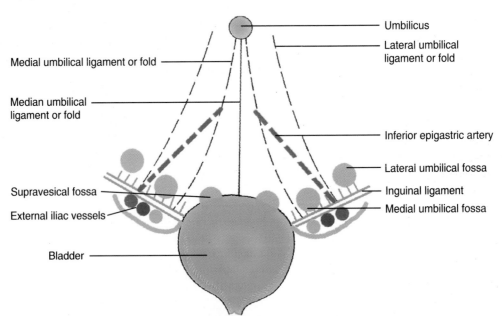

Fig. 4.86. Peritoneal folds and fossae.

Dissection medial to medial umbilical fold during laparoscopic hernioplasty should be avoided as it may cause injury to urinary bladder.
- **Lateral umbilical ligaments or folds or Plica epigastrica**
  - These are two folds, one on either side. These are formed by peritoneal folds covering inferior epigastric vessels. These folds are lateral to medial umbilical folds.

NOTE

Laparoscopic hernioplasty dissection and incision over lateral umbilical fold can cause injury to inferior epigastric vessels which may lead to severe bleeding.
Dissection and cauterisation lateral to lateral umbilical fold must be done with caution as it may damage nerves.

Six Peritoneal Fossae (Fig. 4.87)

The five peritoneal folds divide the lower anterior abdominal wall in the following fossae:
- **Supravesical fossa**
  - It is in between median and medial umbilical ligament on each side. Hernia is rare in this region due to rectus muscle. It is the site of supravesical hernia.
- **Medial fossa**
  - It is between medial and lateral umbilical ligaments. It is the site of direct inguinal hernia and femoral nerve.
- **Lateral fossa**
  - It is lateral to lateral umbilical ligament on both sides. It is the site of internal inguinal ring and so is the site of indirect inguinal hernia. Its medial boundary is formed by inferior epigastric vessels and lateral border of rectus muscle. Its lateral boundary is not properly defined.

Important Anatomical Inguinal Landmarks in Laparoscopic Surgery

Anatomical landmarks are important areas to be identified to avoid complications.

Before incision of peritoneum

- Inferior epigastric vessels
- Medial umbilical ligament (obliterated umbilical artery)
- Spermatic vessels
- Vas deferens

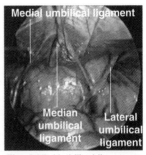

Fig. 4.87. Umbilical ligaments.
Courtesy Dr Pradeep Chowbey,
Chairman Dept. of MAS, SGRH,
New Delhi.

After incision of peritoneum

- Internal inguinal ring
- Iliopubic tract
- Cooper's ligament
- Femoral canal

Important anatomical landmarks are discussed below.

(1) "Trapezoid of Disaster"(Seid) or "Square of Doom"(Annibali and Fitzgibbons) (Figs. 4.88A & B)

Injury to vessels residing in the retroperitoneum is the most feared complication, as the associated mortality rate is significant. These usually occur during initial access to the abdomen or preperitoneal space in the case of a TEP repair.[31]

It is a trapezoid-shaped area which can lead to serious complications. It is further divided in two triangles:
- **Triangle of doom** – It is a medially placed triangular area.
- **Triangle of pain** – It is a laterally placed triangular area (Spaw in 1991).

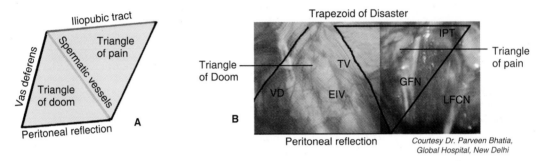

Fig. 4.88A. Trapezoid of Disaster, diagrammatic representation, **B.** Laparoscopic view.

Courtesy Dr. Parveen Bhatia, Global Hospital, New Delhi

Triangle of Doom (Spaw) (Figs. 4.89A & B)
It contains external iliac vessels.

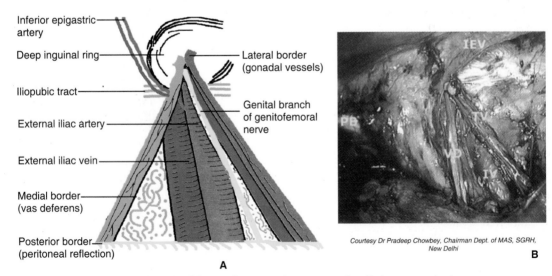

Courtesy Dr Pradeep Chowbey, Chairman Dept. of MAS, SGRH, New Delhi

Fig. 4.89A. Triangle of Doom, diagrammatic representation, **B.** Laparoscopic view.

NOTE

Any dissection in Triangle of Doom can cause injury to external iliac vessels and may lead to severe bleeding. No dissection should be performed in this area and no staple should be applied here.

It contains:
- External iliac artery
- External iliac vein
- Inferior epigastric vessels

It is formed as follows:
- **Apex–** Meeting point of vas deferens and testicular vessels at deep inguinal ring.
- **Medial boundary–** Vas deferens.
- **Lateral boundary –** Testicular vessels.
- **Base –** An imaginary line connecting lower part of the medial border and lateral border (peritoneal reflection).

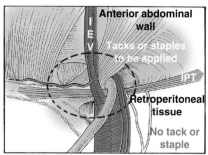

Fig. 4.90. No dissection or staple is done below iliopubic tract.

Triangle of Pain – (Annibali and Fitzgibbons) (Figs. 4.91A & B)

It contains most of the nerves of this area.

It contains:
- Femoral nerve
- Femoral branch of genitofemoral nerve
- Lateral femoral cutaneous nerve

NOTE

Some nerves can be damaged by dissection or application of staples in Triangle of Pain, so no dissection or staple should be applied here (Fig. 4.90).

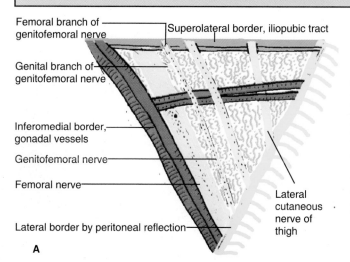

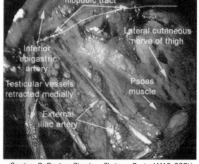

Courtesy Dr Pradeep Chowbey, Chairman Dept. of MAS, SGRH, New Delhi

A **B**

Fig. 4.91A. Triangle of pain, diagrammatic representation, **B.** Laparoscopic view.

During laparoscopic repair, lateral femoral cutaneous and genitofemoral nerves are most often affected, usually best treated by re-exploration with neurectomy. Mesh removal is usually needed as well.[32]

It is formed as follows:
- **Apex** – Meeting point of iliopubic tract and testicular vessels at deep inguinal ring.
- **Inferiomedial boundary** – Testicular vessels.
- **Superolateral boundary** – Iliopubic tract.
- **Base:** An imaginary line connecting iliopubic tract and testicular vessels (peritoneal reflection).

The injury in triangle of doom and triangle of pain can be avoided by not putting any suture or staple below the level of iliopubic tract.

(2) Corona Mortis or Crown of Death or Circle of Death (Figs. 4.92A & B)

Pubic branch of inferior epigastric artery travels down and anastomoses with obturator artery, a branch of internal iliac artery. In 20-30% cases, pubic branch is enlarged and replaces the obturator artery and then it is known as accessory or aberrant obturator artery. The aberrant obturator artery forms an anastomosis between external and internal iliac arteries. The injury to this artery leads to severe hemorrhage. The aberrant obturator artery is present at the neck of femoral hernia sac and it can be damaged if massive bleeding occurs during femoral hernia repair by laparoscopy. Due to this reason, this arterial circle is known as "corona mortis". Injury in this area usually occurs during fixation of mesh in hernioplasty.

Major haemorrhages from Corona Mortis are not common but rare in experienced hands and require urgent laparotomy. There is no place for laparoscopic management of major vessel injury. Wantz GE has reported few cases of major vessel injury haemorrhage, after 4114 Shouldice's hernia repair.[33]

Tributaries of obturator vein can be damaged while dissecting around Cooper's ligament.

The veins in this area also can be troublesome especially iliopubic, obturator and their tributaries as they may be larger than their accompanying arteries.[34]

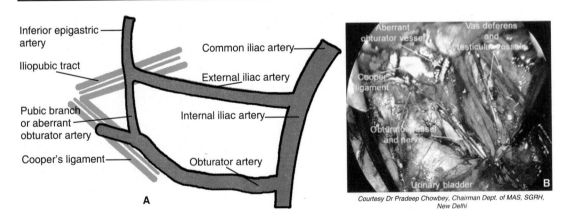

Courtesy Dr Pradeep Chowbey, Chairman Dept. of MAS, SGRH, New Delhi

Fig. 4.92A. Corona mortis, diagrammatic representation, **B.** Laparoscopic view.

(3) Inferior epigastric vessels (Fig. 4.93)

These are the branches of external iliac vessels.

Importance
- Bleeding from their injury during laparoscopic hernia repair is quite brisk and irksome.
- Inferior epigastric artery is most prominent near its origin from medial side of external iliac artery.
- Inferior epigastric artery forms lateral border of Hesselbach's triangle.
- Direct inguinal hernia is identified medial to these vessels and indirect inguinal hernia is identified lateral to these vessels.

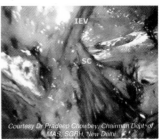

Fig. 4.93. Inferior epigastric vessels, laparoscopic view.

> ## NOTE
>
> *Pubic branch in laparoscopic hernia repair (Fig. 4.94A)*
>
> *Pubic artery goes down vertically on medial side and crosses the Cooper's ligament and anastomoses with obturator artery at obturator foramen. The anterior pubic artery is large in 25-30% individuals and can replace the obturator artery; if it replaces then it is called aberrant obturator artery. This artery passes over lacunar ligament from inside and thus can be damaged during femoral hernia operation when the lacunar ligament is divided.[35]*

The inferior epigastric vessels run upwards at medial to deep inguinal ring raising a peritoneal fold called "lateral umbilical ligament".

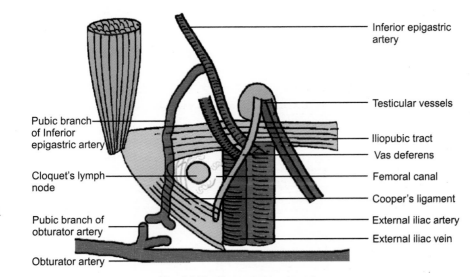

Fig. 4.94A. Aberrant obturator artery.

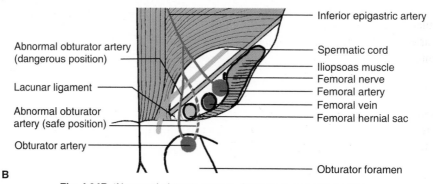

Abnormal obturator artery (dangerous position)

Lacunar ligament

Abnormal obturator artery (safe position)

Obturator artery

Inferior epigastric artery

Spermatic cord

Iliopsoas muscle

Femoral nerve

Femoral artery

Femoral vein

Femoral hernial sac

Obturator foramen

B

Fig. 4.94B. Abnormal obturator artery, dangerous and safe positions.

KEY POINT

The aberrant obturator artery can be damaged during femoral hernia operation while dividing lacunar ligament. It is present in 20% cases.

Medial umbilical ligament (obliterated umbilical artery)

- It can be confused with inferior epigastric artery but can be differentiated by following its course from internal iliac artery towards umbilicus (umbilical port).
- It runs midway between internal inguinal ring and Cooper's ligament.
- Dissection medial to it can damage urinary bladder.

(4) Spermatic vessels (Fig. 4.95)

They descend lateral to external iliac vessels and enter internal inguinal ring. They bisect the "Trapezoid of Disaster" and divide into "Triangle of Doom" and "Triangle of Pain". They are seen crossing from retroperitoneal area from lateral side and entering into deep inguinal ring. They are easily damaged and cause haemorrhage.

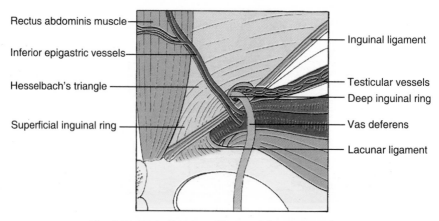

Rectus abdominis muscle

Inferior epigastric vessels

Hesselbach's triangle

Superficial inguinal ring

Inguinal ligament

Testicular vessels

Deep inguinal ring

Vas deferens

Lacunar ligament

Fig. 4.95. Groin anatomy, diagrammatic representation.

Testicular artery originates from abdominal aorta at L2 level below the origin of renal artery. Testicular artery runs along lateral border of ureter and external iliac artery, crosses the iliopubic tract and enters the inguinal canal from lateral side of deep inguinal ring.

(5) Vas deferens (Fig. 4.96)

It can be seen ascending and entering internal inguinal ring from medial and inferior side.

It forms medial boundary of "Trapezoid of Disaster" and "Triangle of Doom".

Injury to vas deferens is unusual.

(6) Internal inguinal ring (Fig. 4.96)

• It is identified by confluence of vas deferens and testicular vessels.
• It is seen just lateral to inferior epigastric vessels.
• The inferior epigastic vessels, the internal inguinal ring with spermatic vessels, and the vas deferens should be identified. These three structures form the so-called "Mercedes-Benz" sign.

Importance

It is the site of indirect inguinal hernia.

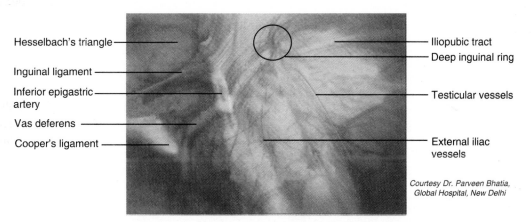

Courtesy Dr. Parveen Bhatia,
Global Hospital, New Delhi

Fig. 4.96. Groin anatomy, laparoscopic view, deep inguinal ring.

(7) Myopectineal Orifice (MPO) of Fruchaud (Figs. 4.97 & 4.98)

Henry Fruchaud, in 1956, gave the theory of aetiology of groin hernia.

> *Fruchaud's Theory*
>
> All groin hernias occur through a weak area in groin, "myopectineal orifice" which is now called "Myopectineal orifice of Fruchaud."

Fruchaud's contribution to inguinal herniology was the explanation of the common anatomic aetiology of direct, indirect and femoral hernias.[36]

Adequate exposure of myopectineal orifice of Fruchaud is required in laparoscopic hernia repair for proper covering and fixation of mesh, most common reason of recurrence is incomplete dissection of MPO.[52]

MPO is divided by iliopubic tract in two compartments:
• Superior compartment.
• Inferior compartment.

Superior compartment

This compartment is further divided in the following two compartments by inferior epigasteric vessels:
• Medial compartment which is prone to direct inguinal hernia.
• Lateral compartment containing deep inguinal ring prone to indirect inguinal hernia.

Inferior compartment

This compartment is also further divided in the following two compartments:
• **Medial compartment or Lacuna vasculorum:** This compartment has femoral vessels and femoral canal which is prone to femoral hernia. It is an area below the iliopubic tract through which external iliac vessels cross the pelvis and reach femoral triangle in thigh. It is a neurovascular compartment through which femoral nerve and iliopsoas muscles reach thigh.
• **Lateral compartment or Lacuna musculorum:** This compartment contains iliopsoas muscle. It is a neuromuscular compartment containing femoral nerve also.

If you see from posterior side, you will find that rectus muscle is attached to pubic bone. The pubic bone forms the centre and below it is urinary bladder. Lateral part of pubic bone is the site of Cooper's ligament which extends laterally. The iliopubic tract is attached to Cooper's ligament medially and then extends along superior pubic ramus, crossing the external iliac vessels, forming inferior border of deep inguinal ring, attaching to iliopsoas fascia and then to ASIS.

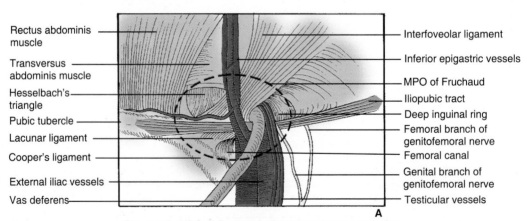

Fig. 4.97A. MPO of Fruchaud, diagrammatic representation.

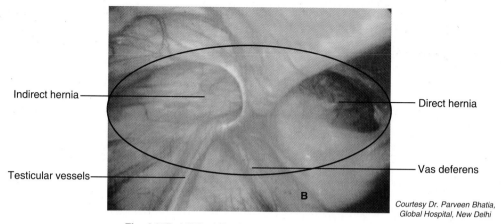

Fig. 4.97B. MPO of Fruchaud, laparoscopic view.

Courtesy Dr. Parveen Bhatia,
Global Hospital, New Delhi

(8) Hesselbach's Triangle (Figs. 4.98A & B)

Laparoscopic view of this triangle is quite different then anterior view. Iliopubic tract forms the base instead the inguinal ligament. Both the old and the new Hesselbach's triangles and their derivatives are clearly identified by laparoscopic view.

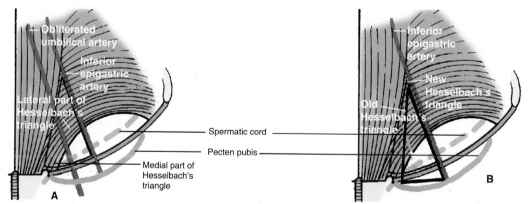

Fig. 4.98A & B. Hesselbach's triangle, old and new, lateral and medial parts, laparoscopic view.

(9) Iliopubic tract

It is a thick tract, which is a lateral extension of fascia transversalis. The area above the iliopubic tract is anterior abdominal wall and the area below the iliopubic tract is retroperitoneal area. The iliopubic tract is visible in laparoscopic hernia repair lateral to inferior epigastric vessels reaching ASIS.

NOTE

- *Iliopubic tract separates internal inguinal ring and femoral canal.*
- *Staples or tacks should never be placed below the iliopubic tract.*

It is anterior to Cooper's ligament and posterior to inguinal ligament and can be seen as white tract.

(10) Cooper's ligament

- It is a condensation of fascia transversalis and periosteum adherent to pubic ramus.
- It joins iliopubic tract and lacunar ligament.
- It is seen as white curvilinear structure.
- The adipose tissue surrounding Cooper's ligament has to be removed to visualise it properly in laparoscopic hernia repair.

(11) Femoral canal

- It is the site of femoral hernia.
- It is behind iliopubic tract.
- It is medial to femoral vein and lateral to lacunar ligament.

> *Important points in relation to the exposure and dissection of anatomical landmarks in groin hernia (Fig. 4.99)*
>
> - *A hernia above iliopubic tract is inguinal hernia and a hernia below it is a femoral hernia.*
> - *Dissection in trapezoid of disaster must be avoided.*
> - *Staples should not be applied below iliopubic tract.*
> - *Following structures must be exposed and identified*
>   - *Inferior epigastric vessels*
>   - *Internal inguinal ring*
>   - *Iliopubic tract*
>   - *Spermatic cord and vas deferens*
>   - *Testicular vessels*
>   - *Cooper's ligament*
>   - *Transversus abdominal arch*

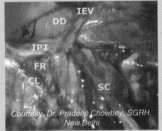

Courtesy, Dr. Pradeep Chowbey, SGRH, New Delhi

Fig. 4.99. Anatomical laparoscopic landmarks in groin hernia.

(12) The lacunar ligament

It can be seen as a triangular ligament between iliopubic tract and Cooper's ligament forming medial border of femoral canal in laparoscopic hernia repair.

(13) Venous circle of Bendavid (R. Bendavid) (Fig. 4.100)

- It is a network of veins.
- It is situated in "Space of Bogros".
- It receives tributaries from:
  - Deep inferior epigastric vein
  - Iliopubic vein
  - Rectusial vein
  - Suprapubic vein

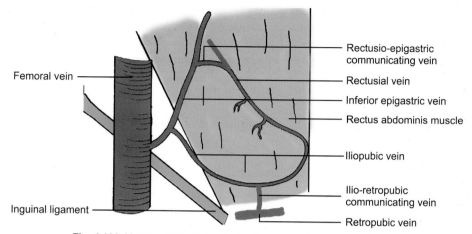

Fig. 4.100. Venous circle of Bendavid, diagrammatic representation.

- Retropubic vein
- Aberrant obturator vein (in 70% individuals)

Importance of Circle of Bendavid

The veins in this area can be troublesome[34].
It is important to know about these minor looking veins as their injury during laparoscopic hernia surgery can lead to haemorrhage and haematoma formation. Sometimes it is difficult to stop such bleeding and resulting panic can cause damage to other important structures.

Rectusial vein
Rectusial vein runs along lateral border of rectus muscle and forms venous anastomosis with iliopubic vein.

Iliopubic vein
Iliopubic vein runs deep to iliopubic tract and joins inferior epigastric vein.

Retropubic vein
Retropubic vein is found on posterior aspect of pubic ramus.

NOTE

These veins can collapse during laparoscopic surgery due to high carbon dioxide pressure and their injury is not visualized at that time but form haematoma later on when carbon dioxide is removed.

Nerves in preperitoneal space

The main nerves in inguinofemoral region are situated in a triangular area called "Triangle of Pain". It contains the following nerves:

- Genitofemoral nerve is on psoas muscle on medial side of "Triangle of Pain".
- Genital branch of genitofemoral nerve crosses the lower part of external iliac artery and pierces the iliopubic tract and enters the deep inguinal ring.
- Femoral branch of genitofemoral nerve runs along distal part of psoas muscle.
- Femoral nerve is lateral to genitofemoral nerve. It lies between psoas and iliacus muscles.
- Lateral cutaneous nerve of thigh is medial to ASIS.

Important Blood Vessels in Laparoscopic Hernia Repair

External iliac vessels

External iliac artery becomes femoral artery when it crosses iliopubic tract. It lies on psoas muscle. External iliac vein lies posterior and medial to it. External iliac artery and vein are the largest vessels in the area. They are seen medial to psoas muscle and going down under iliopubic tract to enter thigh becoming femoral vessels.

External iliac artery gives two branches from its distal part:
- Inferior epigastric artery – from medial aspect of external iliac artery.
- Deep circumflex iliac artery – from lateral aspect of external iliac artery.

Both branches of external iliac artery are given approximately at the same level just before going deep to iliopubic tract.

Pampiniform Plexus of Veins (L. Pampinus = tendril, shaped like a tendril) (Figs. 4.101 & 4.102)

These veins drain into testicular veins which in turn drain into:
- Inferior vena cava on right side.
- Renal vein on left side.

Pampiniform plexus of veins are classified into four groups by Ergun.[37]

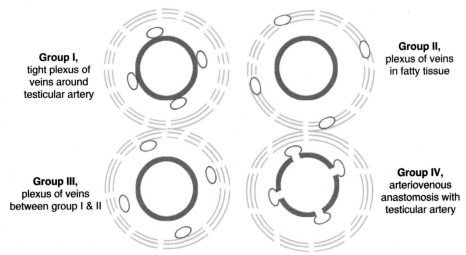

Group I, tight plexus of veins around testicular artery

Group II, plexus of veins in fatty tissue

Group III, plexus of veins between group I & II

Group IV, arteriovenous anastomosis with testicular artery

Fig. 4.101. Grading of pampiniform plexus.

Group I: Tight plexus of veins around testicular artery.

Group II: Plexus of veins in fatty tissue.

Group III: Plexus of veins located between group I and II.

Group IV: Artereovenous anastomosis with testicular artery.

Deferential vessels

Artery of vas deferens arises from inferior vesical artery. It forms network in adventitia of vas deferens.

Vein to vas deferens drains into pampiniform plexus and vesical plexus.

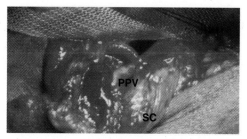

Fig. 4.102. Spermatic cord and pampiniform plexus of veins.

KEY POINT

Anatomical landmarks must be displayed well and identified in laparoscopic hernia repair. No tack or staple should be applied below iliopubic tract and specially in the area of Trapezoid of Doom.

REFERENCES

1. **Norman L. Browse**., (1997). An introduction to the symptoms and signs of surgical disease, 3rd edition, p. 320.
2. **Peter L. Williams, Mary Dyson**., (1989). Gray's anatomy, 37th edition, p. 426.
3. **Chaurasia BD**., (2004). Human anatomy, 4th edition, p. 194.
4. **Panton JA**., (1922). Factors bearing upon the etiology of femoral hernia. *J. Anat.*, 57: 106.
5. **Mc Vay CB**., (1974). The anatomic basis for inguinal and femoral hernioplasty. *Surg. Gynecol. Obstet.*, 139: 1931–45.
6. **Condon RE**., (1971). Surgical anatomy of the transversus abdominis muscle and transversalis fascia. *Ann. Surg.*, 173: 1–5.
7. **Lytle WF**., (1978). The inguinal and lacunar ligaments. In: Nyhus LM, Condon RE, Editors, Hernia, 2nd edition, Philadelphia, JB Lippencott Co. p. 54.
8. **Harold Ellis**., (2006). Eponyms in groin surgery, *Surgery International*, **43**, 257.
9. **Ellis HA**., (2001). History of surgery. Cambridge; Cambridge Universitiy Press.
10. **Rutkow IM**., (2003). A selective history of hernia surgery in the late 18th century: The Treatise of Percivall Pott., Jean Louis Petit, D. August de Gimbernat, and Peter Camper, *Surg. Clin. North Am.*, 83: 1021–44.
11. **Condon RE**., (1989). The anatomy of the inguinal region and its relation to the groin hernia. In Nyhus LM, Condon RE (Eds): Hernia, 3rd edition Philadelphia: JP Lippencott, p. 18.
12. **Nyhus LM**., (1960). An anatomical reappraisal of the posterior inguinal wall, with special consideration of the iliopubic tract and its relation to groin hernias. *Surg. Clin. North Am.*, 44: 1305.
13. **Stoppa RE**., (2002). The midline preperitoneal approach and prosthetic repair of groin hernias, in Fitz Gibbons Jr. RJ: Greenburg AG(Eds): Nyhus and Condon's Hernia, 5th edition, Philadelphia: Lippincott Williams and Wilkins, p. 199.

14. **Cooper A.**, (1804). The anatomy and surgical treatment of abdominal hernia. Philadelphia: LE and Blanchard, p. 26.
15. **Williams PL, Dyson M.**, (1989). Gray's anatomy, 37th edition, p. 604.
16. **Browne D.**, (1938). Diagnosis of undescended testicle, *Br. med. J.* 2: pp. 168–171.
17. **Mahadevan V.**, (2006). Anatomy of the anterior abdominal wall and groin, *Surgery International*, **43**, 221.
18. **Mark A Malangoni** *et al.*, (2004). Hernias, Sabiston textbook of surgery, 17th edition, p. 1201.
19. **F. Charles Brunicardi** *et al.*, (2005). Schwartz; principles of surgery, 8th edition, p. 1359.
20. **Carrol EH, Scott Conner.**, (2006). The SAGES manual, fundamentals of laparoscopy, thoracoscopy and GI endoscopy, 2nd edition, p. 19.
21. **Voitk AJ Tsao SG.**, (2001). The umbilicus in laparoscopic surgery: *Surg. Endose.* 15: 878.
22. **Martein Kurzer, Allan E. Kark.**, (2005). Inguinal hernia repair- An update: Recent advances in surgery, 28, p. 81.
23. **Bay Nielsan M, Norden P, Kehlet H.**, (2004). Chronic pain after TEP repair of inguinal hernia. *Br. J. Surg.* 291: 1372–76.
24. **Annibali R, Quinn TH, Fitzgibbons RJ Jr.**, (1994). Avoiding nerve injury during laparoscopic hernia repair; critical areas for staple placement, in Arregui ME, Nagan RF (Eds): Inguinal hernia: advances or controversies? Oxford: Radcliff Medical Press, p. 41.
25. **Rosenberger RJ, Loeweneck H, Meyer G.**, (2000). The cutaneaous nerves encountered during laparoscopic repair of inguinal hernia: New anatomical findings for the surgeons, *Surg. Endosec.* 14: 731.
26. **Kirk RM.**, (2000). Surgical operations, 4th edition, p. 153.
27. **Wellwood J, Sculpher MJ, Stoker D**. *et al.*, (1998). Randomise controlled trial of laparoscopic versus open mesh repair for inguinal hernia outcome and cost. *Brit. Med. Jour.* 317: 103–10.
28. **Rizk NN.**, (1980). A new description of the anterior abdominal wall in man and mammals, *J. Anat.*, 131: 273–385.
29. **Arnbjornsson E.**, (1982). Development of right inguinal hernia after appendicectomy. *Am. J. Surg.* 143:174.
30. **Bennett DH.**, (2005). A companion to specialist surgical practice, core topics in general and emergency surgery, 3rd edition, p. 57.
31. **F. Charles Brunicardi** *et al.*, (2005). Schwartz; principles of surgery, 8th edition, p. 1389.
32. **Heise CP, Starling JR.**, (1998). Mesh inguinodynia: A new clinical syndrome after inguinal herniorrhaphy. *J. Am Coll Surg.*, 187: 1528.
33. **Wantz GE.**, (1989). The Canadian repair of inguinal hernia. In Nyhus LM, Condon RE (Eds): Hernia, 3rd edition, *Philadelphia*, pp. 236–248.
34. **Bendavid R.**, (1992). The space of bogros and the deep inguinal venous circulation. *Surg. Gynecol. Obstet.* 174: 355.
35. **GAG Decker** *et al.,* (1999). Lee Mc Gregor's, Synopsis of surgical anatomy, Indian edition, 12th edition, p. 129.
36. **F. Charles Brunicardi** *et al.,* (2005). Schwartz; principles of surgery, 8th edition, p. 1358.
37. **Bhatia P.**, (2003). Laparoscopic hernia repair, a step-by-step approach, p. 4-8.
38. **Bendavid R.**, (2007). The shouldice method of inguinal herniorrhaphy, Mastery of surgery, 5th edition, Lippincott Williams & Wilkins, p. 1897.

39. **Fischer JE, Bland KI.**, (2007). Mastery of surgery, 5th edition, Lippincott Williams & Wilkins, pp. 1864–67.

40. **Gilbert AI.**, (2007), Generation of the plug and patch repair: Its development and lesson from history, mastery of surgery, 5th edition, Lippincott Williams & Wilkins, p. 1942.

41. **Fischer JE.**, (2007). Surgery of hernia, Mastery of surgery, 5th edition, Lippincott Williams & Wilkins, p. 1857.

42. **Fruchaud H.**, (1956). Anatomie Chirurgicale des hernies de l' aine. Paris: Doin.

43. **Amid PK.**, (2004). Causes, prevention and surgical treatment of postherniorrhaphy neuropathic inguinodynia: Triple neurectomy with proximal end implantation. Hernia, 8: 343.

44. **Amid PK.**, (2004). Radiologic images of meshoma: A new phenomenon after prosthetic repair of abdominal wall hernias, *Arch. Surg.*, 139: 1297.

45. **King M, Bewes P, Cairns J, Thornton J** *et al.*, (2005). Hernias, primary surgery, non-trauma, **1,** Oxford Publications, p. 200.

46. **Nyhus LM.**, Iliopubic Tract Repair of Inguinal and Femoral Hernias: The Posterior (Preperitoneal) approach, p. 1 http://www.masteryofsurgery.com/pt/re/fischer.

47. **Thomas A.**, (1836). *J. Comm Ed. Pract.*, 4: 137.

48. **Bhatia P.**, (2008). Current status of laparoscopic inguinal hernia surgery, Clinical G.I. surgery, 1st edition, HEF, p. 922.

49. **Skandalakis JE** *et al.*, (2000). Surgical anatomy and techniques, 2nd edition, Springer, p. 132.

50. **Mc Vay CB.**, (1984). Anson and Mc Vay surgical anatomy, 6th edition, Philadelphia: WB Saunders, p. 484.

51. **Bariol** *et al.,* (2003). ANZ *J. Surg.* 3: 649.

52. **Takata MC** *et al.*, (2008). Laparoscopic inguinal hernia repair, *Surg Clin. N. Am.*; 88, 157–178.

53. **Itani KMF,** *et al.*; (2008). *Surg. Clin N. Am.*; 88, 205

54. **Ferzli GS.**, *et al.*, (2008). Post herniorrhaphy groin pain and how to avoid it. *Surg. Clin. N. Am.*, 88, 205.

Section 3
CLINICAL FEATURES

"Tis a lesson you should heed,
Try, Try again.
If at first you don't succeed,
Try, Try again"
-William E Hickson

5

Aetiology of Hernia

*"Let the relation of real knowledge to real life be visible to your pupils, and
let them understand how with knowledge the world could be transformed"*
— **Bertrand Russel**

The two main factors playing role in aetiology of hernia are:
• Weakness of abdominal musculature.
• Increased intra-abdominal pressure, which pushes the abdominal contents out.

WEAKNESS OF ABDOMINAL MUSCULATURE

It may be congenital or acquired.

Congenital Weakness

• **Persistent processus vaginalis (Figs. 5.1 A & B)**
  – It is a preformed sac through which abdominal contents herniate. It causes indirect inguinal hernia.[16] The processus vaginalis if patent, is a potential hernia and not a real hernia. A real hernia contains some abdominal viscera.
• **Patent canal of Nuck**
  – In females it causes indirect inguinal hernia.

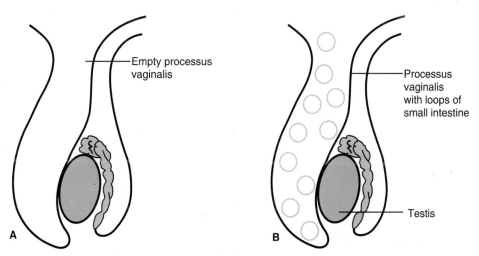

Fig. 5.1A. Preformed sac, a potential hernia, **B.** Preformed sac with loops of intestine, a real hernia.

- **Incomplete closure of umbilicus**
  - It causes infantile umbilical hernia.
- **Collagen abnormalities**
  - Such abnormalities predispose the body to develop hernia.
  - Common collagen changes observed are:
    a) Reduction in oxytalin fibres.
    b) Reduction of polymerised collagen.
    c) Decrease in concentration of hydroxy polypropylene.
    d) Increase in amorphous substance of elastin fibres.
- **Congenital abnormalities** i.e. hydrops foetalis, cryptorchidism (absence of one testis).
- Prematurity, low birth weight and meconium peritonitis.
- **Hereditary disorders**:
  - Mucopolysaccharidosis
  - Connective tissue disorders
    a) Ehler-Danlos Syndrome
    b) Hunter-Hurler Syndrome
- Family history of hernia, familial predisposition plays a role[1] in hernia development.

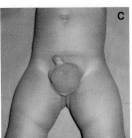

Fig. 5.1C. Congenital left indirect inguinal hernia.
Courtsey, Dr Parveen Bhatia, Global Hospital, New Delhi

It is easy to accept that indirect inguinal hernias have a congenital origin in children or young men, but it is not convincing in well-built adult (Fig. 5.1C).

Acquired Weakness

- **Obesity**
  - Fat acts like a screw driver. It separates muscle fibres and causes muscular weakness. It usually causes the following hernias:
    a) Direct inguinal hernia
    b) Paraumbilical hernia
    c) Hiatus hernia
- **Repeated pregnancies**
  - Repeated pregnancies causes muscular weakness leading to hernia.
- **Surgical incisions**
  - Incisions cause damage to nerves and cause muscle weakness. During appendicectomy, ilioinguinal nerve can be cut leading to weakness of transversus abdominis muscle causing direct inguinal hernia (Figs. 5.2A & B).
- **Infection**
  - Incisional hernia occurs after previous operation due to infection in early post-operative period (Fig. 5.2C).
- Loss of body weight.
- Advance age.
- Lack of physical exercise.
- Chronic Ambulatory Peritoneal Dialysis (CAPD)
- Ascites.
- Connective tissue disorders.

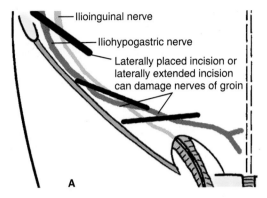

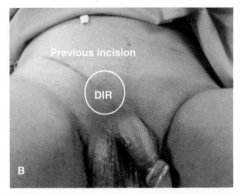

Ilioinguinal nerve

Iliohypogastric nerve

Laterally placed incision or
laterally extended incision
can damage nerves of groin

A

Previous incision

DIR

B

Fig. 5.2A. Injury to nerves causes inguinal hernia, **B.** Direct inguinal hernia developed after previous indirect inguinal
hernia operation, the incision was too long and laterally placed caused injury to ilioinguinal nerve.

INCREASED INTRA-ABDOMINAL PRESSURE

Rise of intra-abdominal pressure is the main cause of production of hernia. Any situation where
intra-abdominal pressure increases may cause hernia such as straining for micturition or defaecation,
chronic cough and intra-abdominal malignancy etc. Common
causes of increased intra-abdominal pressure are given below:

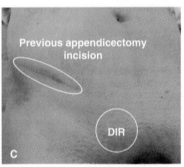

* Whooping cough in children.
* Coughing in bronchitis, tuberculosis, etc.
* Straining
  – Constipation
    a) Habitual constipation.
    b) Rectal stricture, stenosis or tumour.
  – Urinary
    a) Infant-phimosis, meatal stenosis.
    b) Young adult-stricture urethra.
    c) Old age-bladder neck obstruction, BPH (benign
       prostatic hyperplasia) and carcinoma of prostate.
  – Powerful efforts on straining during lifting heavy weight.
* Obesity.
* Smoking.
* Intra-abdominal malignancy.
* Peritoneal dialysis.
* Repeated pregnancy.
* Ascites.
* Upright posture.

Previous appendicectomy
incision

DIR

C

Fig. 5.2C. Direct inguinal hernia
developed after previous
appendicectomy, incision was too long.

Common Causes of Abdominal Wall Hernias

Coughing i.e. whooping cough or chronic cough

Whooping cough in childhood and chronic cough in adults cause hernia.

Straining i.e. micturition or defaecation

Straining at micturition as in prostate hypertrophy and urethral stricture causes hernia. Straining at defecation in chronic constipation may also develop hernia

Obesity (Fig. 5.3)

Obese persons have more chances of developing hernia than persons of average weight.
   Fat leads to the following hernias:
• Paraumbilical hernia
• Direct inguinal hernia

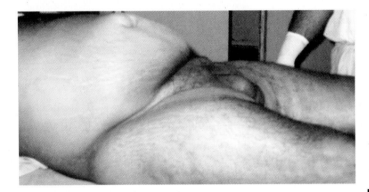

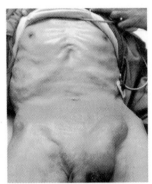

Fig. 5.4. Chronic smoker with cachexia having huge inguinal hernia.

Fig. 5.3. An obese men of 130 kg having paraumbilical hernia.

Smoking (Fig. 5.4)

It causes hernia in two ways:
• It increases intra-abdominal pressure due to cough.
• It causes collagen deficiency which weakens the tissues and thus susceptibility of hernia increases.

NOTE

Defective collagen metabolism in cigarette smokers that causes hernia formation is called "metastatic emphysema". The term "metastatic emphysema" was coined by Cannon and Read[2].

   Nowadays search for aetiology of abdominal wall hernia (AWH) is focused on alterations in connective tissue ultrastructure. The changes in connective tissue ultrastructure lead to thinning of collagen fibres and decrease in general amount of elastic fibres. The elastic fibres are replaced by ground matter which leads to weaknening of connective tissue and causes hernia.
   There is some association between hernia development, cigarette smoking and aneurysm formation. A collagen defect has been demonstrated in these patients.[3]

There is now extensive experimental evidence to support the view that collagen derrangement causes inguinal hernia development.[4]

Peritoneal dialysis

It can cause indirect inguinal hernia by opening the congenital patent processus vaginalis, which was occult earlier.

Intra-abdominal malignancy

Intra-abdominal malignancy raises the intra-abdominal pressure and increases the chances of hernia.

Repeated pregnancy

It is responsible for repeated rise in intra-abdominal pressure causing stretching of pelvic ligaments leading to femoral hernia. Therefore, femoral hernia is rare in men and nulliparous women but more common in multiparous women. Repeated pregnancies is also responsible for umbilical and paraumbilical hernias.

Low birth weight

Low birth weight children are prone to get abdominal wall hernia.
    32% newborn males below 1500 g require hernia operation by the age of 8 years[5].

Hypothesis of Aetiology of Inguinal Hernia

Evolutionary changes are responsible for the inguinal hernia development in man. The evolutionary changes which are responsible for the development of hernia in human beings are:
* Iliac crest grows forward (Figs. 5.5A & B) into external oblique muscle so the inguinal ligament is not operated by fleshy fibres of external oblique muscle but by aponeurosis of external oblique muscle. In other mammals, external oblique is not attached with iliac crest. Muscles are stronger than aponeurosis.
* Internal oblique and transversus abdominis muscles initially originate from anterior border of ilum and sheath of ilopsoas muscle (Figs. 5.6A & B) and acts as a strong sphincter of inguinal canal. Later on their origin shifts to iliac crest and inguinal ligament and their sphincteric action is lost.

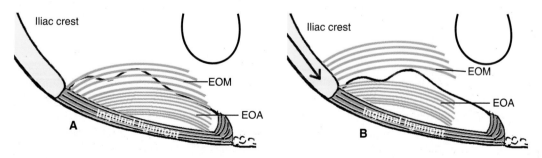

Fig. 5.5A. Hypothesis of aetiology of inguinal hernia, **B.** Iliac crest grows forward.

- "Saccular theory of Russell" of indirect inguinal hernia formation is still relevant. According to Russell, "presence of a developmental diverticulum associated with a patent processus vaginalis, was essential in every case".[6]
  Robert Hamilton Russell (1860-1933) was a surgeon at Alfred Hospital, Melbourn, Victoria, Australia.

Russell's hypothesis does not explain every case of indirect inguinal hernia due to the following reasons:

- A patent processus vaginalis may be found at autopsy without the presence of hernia.[7]
- Obliterated processus vaginalis may be found with abdominal wall defect lateral to inferior epigastric vessels having hernia.

"Weakening of the abdominal wall tissue as one of the causes of inguinal hernia was suspected by Cooper as far back as 1800".[8]

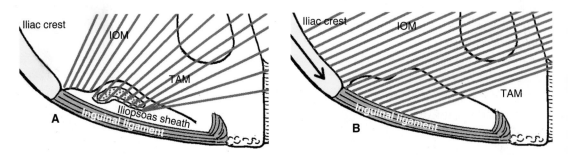

Fig. 5.6A&B. Hypothesis of aetiology of inguinal hernia, internal oblique and transversus abdominis muscles, shift from anterior border of ilium and iliopsoas sheath to iliac crest and inguinal ligament.

Hypothesis of Aetiology of Femoral Hernia

- Due to peculiar growth of pubic bones in humans the space between inguinal ligament and pubic bone (crural passage) becomes wide. The width of this crural passage in man is more than in any mammal. This predisposes man to femoral hernia.
- The mode of insertion of the fibres of transversus abdominis muscle and its sheath to superior pubic ramus is related to the pathogenesis of femoral hernia. If the insertion is through a narrow band, a cone-shaped defect overlying the femoral ring (the femoral cone) results which predisposes to femoral hernia development.

Femoral cone theory (Fig. 5.7)

Preperitoneal fat with or without sac enters the "femoral cone" due to raised abdominal pressure. It is stage I or internal femoral hernia which can only be detected if the preperitoneal space is explored during inguinal herniorrhaphy. At time, the fatty contents of the femoral cone exit from the narrow distal orifice, then a stage II or external femoral (symptomatic) hernia develops. By the time of diagnosis, 16% of stage II femoral hernias are irreducible and 25 to 40 % are present with incarceration or strangulation.

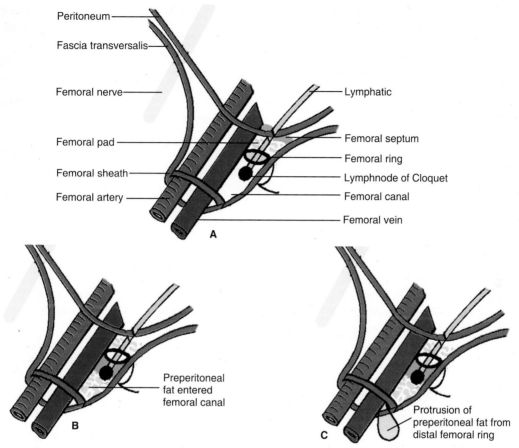

Peritoneum
Fascia transversalis
Femoral nerve
Femoral pad
Femoral sheath
Femoral artery

Lymphatic
Femoral septum
Femoral ring
Lymphnode of Cloquet
Femoral canal
Femoral vein

A

Preperitoneal fat entered femoral canal

B

Protrusion of preperitoneal fat from distal femoral ring

C

Fig. 5.7. Hypothesis of aetiology of femoral hernia, **A.** Normal anatomy, **B.** Stage I or internal femoral hernia, **C.** Stage II or external femoral hernia.

- Femoral hernia sometimes occurs after inguinal herniorrhaphy[9] (Fig. 5.8), and it is due to following reasons:
  - Preperitoneal dissection pushes preperitoneal fat into femoral cone.
  - Missed hernia during procedure.
  - Development of new femoral hernia.

NOTE

It is often difficult to distinguish between normal femoral plug and a true femoral hernia. Increase in incidence of femoral hernia in laparoscopic herniorrhaphy series may be the result of this error. Surgeon should avoid manipulating femoral pad as it may predispose the patient to development of a true femoral hernia.[9]

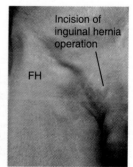

Incision of inguinal hernia operation

FH

Fig. 5.8. Femoral hernia developed after inguinal hernia operation.

HERNIA AND TISSUE HEALING (FIG. 5.9)

The tissue healing after an operation is a complex process more so in hernia surgery as it occurs in various layers. The tissues are also strained and weak at hernia site.

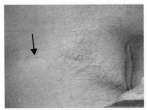

Fig. 5.9. Good tissue healing causes faint scar.

Healing of wound after hernia surgery occurs through the following three processes:

- Hemostasis, inflammation and repair.
- Hernia healing happens in three phases:
  - Lag-phase – Haematoma, inflammation
  - Proliferative phase – Fibroblast number increases, extra cellular matrix deposited, angiogenesis
  - Remodelling phase – Scar maturation, cell number decreases, collagen fiber bundle organization.

Hemostasis

Hemostasis tries to stop bleeding by two processes:

- Vasospasm of vessels
- Platelet plugging.
  - It occurs with help of platelets and coagulation mechanism. Various blood cells rush towards the operation site immediately after surgery. The first cell reaching the hernia operation site is platelet followed by neutrophils, lymphocytes and monocytes.
- Some wound chemicals act like hormones, and these are called cytokinins. These are produced by platelets and other cells to carry on wound-healing process. Common cytokinins are:
  - TGF-B (Transforming growth factor beta)
  - PDGF (Platelet derived growth factor)
  - EGF (Epidermal growth factor)
  - bFGF (Basic fibroblast growth factor)
  - Interleukins
  - Interferons

TGF-B is related to healing of hernia operation wound. It is more important in persons suffering with collagen disorders and smokers where collagen deficiency occurs. Normal TGF-B production is important to avoid recurrence of hernia.

Inflammation

Blood flow increases at the hernia operation site and cellular healing process starts. Inflammation and the process of repair take place simultaneously. Collagen starts synthesising in wound within 12 hours after hernia operation and reaches to maximum production within 5-6 days.

Repair

The process of wound repair involves the following developments:

- Granular tissue formation
- Collagen formation
- Scar formation

Fibroblasts produce collagen as well as matrix.

COLLAGEN

Collagen is a protein containing proline, hydroxyproline and glycine produced by fibroblasts. Collagen is of several types but type I and type III are mainly concerned with the aetiology of abdominal wall hernia and repair of hernia operation wound.

The production of type I and type III collagen increases in the early wound healing.

Also conversion of type III collagen to type I collagen occurs during wound healing

The wound healing increases and continues for 3 to 6 months. The collagen fibres continue to develop and reorient to remodel the scar. Similarly, the wound strength continues to increase till it reaches a normal level.

If there is collagen deficiency by birth or due to smoking, then collagen fibres do not produce normal wound strength and recurrence of hernia occurs.

"There is also a decrement of the index type I collagen compared to type III collagen due to an increased synthesis of collagen III fibres.... This probably causes different physical properties of the collagen matrix of the abdominal wall thus inducing inguinal hernia and late recurrence."[10]

Collagen is a protein and plays an active and important role in wound healing and maintaining elasticity and strength of the tissues. There are more than 18 types of collagens, but type I and type III are important from hernia point of view. Type I is found in extra-cellular matrix of skin and other tissues. Type III collagen is normally present, but becomes prominent during wound healing and smoking. Net production of collagen goes up to 21 days and then loss starts, and type III (immature collagen) changes to type I (mature collagen).

Primary hernias are the result of a connective tissue disorder, whereas secondary hernias (e.g. incisional hernias) are most frequently due to a technical failure. Recurrent hernias likely are a combination of both mechanisms.[11]

Increased proteolytic activity may cause weakness in structural tissue. Matrix metallo-protease (MMP)-2 overexpression was measured in fibroblasts of patients with direct inguinal hernias and MMP-13 overexpression was detected in patients with recurrent inguinal hernias.[12,13]

Growing evidence supports that incisional hernias and recurrent hernias are most often the result of early surgical wound failure ...... in "lag phase" During the initial lag phase of healing the laparotomy wound is mechanically weakest. As surgical patients recover increasing wall loads can cause acute wound failure.[14]

NOTE

Recently, molecular biological investigations have proven the theory of disturbed composition of the extra-cellular matrix in patients with recurrent hernias. In particular, there is a decreased ratio of collagen type I and type III.[15]

KEY POINT

The most common hernia is indirect inguinal hernia and it occurs due to persistence of patent processus vaginalis. Straining by raising intra-abdominal pressure and smoking leading to collagen deficiency cause hernia.

REFERENCES

1. **Abramson JH, Gofin J, Hopp C** *et al.,* (1978). The epidemiology of inguinal hernia: A survery in Western Jerusalem. *J. Epidemiol. Community Health*, 32: 59.
2. **Cannon DJ, Read RC.**, (1981). Metastatic emphysema: A mechanism for acquiring inguinal herniation. *Ann. Surg.*, 194: 270.
3. **Cannon DJ, Casteel L, Read RC.**, (1984). Abdominal aortic anurysm, Leriche's syndrome, Inguinal herniation and smoking. *Arch. J. Surg.*, 19: 387–9.
4. **Peacock EE, Madden JW.**, (1974). A study on the biology and treatment of recurrence of inguinal hernia: Morphological changes. *Ann. Surg.*, 1979: 567–71.
5. **Kitchen WH, Doyle LW, Ford GW.**, (1991). Inguinal hernia in very low birth weight children: A continuing risk to age 8 years. *J. Peadiatr Child Health*, 27: 300.
6. **Russel RH.**, (1906). The saccular theory of hernia and the radical operation. *Lancet*. 3: 1197.
7. **Condon RE.**, (1925). The anatomy of inguinal region and its relation to oblique inguinal hernia. *Surg. Gynecol. Obstet.*, 41: 610.
8. **Amid P.K.**, (2007). Lichtenstein tension-free hernioplasty, Mastery of surgery, Lippincott Williams & Wilkins, 5th edition, pp. 1932–39.
9. **Bendavid R.**, (2002). Femoral pseudo-hernias: Hernia, 6: 141.
10. **Campanelli G, Cavagnoli R, Buratti M.S, Clofri U, Casirani R.**, (2004). The preperitoneal prosthetic approach for the repair of recurrent inguinal hernia, Wantz technique; New procedures in open hernia surgery, p. 85.
11. **Itani K.M.F., Hawn M.T.** (2008). Biology of hernia formation, *Surg. Clin. N. Am.* **88,** 1. p. 2.
12. **Klinge U.** *et al.,* (1999). Synthesis of type I and III collagen, expression of fibro nectin and matrix metallo proteases-I and -13 in hernial sac of patients with inguinal hernia. Int. *J. Surg. Investig.* 1(3): 219–27.
13. **Zheng H, Si Z, Kasperk R.** *et al.,* (2002). Recurrent inguinal hernia: diseases of the collagen matrix? *World J. Surg.* 26(4): 401–8.
14. **Itani K.M.F., Hawn M.T.** (2008). Biology of hernia formation, *Surg. Clin. N. Am.* **88,** 1. 4–5.
15. **Schumpelick V.**, (2006). Light weight meshes in incisional hernia repair, *Journal of Minimal Access Surgery*, **2,** pp. 117–123.
16. **Itani KMF.** *et al.,* (2008). *Surg. Clin. N. Am.*; **88**, 38.

6

Protective Mechanisms of Body Against Groin Hernias

"Anatomy can be a boring subject, clinical anatomy is fascinating."
— **Richard S Snell**

Normally two mechanisms act to prevent hermination through the inguinal canal, **shutter mechanism** and **Sling of Keith**.[1] In addition to these two mechanisms, the body has some other protective and supportive mechanisms against this area of weakness. A few are discussed below.

SHUTTER MECHANISM (Figs. 6.1 A-C)

Internal oblique muscle fibres make an arch forming anterior wall, roof and posterior wall of inguinal canal. When this muscle contracts the roof comes down to floor like downing of the shutter of a shop closing the canal completely. So intra-abdominal viscus cannot protrude.

    The parts of internal oblique muscle and transversus abdominis form an arch over inguinal canal, called "deep inguinal arch". This arch is constantly on alert while standing and walking and contracts immediately on rise of intra-abdominal pressure on straining and prevents the herniation of viscera.

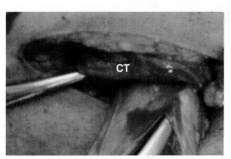

Fig. 6.1A. Shutter mechanism, front view.

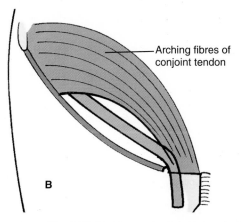

Arching fibres of conjoint tendon

B

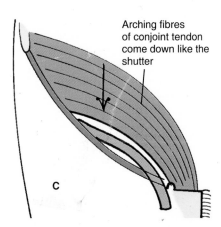

Arching fibres of conjoint tendon come down like the shutter

C

Fig. 6.1B. Shutter mechanism before contraction of muscles, **C.** After contraction of muscles.

FLAP VALVE MECHANISM

Whenever intra-abdominal pressure increases, the anterior and posterior walls of inguinal canal come in contact with each other and thus block the inguinal canal avoiding any protrusion of viscus through it.

BALL VALVE MECHANISM

When intra-abdominal pressure rises suddenly, while coughing or sneezing, the cremasteric muscle contracts and it lifts the spermatic cord upwards which blocks the superficial inguinal ring and thus shuts the door for protrusion of viscus.

SLIT VALVE MECHANISM (Figs. 6.2A & B)

When intra-abdominal pressure increases suddenly, the external oblique muscle contracts and its aponeurosis tightens which pulls two crura of superficial inguinal ring and they approximate together closing superficial inguinal ring. In this mechanism, intercrural fibres help in bringing two crura together.

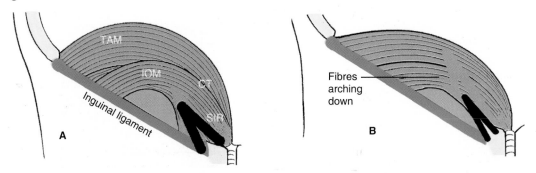

Fig. 6.2A. Slit valve mechanism, superficial inguinal ring opened, **B.** Superficial inguinal ring closed.

GUARDING MECHANISM FOR SUPERFICIAL INGUINAL RING (Fig. 6.3)

Conjoint tendon and reflected part of inguinal ligament guard the superficial inguinal ring from behind. So no protrusion can happen from behind.
Cooper in 1800, described the EOA as the outer barrier to inguinal canal.[2]

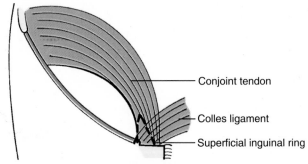

Fig. 6.3. Guarding mechanism for superficial inguinal ring.

GUARDING MECHANISM FOR DEEP INGUINAL RING (Fig. 6.4)

Fleshy fibres of internal oblique muscle guard the deep inguinal ring from front. It prevents protrusion of abdominal contents through deep inguinal ring. In Africans, indirect inguinal hernia incidence is higher than in Europeans[3] due to narrow origin of internal oblique muscle so it cannot guard deep inguinal ring and thus predisposes to hernia.

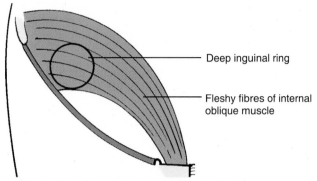

Deep inguinal ring

Fleshy fibres of internal oblique muscle

Fig 6.4. Guarding mechanism for deep inguinal ring.

Hormones

Gonadotrophin hormone helps in maintaining the tone of inguinal musculature which compensates for weakness of abdominal wall.

Obliquity of Inguinal Canal

The slanting direction or obliquity of inguinal canal helps in warding off the protrusion of viscus.

> *Transversalis fascia (Figs. 6.5 A & B)*
>
> • It is firmly adherent to the posterior surface of the transversus abdominis muscle so the contraction of this muscle pulls the deep inguinal ring laterally and upwards avoiding protrusion of viscera (Sling of Keith).[4]
> • Transversalis fascia is thickened in groin which gives some protection against development of groin hernia.

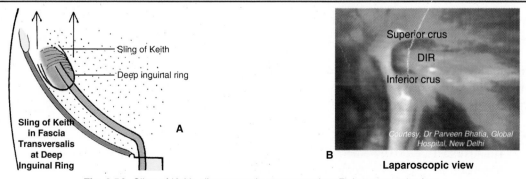

Sling of Keith

Deep inguinal ring

Sling of Keith
in Fascia
Transversalis
at Deep
Inguinal Ring

A

Superior crus

DIR

Inferior crus

Courtesy, Dr Parveen Bhatia, Global Hospital, New Delhi

B

Laparoscopic view

Fig. 6.5A. Sling of Keith, diagrammatic representation, **B.** Laparoscopic view.

SUMMATION EFFECTS OF PROTECTIVE MECHANISMS AGAINST INGUINAL HERNIA

All the above-mentioned factors work together whenever there is rise in intra-abdominal pressure while coughing, lifting weight, sneezing, etc. and leads to:
- Closure of superficial inguinal ring
- Closure of deep inguinal ring
- Obliteration of inguinal canal

Weak spots in anterior abdominal wall are strengthened and herniation of abdominal contents is prevented through inguinal canal.

PROTECTIVE MECHANISMS AGAINST FEMORAL HERNIA

Medial compartment of femoral sheath is known as femoral canal. It is ordinarily less than 2 cm in diameter and contains lymphatic vessels and glands.[5] McVay demonstrated that width of the femoral ring is the main aetiological factor of the femoral hernia.[6] The femoral ring is a sort of safety valve for expansion of femoral vein.[6] When intra-abdominal pressure increases then femoral vein gets dilated and pushes the lateral wall of femoral canal. It accommodates elevated venous pressure and almost blocks the femoral canal thus avoiding protrusion of abdominal contents through femoral canal and development of femoral hernia. Keith demonstrated that under persistent raised intra-abdominal pressure during pregnancy, preperitoneal fat insinuates through the femoral ring to the femoral canal, which leads to the development of a femoral peritoneal sac. It then descends down the femoral canal and out of femoral orifice and forms a femoral hernia. So repeated increase in intra-abdominal pressure (repeated pregnancies) will develop a hernia.[7]

NOTE

Surgeon should avoid manipulating the femoral pad as it may predispose the patient to the development of femoral hernia.[8]

KEY POINT

When intra-abdominal pressure increases, the protective mechanisms come forward to help but if they fail then hernia occurs.

REFERENCES

1. **Cuschieri A,** *et al.,* (2002). Essential surgical practice, 4th edition, p. 174.
2. **Amid PK.,** (2004). Lichtenstein tension-free hernioplasty: Its inception, evolution and principles, Hernia, 8: 1.
3. **Badoe EA.,** (1973). *African J. Med. Sci.,* 4: 51–58.
4. **Keith A.,** (1923-1924). On the origin and nature of hernia. *Br. J. Surg.,* 11: 455–75.
5. **Lichtenstein IL.,** (1986). Femoral hernia. In: Lichtenstein IL, Editor, Hernia repair without disability, 2nd edition, St. Louis, Tokyo: Ishiyaku Euroamerica, p. 130.
6. **McVay CB, Savage LE.,** (1961). Etiology of femoral hernia. *Ann. Surg.,* 154 (Supply): 25.
7. **Hachisuka T.,** (2003). Femoral hernia repair, *Surg. Clin. North Am.,* 83: 1190–91.
8. **Bendavid R.,** (2002). Femoral pseudohernias. Hernia, 6: 141.

7

Classification of Abdominal Wall Hernias

"In surgery, eyes first and most; fingers next and little; tongue last and least"

— **Humphrey George Murray, 1820-1896**

The classification of abdominal wall hernias has become an unending process. For last more than a century surgeons are trying hard to get an ultimate model. They are classifying hernias into inguinal and femoral, inguinal into indirect and direct broadly, for decades. The concept has not changed since the days of Sir Astley Cooper, 1840s.[1]

Rutkow and Robbins did a comprehensive study and summarised the classification of hernias considering new methods of hernia surgery.[2]

Traditional methods of classifying abdominal wall hernias have stood the test of time. Historical details of these traditional classifications are not well traceable but these classifications are still common and popular with surgeons and non-surgeons equally due to their simplicity.

> The first report of groin hernia classification based on anatomy of the defect (i.e., inguinal versus femoral) dates back to the 14th century.[3] For 100 years, surgeons have traditionally classified the groin hernias into indirect, direct, inguinal and femoral. The concept of indirect and direct inguinal hernia was described by Cooper in the 1840s with Hesselbach using the inferior epigastic artery as the defining boundary between these two areas.

Classification of hernias can be summarised as:
- Classificaiton of hernias according to incidence of hernias.
- Classification of hernias according to anatomy.
- Classification of inguinal hernias according to congenital or acquired causes.
- Casten classification (1967).
- Halverson classification (1970).
- Lichtenstein classification (1987)
- Gilbert's classification (1988): Classification of hernias according to type of defect and their suggestive repair.
- Nyhus classification (1993): Classification of hernia according to type of defect.
- Bendavid and Shouldice Hospital classification (1993).
- Schumpelick Aust Arit-Aachen classification (1995).
- Alexandre classification (1998).
- Modified Traditional Classification (2002).
- SGRH (Sir Ganga Ram Hospital) classification for laparoscopic repair of abdominal wall hernias (2004).
- EHS (European Hernia Society) classification.

CLASSIFICATION OF HERNIAS ACCORDING TO INCIDENCE OF HERNIA

Common Hernias (Fig. 7.1)

- Inguinal hernia (73%)
  - Indirect inguinal hernia
  - Direct inguinal hernia
- Femoral hernia (17%)
  - Typical femoral hernia
  - Atypical femoral hernia
    a) Hesselbach's hernia (external femoral hernia)
    b) Narath's or Teale's hernia (prevascular hernia)
    c) Serafini hernia (retrovascular hernia)
    d) De Laugier hernia (lacunar ligament hernia)
    e) Cloquet's hernia (pectineal hernia)
- Umbilical and paraumbilical hernia (8.5%)
- Incisional hernia (1.5%)

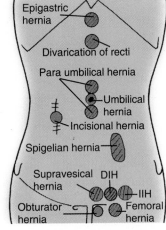

Fig. 7.1. Common and less common hernias.

Less Common Hernias (Fig. 7.1)

- Epigastric hernia
- Lumbar hernia
  - Superior lumbar hernia through superior lumbar triangle (Grynfeltt's triangle)
  - Inferior lumbar hernia through inferior lumbar triangle (Petit's triangle)

Rare Hernias (Fig. 7.2)

- Spigelian hernia
- Obturator hernia
- Gluteal hernia
- Supravesical hernia
- Ogilvie hernia
- Sciatic hernia

CLASSIFICATION OF HERNIAS ACCORDING TO ANATOMY

- Inguinal hernia
- Femoral hernia
- Umbilical and paraumbilical hernia
- Epigastric hernia
- Ventral or incisional hernia
- Spigelian hernia
- Supravesical hernia
- Lumbar hernia
- Obturator hernia

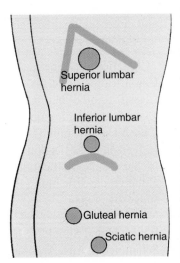

Fig. 7.2. Rare hernias.

- Gluteal hernia
- Sacral hernia

CLASSIFICATION OF HERNIAS ACCORDING TO CONGENITAL OR ACQUIRED CAUSES

- **Congenital causes** – A preformed sac is present through which abdominal contents herniate, e.g., indirect inguinal and umbilical hernia.
- **Acquired causes** – No preformed sac is present and it is acquired, e.g., all direct inguinal hernias are acquired.

CASTEN'S CLASSIFICATION[4] (1967) (Figs. 7.3A-C)

In 1967, Casten F. classified three types of hernias according to normal versus dilated internal ring into the following three groups:
- Small hernias in infants and children with normally functioning internal ring.
- Large indirect hernia with distorted internal ring.
- All direct hernia and femoral hernia.

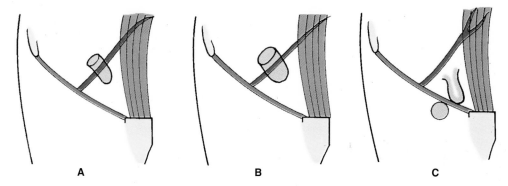

Fig. 7.3. Casten's Classification, **A.** Small indirect hernia with normal internal ring, **B.** Indirect hernia with dilated internal ring, **C.** Direct inguinal hernia and femoral hernia (combined hernia).

HALVERSON AND McVAY CLASSIFICATION[5] (1970) (Figs. 7.4)

In 1970, Halverson K. and McVay C. B. classified inguinal hernia into the following five groups:
- Small hernia – indirect
- Medium hernia – indirect
- Large hernia – indirect or direct
- Femoral hernia
- Combined hernia – any above combination

LICHTENSTEIN CLASSIFICATION (1987)[6] (Fig. 7.5)

In 1987, Lichtenstein I. L. classified hernias as follows:
- Indirect
- Direct

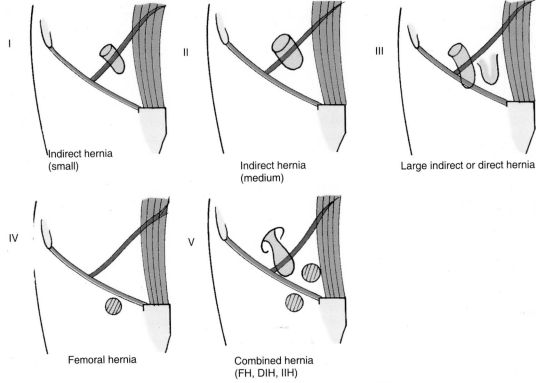

I — Indirect hernia (small)

II — Indirect hernia (medium)

III — Large indirect or direct hernia

IV — Femoral hernia

V — Combined hernia (FH, DIH, IIH)

Fig. 7.4. Halverson and McVay Classification[4] (1970).

- – Whole floor
- – Lateral half of floor
- – Medial half of floor
- – Diverticular
- – Others
- • Femoral
- • Combined (two or more)
- • Others

GILBERT'S CLASSIFICATION (1988) OF HERNIAS ACCORDING TO DEFECT AND SUGGESTIVE REPAIR[7] (Fig. 7.6)

Gilbert's classification is based on the type of defect in posterior wall in direct inguinal hernia and defect in deep inguinal ring in indirect inguinal hernia. He also proposed the repair procedure. Gilbert A.I. described Type I to V types of hernias.

Robbin A.W. modified Gilbert's classification by adding Type VI and VII.

Type I - Tight deep ring
- Does not admit even a finger
- Preperitoneal indirect sac
  [Herniorraphy or hernioplasty]

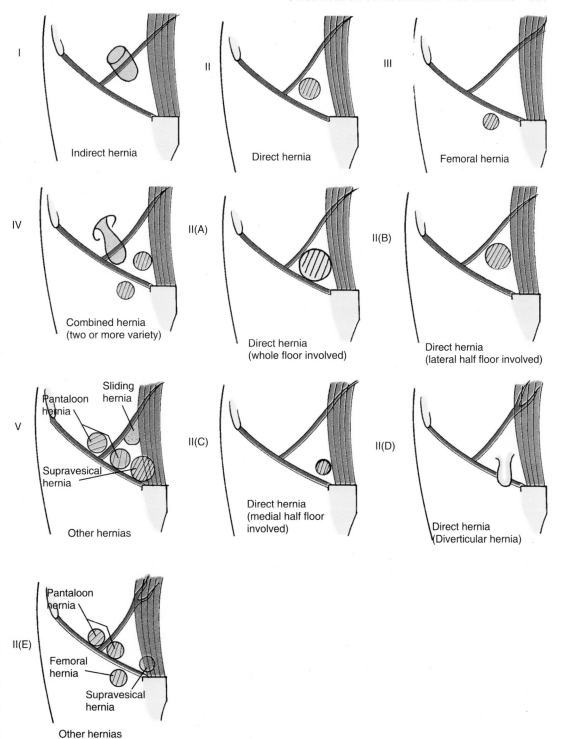

Fig. 7.5. Lichtenstein classification (1987).

Type II - Moderately enlarged deep ring
         - Admits one finger
         - Bubonocele
         [Tightening of deep inguinal ring with herniorrhaphy or hernioplasty]

Type III - Large defect
         - Deep ring 2-3 fingers breadth
         - May be sliding hernia
         [Preperitoneal mesh by slitting transversalis fascia]

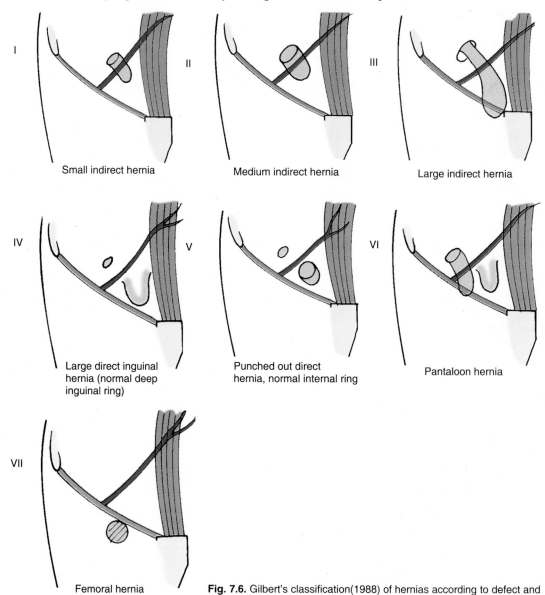

I   Small indirect hernia

II   Medium indirect hernia

III   Large indirect hernia

IV   Large direct inguinal hernia (normal deep inguinal ring)

V   Punched out direct hernia, normal internal ring

VI   Pantaloon hernia

VII   Femoral hernia

Fig. 7.6. Gilbert's classification(1988) of hernias according to defect and suggestive repair.

Type IV   -   Large direct hernia with full defect
           -    Intact deep inguinal ring
              [Mesh repair]
Type V   -   Direct hernia with punched out hole / defect in transversalis fascia
           -    Internal ring is normal
              [Plug the defect or purse string closure of the defect followed by mesh repair]
Type VI   -   Pantaloon hernia
              [Mesh repair]
Type VII   -   Femoral hernia
              [Femoral hernia repair]

NYHUS CLASSIFICATION OF HERNIAS ACCORDING TO DEFECT[8] (1993) (Fig. 7.7)

This classification of inguinal hernia is based on:
- Damage of internal inguinal ring due to hernia
- The defect in Hesselbach's triangle

Type I   –   Indirect inguinal hernia with normal size internal inguinal ring.
Type II   –   Indirect inguinal hernia with dilated internal inguinal ring.
Type III   –   Based on posterior wall defect.
Type IIIA   –   Direct inguinal hernia.
Type IIIB   –   Indirect inguinal hernia with dilated internal inguinal ring which encroaches on inguinal floor. It includes:
         a)   Inguinoscrotal hernia
         b)   Sliding hernia
         c)   Pantaloon hernia
Type IIIC   –   Femoral hernia
Type IV   –   Recurrent hernia
Type IV A   –   Direct
Type IV B   –   Indirect
Type IV C   –   Femoral
Type IV D   –   Combined

BENDAVID AND SHOULDICE HOSPITAL CLASSIFICATION[9] (1993)

Bendavid R classified hernias with the help of Shouldice Hospital. This classification is based on anatomic area, size of hernia defect and length of sac.
    It is also known as TSD classification (T = Type, S = Stage, D = Dimension).

SCHUMPELICK AUST ARIT-AACHEN CLASSIFICATION[10] (1995)

Schumpelick and co-workers used L, M, C and F alphabets for lateral, medial, combined and femoral hernia respectively. They measured abdominal wall defect also.

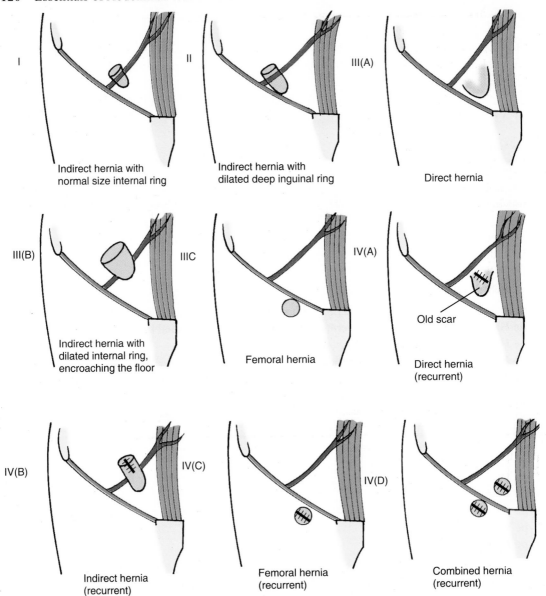

Fig. 7.7. Nyhus classification of hernias according to defect[7] (1993).

L = Lateral
M = Medial
Mc = Medial combined
F = Femoral

Orifice size
Grade I - < 1.5 cm
Grade II - 1.5 -3 cm
Grade III - > 3 cm

ALEXANDRE CLASSIFICATION (1998)[11]

Alexandre J-H advocated this classification with his colleagues. This classification is based on type of hernia, size of orifice and length of hernia sac.

It is also known as TOS classification (T = type, O = orifice, S = sac).
- Type – Indirect / direct / femoral
- Orifice – Maximum diameter in centimeters.
- Sac – Length in centimeters
- Modifiers –   I = Incarcerated
                 B = Bilateral
                 R = Recurrent

MODIFIED TRADITIONAL CLASSIFICATION (2002) (Fig. 7.8)

Robert Zollinger Junior[12] in 1999 gave a unified classification of abdominal wall hernia combining the best features of other types of classification. Later on Nyhus and Condon modified and gave the following classification:

- Indirect
  - Indirect small
  - Indirect medium
  - Indirect large

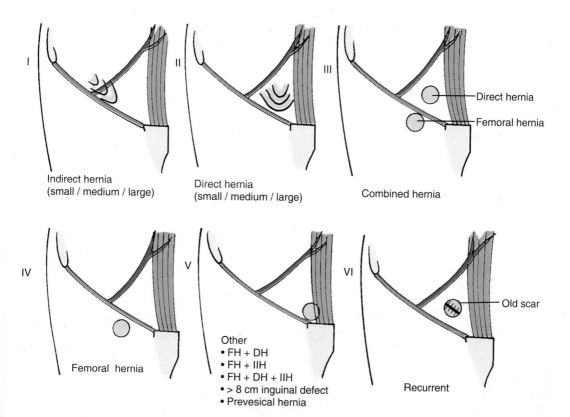

Fig. 7.8. Modified traditional classification (2002).

- Direct
  - Direct small
  - Direct medium
  - Direct large
- Combined
- Femoral
- Others
- Recurrent

SGRH (SIR GANGA RAM HOSPITAL) CLASSIFICATION FOR LAPAROSCOPIC REPAIR OF ABDOMINAL WALL HERNIAS (2004)[15]

After so much work on classification of hernia, no single classification is accepted universally, mostly the traditional classifications are in use.

SGRH classification is a functional classification of groin and ventral abdominal wall hernias. It is based on two factors:
- Preoperative prediction level of difficulty of laparoscopic surgery
- Intraoperative factors that lead to a difficult repair

Factors of Prediction of Grade of Difficulty

- Reducibility
- Degree of descent of the hernia sac
- Previous hernia repair

It divides groin hernia cases into five grades and ventral hernia cases into six grades.

EHS (EUROPEAN HERNIA SOCIETY) CLASSIFICATION OF GROIN HERNIAS

After reviewing the available classifications for groin hernias, the European Hernia Society proposed an easy and simple classification based on Aachen classification.[16]

P = Primary hernia
0 = No hernia detectable
2 = < 3 cm (two finger)
X = Not investigated
M = Medial / Direct hernia

R = Recurrent hernia
1 = < 1.5 cm (one finger)
3 = > 3 cm (more than two fingers)
L = Lateral / Indirect hernia
F = Femoral hernia

NOTE

The best hernia classification should be based on the following factors:
- *Anatomic location*
- *Anatomic function*
- *Reproducibility by both hernia and general surgeon*
- *Suitable for both anterior and posterior approaches*
- *Easy to remember*

KEY POINT

Do not depend and rely on preoperative clinical diagnosis of type of hernia, confirm it at the exploration. Classification of abdominal wall hernias is important from treatment point of view.

REFERENCES

1. **Schumpelick V, Treutner KH.**, (2001). Classification of inguinal hernias. In: Bendavid R, Editor. Abdominal wall hernias: principles and management. New York : Springer-Verlag: pp. 128–30.
2. **Rutkow IM, Robbin AW.**, (1994). Classification of groin hernias. In: Bendavid R, Editor Prostheses and abdominal wall hernias : Austin (TX) : RG Landers, pp. 206–12.
3. **Linner MJ, Asaley SW.**, (2007). Maingot's abdominal operations, 11th edition, McGraw-Hill, p. 103.
4. **Casten DF.**, (1967). Functional anatomy of the groin area as related to the classification and treatment of groin hernias. *Am. J. Surg*, 110: 894.
5. **Halverson K, McVay C.**, (1970). Inguinal and femoral hernioplasty: A 22-year study of the author's methods. *Arch. Surg.*, pp. 101–127.
6. **Lichtenstein IL.**, (1987). Herniorrhaphy: a personal experience with 6321 cases. *Am. J. Surg.*, 153: pp. 553–9.
7. **Gilbert AI.**, (1989). An anatomical and functional classification for the diagnosis and treatment of inguinal hernia, *Am. J. Surg.*, 157: 133.
8. **Nyhus LM, Klein MS, Rogers FB.**, (1991). Inguinal hernia. *Curr. Probl. Surg.*, 28: 417 and 436.
9. **Rutkow IM, Robbins AW.**, (1994). In Bendavid R, Editor. Prostheses and abdominal wall hernias. Austin (TX) : RG Landers.
10. **Schumpelick V, Arit G.**, (1995). *In:* Problems in general surgery, Philadelphia: Lippincot – Raven Publication; pp. 57–8.
11. **Alexandre JH, Bouillot JL, Aovad K.**, (1996). Le Journal de cairo cherugie, 1953–9.
12. **Zollinger RM, Jr.**, (2003). Classification systems for groin hernias, *Surg. Clin. North Am.*, 83: 1053–1063.
13. **Zollinger RM Jr.**, (1993). A unified classification of inguinal hernias. Hernia, 3: 195–200.
14. **Zollinger RM Jr.**, (2002). Classification of ventral and groin hernias. In: Fitzgibbons RJ Jr, Greenburg AG, Editors. Nyhus and condons hernia. 5th edition, Philadelphia, Lippincot, Williams and Wilkins, pp. 71–9.
15. **Chowbey P.**, (2004). SGRH classification for endoscopic repair of hernias, Endoscopic repair of abdominal wall hernia, pp. 34–39.
16. **Misrez M, Alexandre J-H, Campanalli G, Corcione F, Cuccurullo D, Pascual MH, Hocferlin A, Kingsnorth AN, Mandala V, Palt JP, Schumpelick V, Simmermacher RKJ, Stoppa R, Flament JB.**, (2007). The European Hernia Society groin hernia classification: Simple and easy to remember, Hernia, Springer-Verlag, pp. 113–116.

Epidemiology of Abdominal Wall Hernias

"As general rule the most successful man in the life is the man who has the best information."
— **Benjamin Disraeli**

"Between 1995 and 2005, 16,742 Americans died of hernia."[1]

Approximately 20 million inguinal hernia operations are performed every year worldwide. It is estimated that 5% population will develop abdominal wall hernia in their lifetime. Approximately 750,000 inguinal herniorrhaphies are performed every year in United States.[2]

With one in 5 men and one in 50 women have a hernia, it is the most common general surgery operation performed.[15]

Groin hernias constitute 75% of all abdominal wall hernias. Groin lumps are swellings, which account for about 10% of general surgical out patient referrals.[3] Inguinal hernia is the most common hernia among abdominal wall hernias. According to some authorities, 73% are inguinal hernias, 17% are femoral hernias, 8.5% are umbilical hernias (congenital, infant, adult and paraumbilical hernias) and 1.5% are rare hernias (Fig. 8.1). Incisional hernias are excluded.

- Inguinal hernia occurs in 1-3% of all children.
- Processus vaginalis remains patent in 80% of newborns.
- As the age increases, the percentage of patent processus vaginalis diminishes, it is 40-50% at 2 year and 25% in adult.[4]
- 55% inguinal hernia occur on right side (Fig. 8.2) and 45% on left side.
- Bilateral inguinal hernia incidence is 12%.

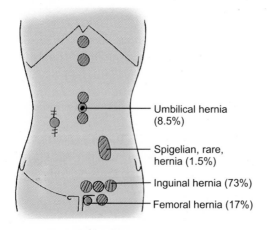

Umbilical hernia (8.5%)

Spigelian, rare, hernia (1.5%)

Inguinal hernia (73%)

Femoral hernia (17%)

Fig. 8.1. Percentage distribution of abdominal wall hernias.

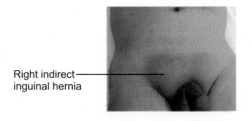

Right indirect inguinal hernia

Fig. 8.2. Right indirect inguinal hernia is the most common hernia of the body.

Indirect inguinal hernia is almost double the number of direct inguinal hernia. Right side groin hernias are more common than left side groin hernias.

The **incidence** of hernia is the development of "new hernias 100,000 per year".

The **prevalence** of hernia is "the percentage of population affected at any given time".

Both are important epidemiological factors.

The incidence of abdominal wall hernias increase with age. It is 50% for men above the age of 75 years.

Lifetime risk for strangulation in an inguinal hernia is commonly quoted 4–6% is perhaps more the result of speculation than fact.[5] To find an accurate picture of the incidence and lifetime risk of strangulation is difficult.

Abramson and colleagues reported that the overall current risk for an adult (40-50 years) male to have an inguinal hernia is 18% and the lifetime risk is 24%. The lifetime risk for the development of bilateral hernia is 39%.[6]

Strangulation is common in indirect inguinal hernia but femoral hernia has the highest rate of strangulation (15-20%).

- Indirect inguinal hernias are uncommon in baby girls compared with boys (ratio 1 : 9)[7]. Male : female ratio of inguinal hernia is 7 : 1 and of femoral hernia is 1 : 4.
- Absolute number of femoral hernia in male and female is same, but there is a lower overall incidence of groin hernia in women.[8]
- Groin hernias are more common in men than women.
- Direct hernia is uncommon in women but femoral and umbilical hernia are more common.
- 10% of women and 50% of men having a femoral hernia will develop an inguinal hernia.
- Less than 10% of all elective hernia repairs are performed in women.[9]
- Incisional hernias are twice common in women as compared to men.[10]

The United States Agency for Healthcare Related Quality of life with American College of Surgeons are sponsoring a comprehensive clinical trial for hernia. A Paris Truss Clinic showed hernia obstruction and strangulation probably 0.0037 per patient per year.[11] The incidence of inguinal herniorrhaphy is much higher in USA than other nations, 2800 per one million population per year.[16]

HERNIA: BURDEN ON NATION

Hernia costs the nation in two ways:
- **Man-hour loss** – It is due to morbidity caused by operation and post-operative complications of hernia.
- **Direct cost of operation** – It is increasing in every nation every year.

In every country, laparoscopic hernia repair costs more than open hernia repair. According to an estimate, in USA[12], the cost of open hernia operation is approximately 3500 US dollars and the cost of laparoscopic hernia repair is 7500 US dollars. In the United Kingdom, the cost varies similarly,[13] open hernia repair cost is approximately half the cost of laparoscopic hernia repair.

> **NOTE**
>
> *Annual burden of hernia on US government is approximately more than 3 billion US dollars. In India Employee's State Insurance Corporation is bearing healthcare costs since 1952 of 2.8% workforce of India.[14] One can imagine the massive cost of this huge task.*

> **KEY POINT**
>
> *Five percent of world population will develop abdominal wall hernia in their lifetime.*

REFERENCES

1. **Blackbourne LH.**, Surgical recall, 2nd edition, Lippincott, William & Wilkins.
2. **Rutkow IM.**, (1996). Epidemiological, economic and sociologic aspects of hernia surgery in the United States in the 1990s, *Surg. Clin. North Am.*, 78: 941.
3. **H. George Burkitt.**, (2001). Essential surgery, 3rd edition, p. 339.
4. **Lawrance WW** *et al.,* (2003). Inguinal and scrotal disorders, current surgical, 11th edition, pp. 1336–1338.
5. **Report of a working party convened by the Royal College of Surgeon of England.**, (1993). Clinical guidelines on the management of groin hernia in adults. London; Royal College of Surgeons of England.
6. **Abramson JH, Gofin J, Hopp C.** *et al.,* (1978). The epidemiology of inguinal hernia. A survey in Western Jerusalem, *J. Epidemiol. Community Health*, 32: 59.
7. **Kevin G. Burnand** *et al.,* (2005). The New Aird's Companion in surgical studies, 3rd edition, p. 541.
8. **Mc Intosh A, Hutchinson A, Roberts A**, *et al.,* Evidence based management of groin hernia in primary care–a systematic review. *Fam. Pact.* 17: 5, 442.
9. **Bendavid R.**, (1994). Femoral hernias in females : Facts, figures and fallacies in Bendavid R (Ed): Prostheses and abdominal wall hernias, Austin, TX : Lander Publishing, p. 82.
10. **Townsend CM** *et al.,* (2004). Sabiston textbook of surgery, 17th edition, **2**, p. 1201.
11. **Neuhauser D.**, (1997). Elective inguinal herniorrhaphy versus truss in the elderly, Bunkers JP, Barnes BA, Mosteller F (Eds): Costs, risks and benefits of surgery. New York: Oxford University Press, p. 233.
12. **Swanstorm LL.**, (2000). Laparoscopic hernia repair, the importance of cost as an outcome measurement at the century's end, *Surg. Clin. North Am.*, **20**, M04, 1341–1351.
13. **Wellwood J** *et al.,* (1998). Randomized controlled trial of laparoscopic versus open mesh repair for inguinal hernia; Outcome and cost, *Br. Med. J.*, 317: 103–110.
14. **Bhatia P and John SJ.**, (2003). Laparoscopic hernia repair, a step by step approach, pp. 2.1–2.8.
15. **Bhatia P.**, (2008). Current status of laparoscopic inguinal harnia surgery, clinical G.I. Surgery, 1st edition, *HEF*, p. 922.
16. **Turaga K., Fitzgibbons RJ.** *et al.,* (2008). Inguinal hernias: should we operate, *Surg. Clin. N. Am.*; **88,** 127–38.

Inguinal Hernia

9

"God gave you ears, eyes and hands; use them on the patient in that order."

— **William Kelsey, 1889-1963**

Inguinal hernia is the protrusion of the abdominal contents through the inguinal region of abdominal wall.

The inguinal region is a weak area in anterior abdominal wall. The following structures are present in inguinal area (Fig. 9.1):
- Inguinal canal
- Deep inguinal ring
- Superficial inguinal ring

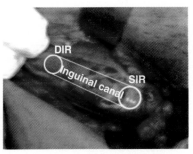

Fig. 9.1. Weak area of groin, "Achilles heel of groin".

> A semilunar D-shaped gap (Fig. 9.2) exists beneath the arched fibres of internal oblique muscle. This area is filled with only transversalis fascia, preperitoneal tissue and peritoneum. It is the weak spot in inguinal region. Here, transversalis fascia is the only restraint to herniation of the abdominal contents.[1] Direct inguinal hernia occurs here.

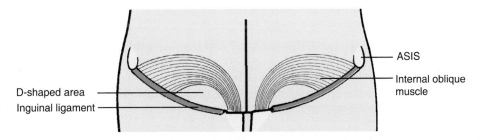

Fig. 9.2. D-shaped weak areas in inguinal regions, Achilles heel of groin.

75% of all abdominal wall hernias occur in the groin.

Inguinal hernia is the most common form of hernias. It is more common on the right side. It is due to delayed descent of right testis and so delayed closure of processus vaginalis.
- 65% inguinal hernias are indirect hernias.
- 35% are direct inguinal hernia.

The difference between indirect and direct inguinal hernias are shown in Fig. 9.3A.

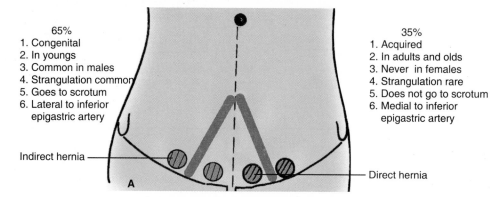

65%
1. Congenital
2. In youngs
3. Common in males
4. Strangulation common
5. Goes to scrotum
6. Lateral to inferior
   epigastric artery

35%
1. Acquired
2. In adults and olds
3. Never in females
4. Strangulation rare
5. Does not go to scrotum
6. Medial to inferior
   epigastric artery

Indirect hernia

Direct hernia

A

Fig. 9.3A. Difference between indirect and direct inguinal hernias, diagrammatic view.

- Bilateral inguinal hernia incidence is 12%. (Fig. 9.3B)
- 5% cases have both direct and indirect inguinal hernia (pantaloon hernia).
- 22% will develop contralateral hernia, as confirmed by laparoscopy.
- In infants with one-sided inguinal hernia, the processus vaginalis is patent on contralateral side in 60% cases, if the other side is explored.[2]
- Males are more than 10 times affected by inguinal hernia than females.
- Indirect inguinal hernia is common in youngs and direct inguinal hernia is common in adults and olds.
- Inguinal hernia in females is usually indirect hernia and direct hernia in females is rare.
- Lifetime prevalence of inguinal hernia is 25% in males and 2% in females.
- Inguinal hernia has approximately 10% incidence of incarceration.
- In children, the recurrence rate is less than 10%.
- Indirect inguinal hernia is uncommon in baby girls as compared to boys (ratio 1 : 9).

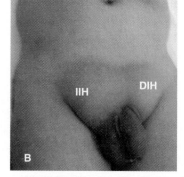

IIH   DIH

B

Fig. 9.3B. Direct and indirect inguinal hernias.

- Inguinal hernia incidence is much more in Africans than in Europeans and others. It is due to following three factors:[29]
  - Pelvis in Africans is more oblique.
  - Pubic arch is lower.
  - Narrow origin of internal oblique muscle from inguinal ligament and it fails to protect deep inguinal ring.

In a general hospital, inguinal hernias account for about 7% of surgical outpatient consultation and 12% of operating theatre time.[3]

- **Prince Charles** *of Great Birtain suffered from sport's hernia and was operated at King Edward VII Hospital, London, in March 2003.*
- **Harrison Ford**, *Hollywood actor, developed hernia while shooting of* **"Indiana Jones and Temple of Doom".**
- **Pop star Madona**, *47, developed a hernia while performing a dance routine at the Grammy Award Show. She was operated at Cedars Medical Center, New York, in 2006.*

COMPOSITION OF HERNIA

A hernia consists of three parts (Figs. 9.4 A-C):
- Sac of hernia
- Contents of the hernia sac
- Coverings of the hernia sac

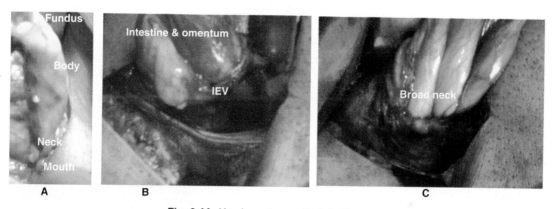

Fig. 9.4A. Hernia parts sac, **B.** & **C.** Contents.

Sac of Hernia

Sac is a pouch or a diverticulum of peritoneum, which contains the viscus or viscera protruding from the weak spot. Sac of hernia has the following four parts (Figs. 9.4 A-G):
- Mouth of sac
- Neck of sac
- Body of sac
- Fundus of sac

Mouth of sac

- It is the opening of the sac through which abdominal contents enter.

Neck of sac

- It is that part of the sac, which passes through the abdominal musculature or through the weak area of the abdominal wall. It is the most constricted or narrow part of hernia. Narrow-necked hernias develop strangulation.

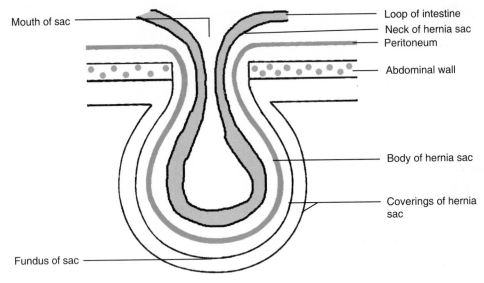

Fig. 9.4D. Parts of the hernia sac.

Femoral, paraumbilical and indirect inguinal hernias are narrow-necked hernias.

Wide-necked hernias usually do not strangulate. Some wide-necked hernias are so big that they do not have any neck.

Some incisional hernias and some direct inguinal hernias are wide-necked hernias.

Body of sac

It is the main portion of the sac. The size of body of sac differs in each case according to the contents. Sac wall may be transilluminant in infants and children, but not in adults. In long standing cases, it may get thickened due to repeated friction.

Fundus of sac

It is the most redundant part of the sac.

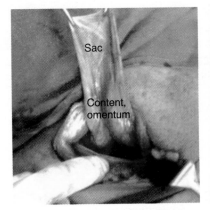

Fig. 9.4E. Hernia sac and contents.

Head, neck and shoulders of the sac (Figs. 9.4 F & G)

With the introduction of prosthetic mesh repair of groin hernia, the anatomy of groin area is studied in more detail. The peritoneal sac is divided in the following three parts as per the requirements of prosthetic mesh placement:

• Head
• Neck
• Shoulders

Head of the sac is the portion distal to the neck of the sac.[22]

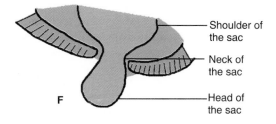
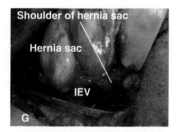

Fig. 9.4.F. Head, neck and shoulders of hernia sac, digrammatic representation, **G.** Laparoscopic view.

The shoulder of the sac is the portion of peritoneum going inside the abdominal cavity from the neck. The shoulders of the sac have to be clearly dissected and separated from fascia transversalis to make a space for prosthetic mesh.

Contents of Hernia Sac

The contents of the hernia sac are the viscera or the part of viscus which protrude through the weak area of abdominal wall and lie within the sac of hernia.

A hernia may contain any of the following structures:

- **Omentum**
  - A hernia containing omentum is called "omentocele" or "epiplocele".
- **Intestine**
  - A hernia containing intestine is called "enterocele". Most common part found in hernia sac is small intestine. Enterocele may contain large bowel and even appendix (Amyand hernia).
- A hernia containing part of **circumference of intestine** is called Richter's hernia (Fig. 9.5A). Richter's hernia is commonest in femoral hernia.
- A part of **urinary bladder** may be present in a hernia. A hernia containing part of urinary bladder or a diverticulum of bladder is called "cystocele". This hernia enlarges just before micturition and becomes smaller after micturition. Pressure on hernia induces a desire to micturate. A few examples of hernias containing urinary bladder are:
  - Direct inguinal hernia
  - Sliding inguinal hernia
  - Femoral hernia

Courtesy Dr. A K Bose, Surgeon & Director Umkal Hospital, Gurgaon.

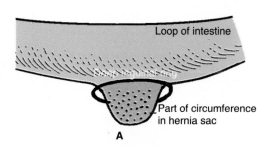
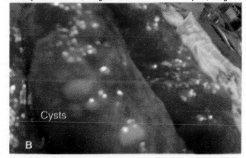

Fig. 9.5A. Richter's hernia.

Fig. 9.5B. Pneumatosis cystoides intestinalis in inguinal hernia sac.

- **Ovary or fallopian tube or both**
  - These may be found in hernia sac.

Meckel's diverticulum (Figs. 9.6 A & B)

A hernia containing Meckel's diverticulum is called "Littre's hernia", after Alexis Littre, 1658-1726, Surgeon and Lecturer of Anatomy, Paris, France. He was the first surgeon to report a case of Meckel's diverticulum in a hernia sac in 1700, much before the birth of Meckel. Meckel's diverticulum was named after Johann Friedrich Meckel, 1781-1833, Professor of Anatomy and Surgery, Halle, Germany, who described it.

- **Peritoneal fluid**
  - It may be ascitic fluid or peritoneal dialysis fluid. Small quantity of peritoneal fluid is always present. It may be blood-stained in strangulated hernia.
- Hernia sac contains any pathology involving the content i.e. Pneumatosis cystoides intestinalis (Fig. 9.5B).

Common contents of hernia

- *Omentum – omentocele or epiplocele*
- *Circumference of intestine — Richter's hernia*
- *Ovary / Fallopian tube*
- *Peritoneal fluid*

- *Intestine – enterocele*
- *Bladder – cystocele*
- *Meckel's diverticulum (Littre's hernia)*

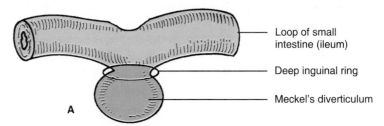

Loop of small intestine (ileum)

Deep inguinal ring

Meckel's diverticulum

A

Fig. 9.6A. Meckel's diverticulum, diagrammatic representation.

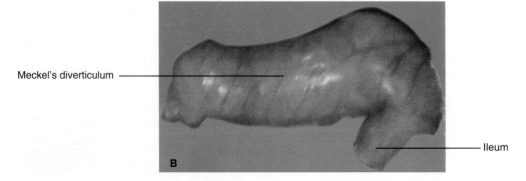

Meckel's diverticulum

Ileum

B

Fig. 9.6B. Meckel's diverticulum, laparoscopic view.

Entero-omentocele

When both the intestine and omentum are present in hernia sac, it is called entero-omentocele.

Amyand's hernia (Figs. 9.7 A-C)

When appendix is present in inguinal hernia, it is known as "Amyand's hernia". The true anatomical name is "Appendicocele". It is a rare entity. Claudius Amyand (1685-1740), Surgeon at St. George's Hospital, London, England, was surgeon to King George II, was the first who described a perforated appendix within the inguinal hernia sac in an 11-year-old boy and performed a successful trans-herniotomy appendicectomy in 1735.[32] The status of appendix present in hernia sac determines the type of hernia repair required:

• If appendix is normal then mesh hernioplasty is done.
• If appendicitis is found then Bassinis' repair is done. No mesh is used.[4]

Pathophysiology of Amyand's hernia

It is found approximately in 1% of adult inguinal hernia repair as uninflammed[33]. D'Alia observed once (0.08%) in 1341 inguinal hernia operations.[34]

Appendix enters the hernia sac, the sac ring compromises with the circulation and lumen of appendix leading to a localised inflammatory process similar to the one created by a faecolith.[5]

Contraction of abdominal muscles and increased intra-abdominal pressure compress the appendix and cause inflammation.

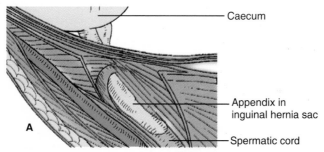

Fig. 9.7A. Amyand's hernia, diagrammatic representation.

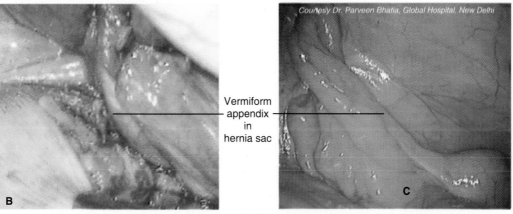

Fig. 9.7B. Amyand's hernia in open repair, **C.** In laparoscopic repair of inguinal hernia.

Richter's hernia (Fig. 9.8)

It is also called "partial enterocele".
"A portion of circumference of the bowel becomes herniated in any kind of abdominal wall hernia." Usually antimesenteric border is involved.
It is described by August Gottlieb Richter, (1742 – 1812), Lecturer of Surgery, Gottengen, Germany.

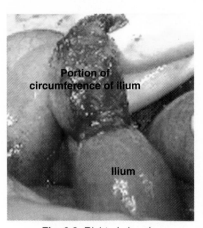

Richter's hernia is commonly seen in:
* Femoral hernia
* Obturator hernia
    It usually undergoes strangulation producing obstruction to the lumen of loop of intestine.
    Intestinal obstruction is not present until half of the circumference of the bowel is involved.

Fig. 9.8. Richter's hernia.

In this, the diagnosis is delayed as the clinical features mimic gastroenteritis as:
* Intestinal colic is present.
* Bowels open normally or diarrhoea is present.
* There may not be vomiting.
* Absolute constipation is delayed until paralytic ileus develops or total obstruction develops.

Problems with strangulated Richter's hernia (Fig. 9.9)
* Diagnosis is delayed due to abnormal clinical features.
* Treatment is delayed as the diagnosis is delayed.
* Gangrene develops at the apex of loop of intestine and peritonitis develops.

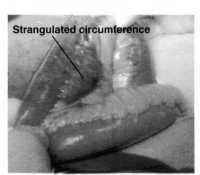

COVERINGS OF HERNIA

The sac passes through the abdominal wall, so the structures of abdominal wall from skin to preperitoneal connective tissue make the coverings of hernia. In long standing and big hernias, different layers of the coverings of hernia become adherent and atrophied and sometimes amalgamate with each other and become indistinguishable from each other.

Fig. 9.9. Strangulated mesenteric hernia.

Coverings of indirect inguinal hernia (Fig. 9.10)

From inside to outside, the following coverings are present in indirect inguinal hernia:
* Peritoneum
* Extraperitoneal fat
* Internal spermatic fascia (derived from transversalis fascia at deep inguinal ring)
* Cremasteric fascia and muscles (derived from internal oblique and transversus abdominis muscles)
* External spermatic fascia (derived from external oblique aponeurosis at superficial inguinal ring)
* Superficial fascia
    – Camper's fascia

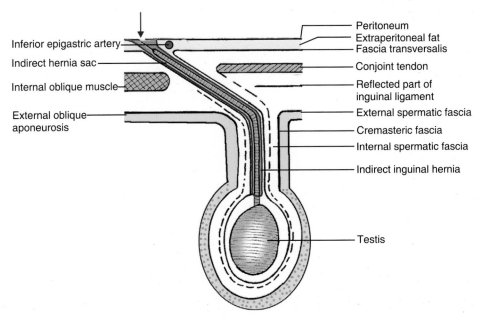

Fig. 9.10. Coverings of indirect inguinal hernia sac.

- Scarpa's fascia
- It also includes dartos muscle of scrotum.
- Skin

Coverings of direct inguinal hernia (Fig. 9.11)

From inside to outside, following coverings are present in direct inguinal hernia:
- Peritoneum
- Fascia transversalis

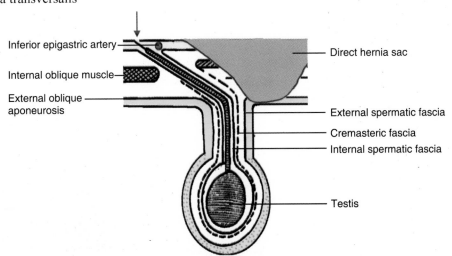

Fig. 9.11. Coverings of direct inguinal hernia sac.

- Conjoint tendon
- External oblique aponeurosis
- Superficial fascia
  - Camper's fascia
  - Scarpa's fascia
- Skin

STATES OF HERNIA

- Reducible hernia
- Irreducible hernia
- Obstructed hernia
- Strangulated hernia
- Inflamed hernia
- Incarcerated hernia

Reducible Hernia (Figs. 9.12 A & B)

It is simple and uncomplicated hernia, which usually reduces itself when a person lies down or reducible by patient himself or by surgeon.
- Reducibility and expansile impulse on coughing are two most important clinical features of hernia.
- A reducible hernia gives an expansile impulse on coughing.
- Common contents are intestine or omentum or both.
- When intestine is the content, first part is more difficult to reduce than the last part.
- When omentum is the content, last part is more difficult to reduce than the first part.
- Intestine reduces with gurgling sound. Omentum reduces without gurgling sound.
- Omentum gives a doughy and granular feel.

Expansile impulse on coughing

It is a classical sign of reducible hernia. It is present in following conditions also:
- Meningocele
- Laryngocele
- Lymphatic cyst in children
- Empyema neccessitans
- Dermoid cyst with intracranial connection

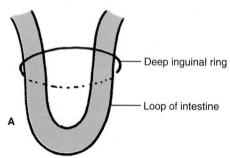
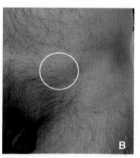

Fig. 9.12A. Reducible hernia, **B.** Left indirect inguinal hernia.

Irreducible Hernia (Figs. 9.13A & B)

In this case, the contents of hernia cannot be completely returned to the abdomen but there is no associated complication. Irreducibility predisposes to strangulation. So irreducible hernia must be operated to avoid strangulation. Irreducibility occurs due to the following reasons:
– Adhesions between the sac and its content
– Adhesions between contents
– Adhesions between one part of the sac to other
– Sliding hernia
– Narrowing of neck of the sac which occurs due to fibrosis or continuous use of truss
– Omentum in the sac (asymptomatic irreducibility indicates an omentocele)
– Incarcerated hernia with large intestine in sac
– Massive hernia inside scrotum (scrotal abdomen) or "wheel barrow hernia"

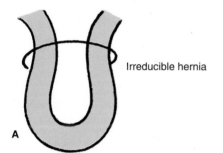
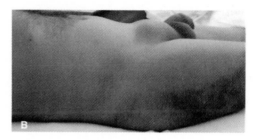

Fig. 9.13A. Irreducible hernia, **B.** Right indirect inguinal hernia.

Common irreducible hernias

• Femoral hernia
• Umbilical hernia

Irreducible hernias are reduced through a method known as Taxis.

Taxis

"Vigorous taxis has no place in modern surgery, and it is only mentioned to be condemned".[5]
    It is a method of reduction of hernia for irreducible, non-obstructed and non-strangulated hernia.

Method of taxis (Figs. 9.14 A-C)

The patient is asked to lie down. Thigh of hernia side is flexed, adducted and medially rotated. This relaxes the muscles as well as the superficial inguinal ring. The fundus of sac is held gently and pressed to squeeze the contents in abdomen.

    In right-sided inguinal hernia, the sac is held with right hand and squeezed gradually over scrotum. At the same time, the proximal portion of hernia sac is guided into inguinal canal by left hand.

Indication of taxis
Irreducible hernia

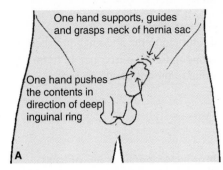

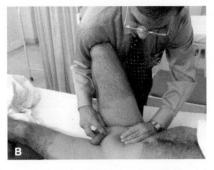

Fig. 9.14A. Method of taxis, diagrammatic representation, **B.** On patient, note flexed, adducted and medially rotated thigh of hernia side.

Contraindication of taxis

Strangulated hernia

If extra force is applied during taxis then following damages can occur:

- Contusion of intestinal wall
- Rupture of intestine
- Reduction en mass (the whole sac with strangulated contents is reduced inside the abdominal cavity and the strangulation continues).

Ideally maximum two attempts should be made for reduction of hernia, if unsuccessful, then abandon the taxis and it should be operated.

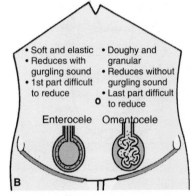

- Soft and elastic
- Reduces with gurgling sound
- 1st part difficult to reduce

- Doughy and granular
- Reduces without gurgling sound
- Last part difficult to reduce

Enterocele   Omentocele

Fig. 9.14C. Difference on taxis between enterocele and omentocele.

Obstructed Hernia (Fig. 9.15)

It is an irreducible hernia containing intestine with obstruction of lumen from within or from outside without affecting the blood supply of intestine.

- It is irreducible and has intestinal obstruction.
- It causes colicky abdominal pain and local tenderness.
- Expansile impulse on coughing is not present.
- Hernia is not reducible.
- Hernia is lax and non-tender.
- The acute intestinal obstruction leads to:
  - Pain in abdomen
  - Vomiting
  - Distension of abdomen
  - Absolute constipation
- Sometimes it is difficult to distinguish obstructed hernia from strangulation clinically, so treat obstructed hernia like strangulation.

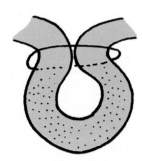

Fig. 9.15. Obstructed hernia.

- Obstructed inguinal hernia occurs due to the following reasons:
  - Narrow neck of the hernia sac.
  - Irreducible hernias are prone to get obstructed.
  - Overcrowding of contents in hernial sac.

Strangulated Hernia (Figs. 9.16 A & B)

"In doubtful cases do not wait too long before exploring, for it is quite wrong to act upon the slogan "Wait and See", When looking may provide the remedy."

- Zachary Cope (1881-1974)

It is an obstructed inguinal hernia with impairment of blood supply of its contents.
- It occurs at any time in either sex and at any age.
- Indirect inguinal hernia strangulates commonly.
- Direct inguinal hernia strangulates rarely except the funicular variety which strangulates more commonly due to its narrow neck.
- Ischaemia and gangrene occur within six hours from first symptom.

NOTE

- *Inguinal hernia is 10 times more common than femoral hernia.*
- *Femoral hernia is 10 times more prone to strangulation than inguinal hernia due to tough and narrow femoral ring.*

- The incidence of strangulated hernia is diminishing due to gradually increasing trend of elective operations for asymptomatic inguinal hernias.

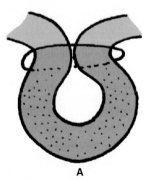
A

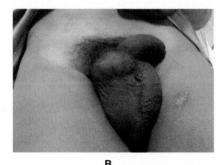
B

Fig. 9.16A. Strangulated hernia, diagrammatic representation, **B.** Strangulated right indirect inguinal hernia.

- Strangulated inguinal hernia without intestinal obstruction is seen in:
  - Omentocele
  - Richter's hernia
  - Littre's hernia

Inflamed Hernia (Figs. 9.17 A & B)

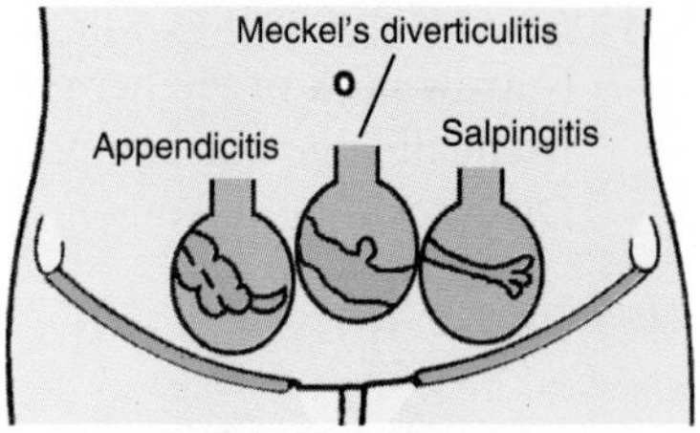

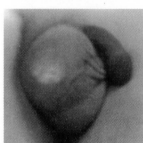

Fig. 9.17A. Conditions causing inflamed hernia.

The inflammation may start inside the hernia sac due to inflammation of its contents.
- It occurs in the following conditions:
  – Acute appendicitis
  – Acute salpingitis
  – Meckel's diverticulitis
- The inflammation may start from outside due to:
  – Trophic ulcer of dependent part of hernia.
  – Trauma which is due to repeated friction in umbilical and incisional hernia. Hernia becomes painful, tender and swollen.
  – Ill-fitted truss.
- Differentiation from strangulation:
  – It is not tense.
  – There is no sign of acute intestinal obstruction.
- Inflamed hernia is diagnosed by the presence of contributory symptoms with local signs of inflammation and oedematous skin.

Incarcerated Hernia

Fig. 9.17B. Inflamed hernia due to Meckel's diverticulitis.

It occurs when a portion of lumen of colon which is in hernial sac is blocked with faeces. It shows the sign of indentation when pressed.

NOTE

Incarcerated hernia is basically an irreducible hernia.
The term "incarceration" is a confusing term and it is better if it is replaced with "irreducible".

KEY POINT

Every irreducible, incarcerated and obstructed hernia should be treated as strangulation and urgent operation is advised.

TYPES OF INGUINAL HERNIA

"A knowledge of healthy and diseased actions is not less necessary to be understood than the principles of other sciences."

— **John Hunter, (1728-1793)**

Inguinal hernia can be classified in the following ways (Fig. 9.18):

- **According to the extent of hernia**
  - Incomplete inguinal hernia
    a) Bubonocele
    b) Funicular hernia
  - Complete or inguinoscrotal hernia
- **According to the site of exit of hernia sac**
  - Indirect or oblique inguinal hernia
  - Direct inguinal hernia
- **According to the contents of hernia sac**
  - Enterocele
  - Omentocele or epiplocele
  - Cystocele
- **According to the time of development**
  - Congenital inguinal hernia
  - Acquired inguinal hernia. (It develops gradually but less commonly suddenly after a muscular effort.)

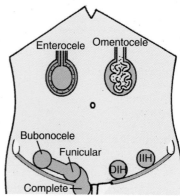

Fig. 9.18. Classification of inguinal hernia.

Indirect or Oblique Inguinal Hernia (Figs. 9.19 A & B)

It occurs due to patent processus vaginalis. Processus vaginalis gets obliterated at or after birth. It occurs first at deep inguinal ring and then just above the testis and finally the remaining part is obliterated to a fibrous cord. If the obliteration does not happen then hernia develops. The contents in hernia travel through the inguinal canal and enter the deep inguinal ring and come out of superficial inguinal ring. Sac runs lateral and anterior to spermatic cord.

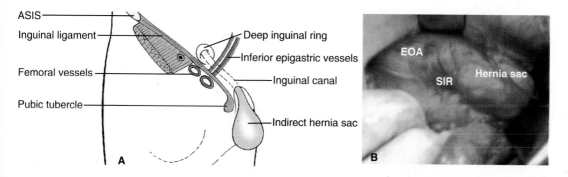

Fig. 9.19A. Indirect inguinal hernia, relations, diagrammatic representation, **B.** Open view.

Important features of indirect inguinal hernia are:

- Commonest of all hernias
- Common in young
- More common in males than females
- Expansile impulse on coughing
- Prone to get obstruction and strangulation
- Congenital due to patent processus vaginalis
- Collagen tissue abnormality in adults

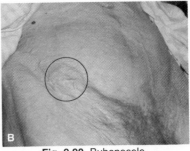

Fig. 9.20. Bubonocele.

It is incomplete or complete hernia.

Incomplete hernia

- Bubonocele
- Funicular

Bubonocele (Figs. 9.20 & 9.23A)
Hernia sac protrudes only in inguinal canal and does not descend further down as the inguinal canal is closed at superficial inguinal ring. *Bubon* is a Greek word and means "groin". It is present as swelling in groin. History is usually short. Most of the patients are adults.

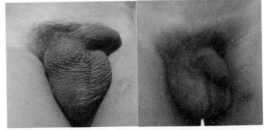

Fig. 9.21. Funicular hernia.   **Fig. 9.22.** Inguinoscrotal indirect hernia.

Funicular (Figs. 9.21 & 9.23B)
Sac comes upto upper end of scrotum but is separated from testis as the processus vaginalis is closed just above the epididymis. Hernia sac lies above the testis and both are separate. Testis can be separately palpated. *Funiculus* is a Latin word and means a "small cord". It occurs in adults with long standing history.

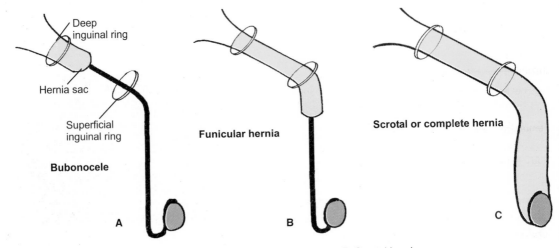

Fig. 9.23A. Bubonocele, **B.** Funicular and **C.** Scrotal hernia.

Complete or scrotal hernia (Figs. 9.22, 9.23C & 9.24))

Hernia reaches upto lower part of scrotum and testis lies within it. The testis can be palpated posteriorly but with difficulty. The inguinal canal is patent throughout its length. The hernia sac is continuous with tunica vaginalis and lies in front and at the sides of testis. It is not seen at birth but present in infancy, adolescent and adult.

Indirect hernia is a congenital hernia and occurs in children and may not appear until adolescent or adult life.

Congenital Indirect Inguinal Hernia

Vaginal (Fig. 9.25)

The processus vaginalis does not occlude so hernia descends upto base of scrotum. Testis lies behind and is difficult to palpate separately.

Funicular (Fig. 9.26)

The processus vaginalis is occluded just above the testis so hernia comes above the level of testis and testis can be palpated separately.

Infantile (Fig. 9.27)

It is similar to funicular hernia except a process of processus vaginalis is formed in front of hernia which reaches as high as superficial inguinal ring. So while operating, a peritoneal sac is found in front of hernia sac, due to the stucking of diverticulum of processus vaginalis at external inguinal ring during its development.

Encysted (Fig. 9.28)

A peritoneal process is present in front of the hernia sac. It also runs upto external inguinal ring. It is also due to sticking of diverticulum of processus vaginalis to superficial inguinal ring.

Interstitial

A diverticulum develops which gets caught between layers of anterior abdominal wall. This is of three types:

• **Superficial extraparietal interstitial hernia** (Fig. 9.29)

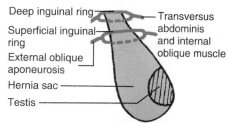

Fig. 9.24. Scrotal hernia.

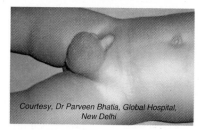

Courtesy, Dr Parveen Bhatia, Global Hospital, New Delhi

Fig. 9.25. Vaginal inguinal hernia.

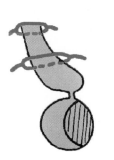 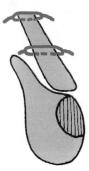

Fig. 9.26. Funicular inguinal hernia.

Fig. 9.27. Infantile inguinal hernia.

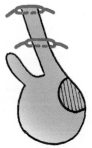

Fig. 9.28. Encysted inguinal hernia.

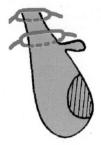

Fig. 9.29. Superficial extraparietal interstitial hernia.

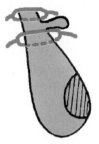

Fig. 9.30. Interparietal or intramuscular hernia.

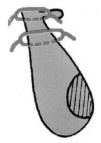

Fig. 9.31. Properitoneal or preperitoneal hernia.

    – It occurs between superficial fascia and external oblique aponeurosis.
- **Interparietal or intramuscular** (Fig. 9.30)
  - It occurs between internal and external oblique muscles.
- **Properitoneal or preperitoneal** (Fig. 9.31)
  - It occurs between fascia transversalis and peritoneum.

Direct Inguinal Hernia

A direct inguinal hernia is a protrusion of abdominal viscera through the posterior wall of inguinal canal, medial to inferior epigastric vessels through Hesselbach's triangle (Figs. 9.32 A-C). It does not descend to scrotum.

    Hesselbach's triangle is divided into lateral and medial part by obliterated umbilical artery (medial umbilical ligament) and in this way direct hernia is also divided into two parts:
- Lateral direct inguinal hernia
- Medial direct inguinal hernia

    Obliteration of deep inguinal ring with thumb does not allow indirect hernia to pop out but direct inguinal hernia comes out.
- Direct inguinal hernia is always acquired. It is never congenital.
- Bilateral direct inguinal hernias are four times more common than indirect hernia.

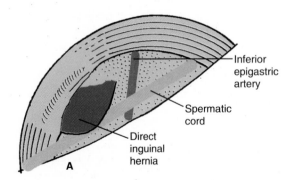

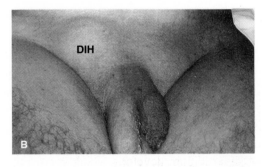

Fig. 9.32A. Direct inguinal hernia, diagrammatic representation, **B.** Right direct inguinal hernia.

- It comes out through the anterior abdominal wall via the weak area in fascia transversalis in posterior wall of inguinal canal. Fascia transversalis progressively weakens in adults, but direct inguinal hernias are uncommon in females.
- According to Francis Brown, Surgeon, Royal Infirmary, Dundee, Scotland, women particularly never develop direct inguinal hernia.[6]
- Occasionally, a direct inguinal hernia occurs suddenly after an awkward sudden physical effort which causes sudden rise of intra-abdominal pressure. It causes split of fascia transversalis leading to sudden appearance of direct inguinal hernia, known as "rupture". The "cause-and-effect" relationship between a specific lifting episode and the development of inguinal hernia is presented in less than 10% of patients.[7]
- The incidence in females is 0.2% of all abdominal wall hernias.
- Direct inguinal hernia does not descend to scrotum.

Aetiology of direct inguinal hernia

- Raised intra-abdominal pressure
- Weakness of posterior wall of inguinal canal and iliopubic tract
- An abnormally high transversus arch
- Limited insertion of transversus abdominis muscle on pubis
- Limited insertion of iliopubic tract to Cooper's ligament

The direct inguinal hernia usually does not increase in size. Sac in direct inguinal hernia lies posterior to or above or below spermatic cord while in indirect inguinal hernia the sac lies anterior and lateral to spermatic cord. Sometimes the sac lies within the spermatic cord, covered with cremasteric muscle fibres.

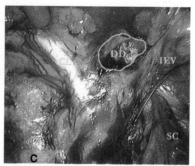

Fig. 9.32C. Right direct inguinal hernia defect, laparoscopic view, DD = Direct Defect.

- Direct inguinal hernia neck is usually wide (Figs. 9.32 A-C).
- Direct inguinal hernia does not strangulate due to wide neck.
- Direct inguinal hernia is most common in male adults.
- Conjoint tendon is attached to pubic tubercle and laterally to pecten pubis but when its lateral extension is not present it fails to protect posterior wall and a direct inguinal hernia occurs.
- Cigarette smoking, direct inguinal hernia and aortic aneurysm have one common thing and that is collagen defect which has been demonstrated.

Important features of direct inguinal hernia

- *All acquired, never, congenital*
- *Usually does not go to scrotum*
- *Rare in females*
- *Common in older males*
- *Rarely strangulates*

Predisposing causes of direct inguinal hernia

• *Straining*   • *Smoking*   • *Surgery, ilioinguinal nerve injury in previous appendicectomy*

KEY POINT

Direct inguinal hernia does not descend to scrotum as it has to push inguinal canal through its posterior and anterior walls.

Funicular Direct Inguinal Hernia (Ogilvie Hernia) (Figs. 9.33 A & B)

• It is also called "prevesical hernia", occurs in elderly males.
• It contains prevesical fat and part of urinary bladder.
• It protrudes through a small defect in medial part of conjoint tendon and above the pubic tubercle.
• It is a narrow-necked hernia hence, prone to strangulation.

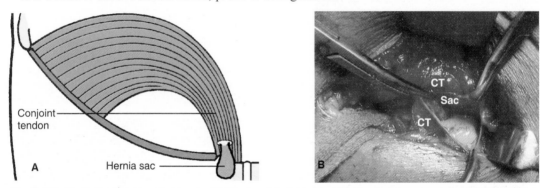

Fig. 9.33A. Funicular direct inguinal hernia (Ogilvie hernia), right side, diagrammatic representation, **B.** Open view.

BASUGA HERNIA

It is Ogilvie hernia, found in Basuga area of Uganda and some other parts of Africa.[35]

Pantaloon or Saddlebag or Dual or Romberg Hernia (Figs. 9.34 & 9.35 A-C)

• It is a combination of both direct and indirect inguinal hernias.
• It has two sacs, striding over inferior epigastric vessels.

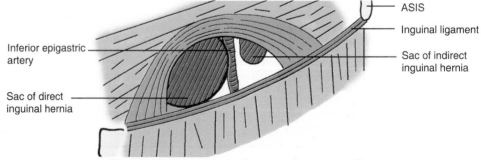

Fig. 9.34. Pantaloon hernia, diagrammatic representation.

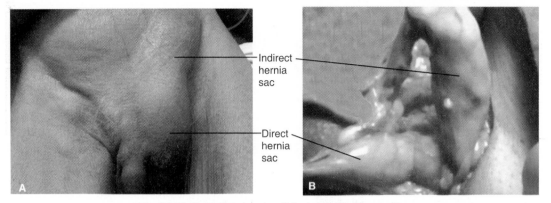

Fig. 9.35A. Pantaloon hernia, clinical view, **B.** At operation.

- It occurs in 5% of all inguinal hernias.
- Sometimes one sac of it is overlooked during the operation and recurrence occurs.

Maydl's Hernia (Hernia-en-W) (Figs. 9.36 A & B)

Two loops of small bowel form a 'W'. The outer loops remain in sac and the connecting loop remains within the abdomen and often strangulates.

- Intestinal obstruction is observed and tenderness is found above the inguinal ligament.
- On operation, the loops of intestine in the hernia sac are found normal and strangulated loop lies within the abdomen. So traction brings out the strangulated loop in the sac. The spread of peritonitis is early as strangulated loop lies inside the abdomen.
- Maydl's hernia is also called "Retrograde strangulation".
- Strangulated loop of 'W' lies within the abdomen and normal loop in hernia sac.

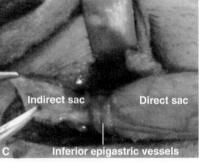

Fig. 9.35C. Pantaloon hernia, inferior epigastric vessels between direct and indirect sac.

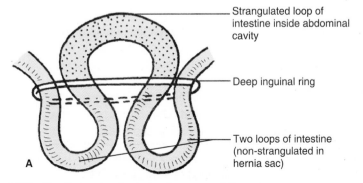

Fig. 9.36A. Maydl's hernia, diagrammatic representation.

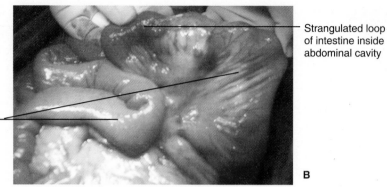

Strangulated loop
of intestine inside
abdominal cavity

Two loops of intestine
(non-strangulated in
hernia sac)

B

Fig. 9.36B. Maydl's hernia, open view.

Clinical features of inguinal hernia (Fig. 9.37)

- General considerations
- History
- Examination

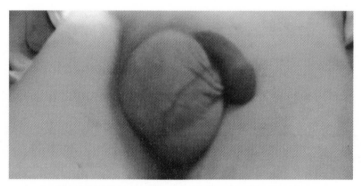

Fig. 9.37. Right inguinoscrotal indirect inguinal hernia.

GENERAL CONSIDERATIONS

- Indirect inguinal hernia is more common than direct inguinal hernia.
- Indirect inguinal hernia is more common especially in children on right side due to later descent of right side testis (Fig. 9.37).
- One-third cases are bilateral (Fig. 9.38).
- Left side is prevalent in 25% men and 20% in women.
- Two-thirds inguinal hernias are indirect.
- Two-thirds of recurrent inguinal hernias are direct.

The accuracy of clinically diagnosing a direct hernia is little more than 50% while an indirect hernia can be correctly diagnosed in 90% of patients.[8,9]

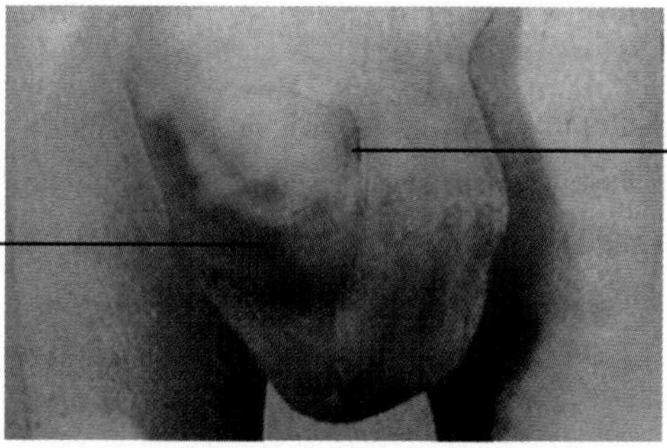

Fig. 9.38. Bilateral inguinoscrotal indirect inguinal hernia.

HISTORY

Age

- It can occur at any age, even may be present at the time of birth.
- Indirect inguinal hernia occurs in children, teens and adults. In males, it is common before the age of five years and peak occurs in early twenties.
- Direct inguinal hernia occurs in elderly men.
- Almost all congenital hernias in children are indirect inguinal hernia and much less commonly direct inguinal and femoral hernias.
- Inguinal hernias are common in premature infants. Specially those with low birth weight, below 1500 g.

Sex

- Inguinal hernia occurs in both males and females.
- Indirect inguinal hernia is common in males but occurs in females also.
- Direct inguinal hernia does not occur in females.
- In infants and children, 90% inguinal hernia occur in boys and 10% in girls.
- Although femoral hernias are found more often in women, the inguinal hernia is still the most common hernia in women.

Occupation

- It is common in workers with strenuous work and heavy weight lifting. It causes strain on abdominal muscles leading to hernia.
- Workmans' Compensation Act in most countries accept that the hernias can be caused by heavy work.

> The exact relationship between direct inguinal hernias and heavy lifting or straining remains unclear and some studies suggest that the incidence of direct hernia is no greater in people in professions that routinely involve heavy manual labour.[23]

- **Side**
  - Indirect inguinal hernia occurs more commonly on the right side due to late descent to right testis and late closure of right processus vaginalis.

- **Presentation**
  - In infants bulge appears when the child cries.
  - It is translucent in infants but never in adults.
  - Initially, a swelling or bulge appears in groin which shows expansile impulse on coughing.
  - Swelling first appears on straining e.g. coughing but gradually it starts coming out even on standing without straining.
  - Gradually, the bulge appears on standing alone and disappears on lying down.
  - Gradually, swelling increases, which disappears on lying down.
  - Gradually, swelling does not disappear on lying down and has to be reduced.
- **Pain**
  - There may be no pain but only discomfort or a lump in the groin is noticed or may be a dragging pain which gets worse as the day passes.
  - Commonest pain in hernia is a dragging sensation which is common in inguinoscrotal hernia. The dragging sensation is felt due to drag on mesentery or omentum. It may cause epigastric pain also.
  - Severe pain indicates strangulation.
  - In some patients pain starts before hernia starts and continues as hernia progresses and then disappears when hernia is fully formed.
  - Pain may be in the groin or in testis on straining.
  - Referred pain is felt in scrotum.
- **Symptoms of intestinal obstruction** (pain, absolute constipation, distension and vomiting)
  If these are present then think of:
  - Obstructed hernia
  - Strangulated hernia
- **Symptoms of causative factors, especially of straining**
  Ask history of:
  - Chronic cough.
  - Dysurea and frequency of micturition for BPH, bladder neck obstruction, urethral stricture.
  - Constipation.
  - Patient will not mention in his/her complain about these symptoms so ask leading questions about these symptoms, so that you can tell them the cause of hernia too.
- **Past history**
  - History of appendicectomy: It is important in direct inguinal hernia because in appendicectomy subcostal or ilioinguinal nerve may be damaged.
  - History of previous hernia surgery as this hernia may be recurrent.
  - History of caesarian section.
  - History of surgical removal of lower ureteric stone.
  - History of lumbar sympathectomy.
- **Family history of hernia**
  - It is important as it may be due to genetic protein and collagen disease i.e. prune belly syndrome.
- **Pregnancy**
  - The increasing intra-abdominal pressure is due to growing fetus and enlarging uterus may make groin hernias symptomatic.[24]

Natural history of inguinal hernia (Fig. 9.39)

- Inguinal hernias usually develop gradually but are exacerbated by any condition like obesity, coughing and straining at micturition and constipation which increases intra-abdominal pressure.
- Initially, the contents of hernia are completely reducible in abdominal cavity. Reduction occurs spontaneously when the patient lies, but gradually the patient needs some manipulation to reduce it. The longer a hernia remains and the larger it becomes, the more difficult it is to reduce.
- Swelling may be present since birth.
- Spontaneous development of a swelling in inguinal area occurs after heavy strenuous work in a young male patients. A young man may give history of precipitation of groin swelling after performing sudden unaccustomed movement with exertion.
- Elderly male may present with a painless swelling in inguinal region following strain for passing urine due to BPH for some time.
- In infants, severe coughing can precipitate an attack of inguinal hernia which may become irreducible.
- Very large "wheel barrow" hernias are usually of long standing and are found in elderly males.
- Some patients give history of episodes of hernia becoming irreducible. They require urgent surgery to avoid strangulation.

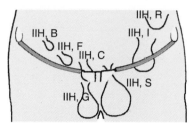

Fig. 9.39. Natural history of inguinal hernia, IIH = indirect inguinal hernia, B=bubonocele, F= funicular, C= complete, G= giant, R = reducible, I = irreducible and S = strangulated.

METHOD OF EXAMINATION

- The patient is examined first in standing and then in supine position (Figs. 9.40 A & B).
- Clothes are removed from umbilicus to mid-thigh.
- A swelling may be present in inguinal region, which may be reaching upto scrotum.
- Location of ASIS and pubic tubercle is important before proceeding further.
- First examine from front and then examine from side (Figs. 9.41, 9.42 A & B).
  - Stand on hernia side of patient. Place one hand on patient's back to support and other hand on lump.

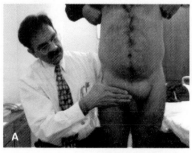

Feeling right groin for impulse on coughing

Palpating right anterior superior iliac spine and pubic tubercle

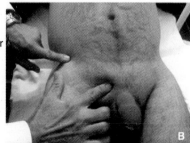

Fig. 9.40A. Examining a hernia patient in standing position, **B.** In supine position.

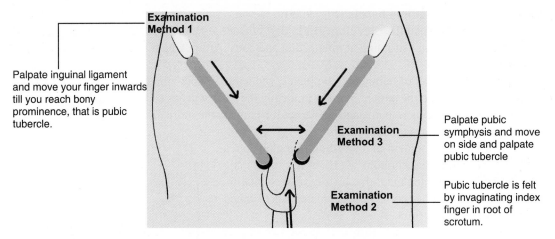

Fig. 9.41. Palpation of pubic tubercle.

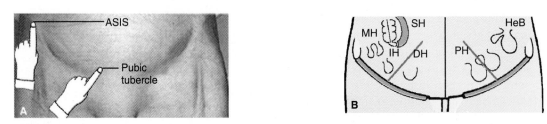

Fig. 9.42A. Palpation of ASIS and pubic tubercle, **B.** Various groin hernias can be diagnosed or suspected by clinical examination.
SH= sliding hernia, MH= Maydl's hernia, IH= indirect hernia, DH= direct hernia, HeB= hernia-en-bissac, and PH= pantaloon hernia.

• Now find the following facts about the lump:
  – Site
  – Size
  – Shape
  – Position
  – Colour
  – Temperature
  – Surface
  – Tenderness
  – Composition (gas / solid / fluid)

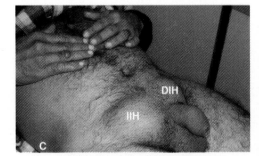

Fig. 9.42C. Hernia becomes prominent on straining.

Site

Site of the lump gives an idea about direct or indirect hernia or femoral hernia. Site in relation to pubic tubercle and inguinal ligament is estimated.

Size

Usually, it is a small bulge, but it may become very big.

Shape

It is a globular lump if it only occupies inguinal canal. It becomes pear-shaped if it comes out of superficial inguinal ring. It may become hourglass-shaped due to narrowing in the middle of the lump due to superficial inguinal ring.

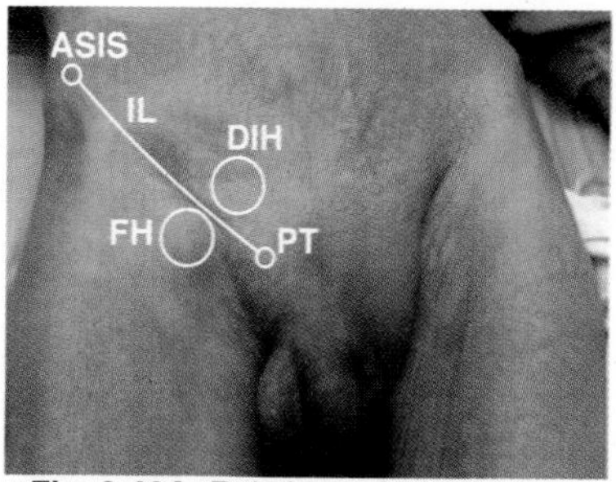

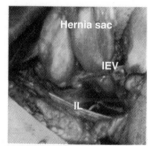

Fig. 9.43A. Relations of inguinal and femoral hernias with groin landmarks.

Position

The lump is above inguinal ligament in inguinal hernia and below in femoral hernia. Indirect inguinal hernia may go to scrotum, but direct inguinal hernia usually does not reach scrotum.

> **NOTE (Figs. 9.43 A & B)**
> * *Neck of the sac in indirect inguinal hernia lies lateral to inferior epigastric vessels.*
> * *Neck of the sac in direct inguinal hernia lies medial to inferior epigastric vessels.*
> * *In inguinal hernia, the neck of the sac is above and medial to pubic tubercle.*
> * *In femoral hernia, the neck of the sac is below and lateral to pubic tubercle.*

Colour

Skin over the uncomplicated inguinal hernia should be normal. It may be tense and red in strangulated hernia, if truss was used then skin may be white and scarred due to the pressure of the pad of truss.

Temperature

The temperature of skin should be normal over the hernia except when the hernia is strangulated or inflamed then it becomes warmer.

Surface

Usually, it is smooth but may be bosselated.

Tenderness

An uncomplicated hernia is non-tender. It may be uncomfortable on applying the pressure. An obstructed and irreducible hernia is painful to squeezing.

Fig. 9.43B. Relations of indirect inguinal hernia neck with inferior epigastric vessels.

Composition

A hernia may contain bowel or omentum. If it contains bowel, then it is soft, fluctuant, resonant and may have bowel sounds and even peristalsis is visible in big hernias. If the hernia sac contains omentum, then it may be firm, rubbery, non-fluctuant and dull on percussion.
* Observe an expansile impulse on coughing which is diagnostic of hernia.
* Scar indicates recurrence. Ragged scar indicates infection in previous surgery.
* Peristalsis may be seen in giant hernia.
* Always examine both inguinal areas. Bilateral inguinal hernias are common.

DIAGNOSTIC SIGNS

Some common diagnostic signs of abdominal wall hernia are:
- It occurs at congential or acquired weak area.
- Reducibility.
- Expansile cough impulse.

> Reducibility and expansile cough impulse may be absent in irreducible or strangulated hernia, but it does not exclude the diagnosis of hernia.

A swelling in loin

Most hernias are best examined in standing position and one can notice a lump or a swelling, if not seen then ask the patient to cough, hernia may pop out.

Reducibility

A lump may disappear when person lies down but if it does not disappear then it is tested by manipulation. First press firmly and then squeeze the lower part of the lump and lift it upwards towards the external inguinal ring. Now observe the point of reduction. If the point of reduction is above and medial to public tubercle, then it is inguinal hernia and if it is below and lateral to pubic tubercle, then it is femoral hernia.

Expansile impulse on coughing (Fig. 9.44 A & B)

Impulse on coughing can be well demonstrated by placing a finger on superficial inguinal ring or holding the root of scrotum with index finger and thumb and asking the patient to cough. An expansile impulse on coughing is felt as the content of hernia sac will try to come out of superficial inguinal ring.
- Swelling may not be present – It appears on coughing.
- Swelling may be present – It will expand in all directions on coughing.
- There will be visible expansile impulse on coughing – There will be palpable expansile cough impulse on holding root of scrotum.

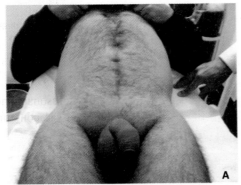 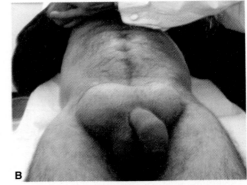

Fig. 9.44A. Bilateral hernia before coughing, **B.** Hernias appeared on coughing showing expansile impulse on coughing.

- The lump must become larger and tense in expansile cough impulse and not merely tense on moving.
- Expansile impulse on coughing must be visible as well as palpable.

> **The impulse on coughing will be absent in:**
>
> – Strangulated hernia
> – Obstructed hernia
> – Irreducible hernia
> – Incarcerated hernia

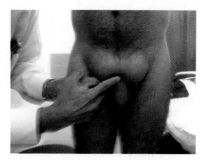

Fig. 9.45. Getting above the swelling test with two index fingers in bilateral inguinal hernia and right hydrocele.

Getting above the swelling (Fig. 9.45)

Hold the spermatic cord with thumb and index finger or by two index fingers above the scrotum.

- It is used to differentiate a scrotal swelling from inguinoscrotal hernia.
- In inguinoscrotal hernia, one cannot get above the swelling.
- In hydrocele or scrotal swelling, one can get above the swelling and spermatic cord can be felt between finger and the thumb. But in inguinoscrotal hernia one cannot get above the swelling.

Malgaigne's Bulge (Figs. 9.46 A & B)

Weakness of abdominal muscles below umbilicus and in inguinal region is shown by raising both the legs simultaneously. It was described by Joseph Francois Malgaigne (1806–1865), Professor of Surgery, Paris, France.

- Ask the patient to raise head or raise legs keeping them straight. Bulgings develop in inguinal area which indicate weak abdominal musculature. Direct inguinal hernia may be associated with Malgaigne's bulges.

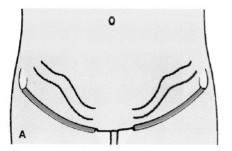 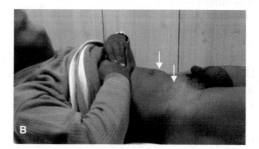

Fig. 9.46 A & B. Malgaigne's Bulge, on raising head or legs.

> **KEY POINT**
>
> *Malgaigne's bulge associated with hernia is an absolute indication for hernioplasty.*

DIAGNOSTIC TESTS FOR INGUINAL HERNIA

The accuracy with which indirect and direct inguinal hernia are clinically distinguished is low.[9]

Zieman's Technique (After Stephen A Ziemann, Surgeon, Providence Hospital, Mobile, Alabama, USA) (Fig. 9.47)

Aim

It is used to differentiate and diagnose indirect inguinal, direct inguinal and femoral hernias.

Method

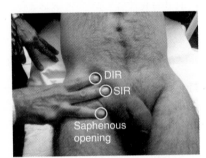

Fig. 9.47. Zieman's technique.

- Ask the patient to lie in supine position and reduce the hernia, then keep
  - Index finger over deep inguinal ring.
  - Middle finger over superficial inguinal ring.
  - Ring finger over saphenous opening.
- Then ask the patient to cough and feel the expansile impulse on coughing and diagnose the hernia according to the site of impulse.

Interpretation

- Impulse felt by index finger – indirect inguinal hernia
- Impulse felt by middle finger – direct inguinal hernia
- Impulse felt by ring finger – femoral hernia

Deep Inguinal Ring Occlusion Test (Fig. 9.48)

Aim

It is done to differentiate indirect inguinal hernia from direct inguinal hernia. Deep inguinal ring occlusion test is the only confirmatory test.

Method

Before starting the test, surface marking is required, mark the following landmarks:

- ASIS – It is the first bony prominence felt while tracing inguinal ligament from medial to lateral side.
- Deep inguinal ring, half inch above mid inguinal point.
- Pubic symphysis.
- Mid inguinal point – It is the middle point between ASIS and pubic symphysis.
  - Ask the patient to lie in supine position.
  - Reduce the hernia.
  - Occlude the deep inguinal ring by thumb just above mid-inguinal point.
  - Ask the patient to cough.

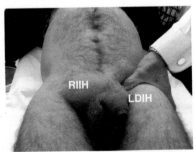

Fig. 9.48. Deep inguinal ring occlusion test.

Interpretation

- Deep inguinal ring blocked and swelling appeared – Direct inguinal hernia.
- Deep inguinal ring blocked and swelling did not appear – Indirect inguinal hernia.

Fallacies of occlusion test

- In pantaloon hernia, indirect hernia component will be occluded but direct hernia will pop out.
- If this test is not done properly, then it will cause confusion.

Finger Invagination Test (Fig. 9.49)

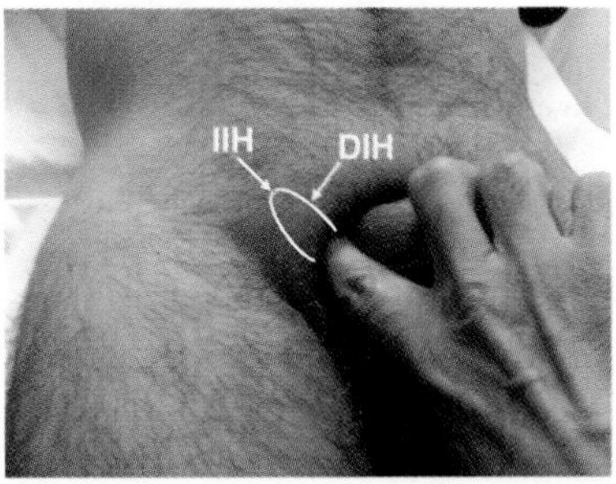

Aim

This test is used to differentiate indirect inguinal hernia from direct inguinal hernia.

Fig. 9.49. Finger invagination test.

Method

- Ask the patient to lie in supine position.
- Reduce the hernia.
- Invaginate skin of scrotum with little finger from bottom of scrotum and push upto pubic tubercle. Rotate the finger and pulp of finger faces towards abdomen of the patient and now feel the superficial inguinal ring by pushing the pulp of your finger in inguinal canal. Now ask the patient to cough and feel the impulse on finger.

Interpretation

- If the impulse is felt at tip of the finger, it is indirect inguinal hernia.
- If the impulse is felt at pulp of the finger, it is direct inguinal hernia.

Inguinal hernia in females

- Labium majus is found thickened on palpation in inguinal hernia.

Fallacy

It cannot be done properly in females as skin of labia is thick and not lax.

KEY POINT

"Getting above the swelling" is a sign which differentiates scrotal swelling from inguinoscrotal swelling or a hydrocele from inguinoscrotal hernia.

Ladd method in children

"When spermatic cord is rolled transversely beneath the gentle pressure of index finger thickening of the cord denotes presence of a hernia." **- Ladd W.E.**

It is named after William Edwards Ladd, American physician (1880-1967). Roll the spermatic cord forth and back transversely between thumb and index finger. Thickening of spermatic cord is demonstrated in this way. It is done in infants and children to diagnose inguinal hernia.

COMPLETE CLINICAL DIAGNOSIS

The complete clinical diagnosis of hernias as follows:
- Whether the lump is hernia or not.
- Right-sided or left-sided.
- Inguinal or femoral.
- Indirect inguinal or direct inguinal.
- Incomplete or complete.
- Enterocele or omentocele.
- Complicated or uncomplicated.

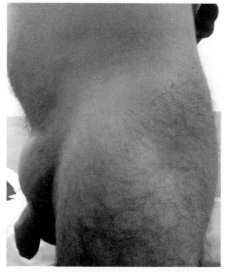

Fig. 9.50. Left inguinal, indirect, incomplete, uncomplicated, enterocele.

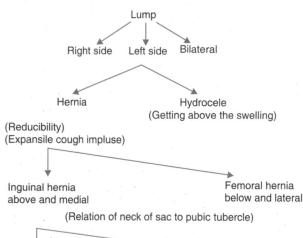

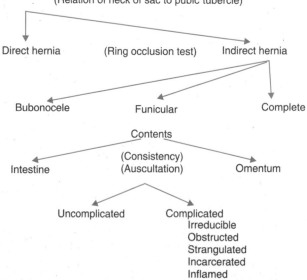

Left inguinal, indirect, incomplete, uncomplicated, enterocele

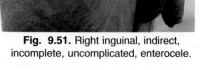

Fig. 9.51. Right inguinal, indirect, incomplete, uncomplicated, enterocele.

GENERAL EXAMINATION

- Examine the other side
- Examine the abdominal wall muscle tone and any previous operation scar
- Examine the chest for infection and abdomen for mass
- Do DRE for prostate
- Examine – for the stricture of urethra

Differences Between Enterocele and Omentocele

Enterocele	*Omentocele*
1. Peristalsis may be seen	1. Peristalsis is never seen
2. Consistency is elastic	2. Consistency is doughy and granular
3. Reduces easily	3. Reduces with difficulty
First part is difficult to reduce than last part	First part is easy than last part
4. Gurgling sound while reducing	4. No gurgling sound while reducing
5 Produces a resonant note on percussion	5. Produces a dull note on percussion
6. Peristalsis may be heard with stethescope	6. Peristalsis cannot be heard

Differences Between Indirect and Direct Inguinal Hernia

	Difference	Indirect inguinal hernia	Direct inguinal hernia
1	**Age**	Common in young people and children	Common in elderly people
2	**Side**	Usually unilateral	Usually unilateral
		1/3rd cases bilateral	50% cases are bilateral
		Common on right side especially in children due to later descent of testis of right side.	
3	**Site of defect**	Deep inguinal ring	Hesselbach's triangle
		Lateral to inferior epigastric artery	Medial to inferior epigastric artery
4	**Relation to spermatic cord**	Lies within covering of or anterior to spermatic cord	Lies outside covering of or posterior to spermatic cord
5	**Shape**	Pear-shaped or pyriform when complete and oval-shaped when incomplete	Globular or spherical in shape. Always incomplete
6	**Relation to pubic tubercle**	Above and medial to pubic tubercle	Below and lateral to pubic tubercle
7	**Reducibility**	Requires manipulation	Spontaneous
8	**Direction of bulge on coughing**	Forward	Forward
		Downward	Downward
		Medially	
9	**Sex**	Males are affected 20 times more	Females are not affected usually
10	**Zieman's technique**	Impulse is felt at the index finger	Impulse is felt at middle finger
11	**Invagination test**	Impulse is felt on the tip of the finger	Impulse is felt on the pulp of finger
12.	**Ring occlusion test**	Hernia will not show a bulge	Hernia will show a bulge
13	**Cause**	Preformed sac	Weakness of posterior wall of inguinal canal
14	**Malgaigne's Bulging**	Absent	May be present
15	**Complications**	Common due to narrow neck	Uncommon due to wide neck

INVESTIGATIONS IN INGUINAL HERNIA

"We all have to confess though with a sigh, on complicated tests we much rely and use too little hand and ear and eye."

— **Zachary Cope (1881-1974)**

Numerous authors have shown that the accuracy with which direct and indirect inguinal hernia can be distinguished clinically before surgery is low.[25]

Plain X-Ray of Abdomen (Figs. 9.52 A & B)

It is useful in obstructed inguinal hernia. The hernia on X-ray may have the following features:
- Shadow of loop of bowel continues up to pelvis.
- Loop of bowel filled with gas seen below inguinal ligament.
- Cut-off segment of loop of bowel is seen in obstructed and strangulated hernias.

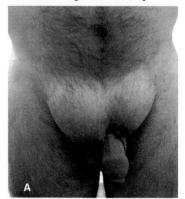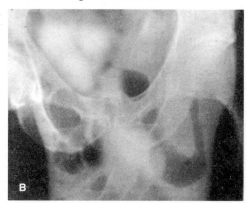

Fig. 9.52A. Bilateral inguinal hernia, **B.** Plain X-ray of abdomen in bilateral inguinal hernia.

Ultrasonography

Ultrasound is the most appropriate investigation with a high degree of sensitivity and specificity in experienced hands.[10]

It is helpful for diagnosing contralateral occult hernia.

CT Scan

It may be useful in diagnosing occult hernia in obese patients especially by contrast enhanced scan.

CT scan of abdomen and pelvis may be useful for the diagnosis of obscure and unusual hernias as well as atypical groin masses.[11]

Colour Doppler Study

It is helpful in obese patients and patients with chronic groin pain.

Herniography

It is a procedure of taking X-rays in supine position after injecting contrast media in peritoneal cavity.

- It shows even small peritoneal protrusion.
- It is not a routinely performed investigation due to its invasive nature.
- It is used in the following selected cases:
  - Undescended testis.
  - Occult inguinal hernia.
  - Unexplained chronic groin pain (inguinodynia) in young men.
  - Recurrent hernia not demonstrated on clinical examination.

MRI

It is helpful in obscure cases when other investigations may not diagnose a hernia.

Diagnostic Laparoscopy

It is required to diagnose a doubtful hernia or hernia in early stage and especially a contralateral hernia.

DIFFERENTIAL DIAGNOSIS OF INGUINOSCROTAL SWELLING (Fig. 9.53)

- Infantile hydrocele
- Varicocele
- Funiculitis
- Torsion of testis
- Tubercular lymphadenitis
- Encysted hydrocele of cord
- Lymph varix or lympangiectasis
- Diffuse lipoma of cord
- Retractile testis
- Malignant extension to cord from tumour of testis

> **NOTE**
>
> *Edward Gibbon (1737-1794), English historian, who is best known for his, "History of Decline and Fall of Roman Empire" was greatly embarrassed by a large hydrocele. The second time this was tapped the hydrocele became infected, and Gibbon died a few days after the operation. The hydrocele was associated with a large scrotal hernia which probably was punctured.*[30]

Infantile Hydrocele

Tunica vaginalis and processus vaginalis are distended upto deep inguinal ring.
- It does not necessarily appear in infants.
- It is not reducible.
- There is no expansile impulse on coughing.

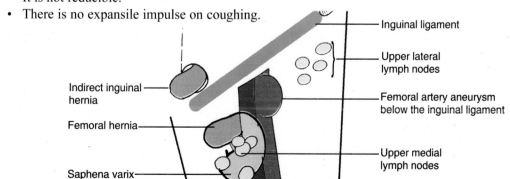

Fig. 9.53. Differential diagnosis of inguinal hernia.

Encysted Hydrocele of Cord

A portion of funicular processus vaginalis remains patent but closes from tunica vaginalis below and peritoneal cavity above.
- It is a cystic swelling which is fluctuant and translucent.
- One can get above the swelling.
- Traction test is positive i.e. if testis is pulled down then swelling comes down.
- Testis can be felt separately.

Varicocele (Fig. 9.54)

It is due to dilated and tortuous veins of pampiniform plexus.

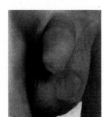

Fig. 9.54. Left varicocele.

> *It usually affects left side because:*
>
> – Left spermatic vein is larger than right spermatic vein.
> – Left spermatic vein enters left renal vein at right angle.
> – Left testicular artery arches over left renal vein at a right angle causing pressure on it.
> – Loaded left colon presses left testicular vein.

- Patient feels an ache or dragging pain on long standing.
- Swelling becomes prominent on standing and disappears on lying down and on elevation of scrotum.
- A thrill or impulse on coughing is felt.
- Swelling feels like a "bag of worms".
- If varicocele is emptied on lying then superficial inguinal ring is occluded. When the patient is asked to stand, the varicocele fills slowly from below.
- In all cases of left-sided varicocele, a carcinoma kidney should always be excluded. In carcinoma of kidney, malignant cells enter renal vein by permeation and block the opening of left spermatic vein. On right side, the spermatic vein enters inferior vena cava which is affected very late.

Lymph Varix

Lymphatic vessels become dilated and tortuous due to obstruction, commonly by filariasis.
- Past history of attacks of fever, pain and swelling in inguinoscrotal area.
- Swelling increases on standing and disappears on lying.
- Thrill-like impulse on coughing is felt.
- Soft, cystic and doughy swelling.
- Eosinophilia is present.
- Microfilariae are seen in blood smear at night.

Funiculitis

- Inguinoscrotal region becomes inflamed.
- Sometimes it is difficult to differentiate from strangulated indirect inguinal hernia. In strangulated hernia, swelling is felt at deep inguinal ring also.
  In India, funiculitis is usually caused by:

- Gonococcal infection
- Filariasis

Diffuse Lipoma of Spermatic Cord (Figs. 9.55 A-C)

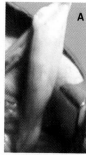

Fig. 9.55A. Lipoma of spermatic cord.

- Spermatic cord is felt soft and lobulated.
- Not reducible.
- No expansile impulse on coughing.
- It can cause symptoms of hernia.
- Sometimes it is difficult to distinguish it from indirect inguinal hernia.

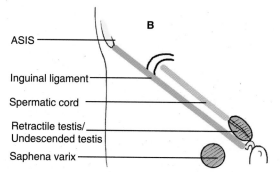
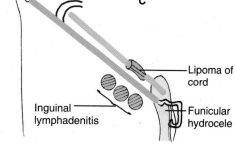

Fig. 9.55 B & C. Differential diagnosis of inguinal hernia.

Torsion of Testis (Fig. 9.56)

- Undescended testis is commonly affected by torsion.
- Tense and tender swelling is present without an impulse on coughing.
- Simulates of strangulated hernia.
- Pain in torsion of testis starts in the groin and not in the testis.

> **NOTE**
>
> *Brown's law (Francis Robert Brown), 1889-1967, Surgeon Royal Infirmary, Dundee, Scotland. "Pain produced in an organ" which has migrated from its primary position, and which has not acquired an additional nerve supply in its secondary or permanent position, is invariably located in the primary position of that organ.*[31]

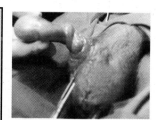

Fig. 9.56. Torsion of testis.

Retractile Testis

- Most commonly lies in superficial inguinal pouch.
- Common in children.
- Testis and scrotum are normally developed.
- Testis can be brought down to the scrotum.

Tuberculosis of Epididymis and Spermatic Cord

- Cord is tender, indurated and nodular.

- Indurated seminal vesicles on DRE.
- Cold abscess and sinuses may develop at the backside of scrotum.
- Symptoms of tuberculosis may be present.

Malignant Extension to Cord from Tumour of Testis

- Cord is hard and nodular.
- Testis shows a tumour.
- Left supraclavicular lymph nodes and para-aortic lymph nodes may be enlarged.

Differential diagnosis of inguinal hernia or groin swelling

In males
- Femoral hernia
- Saphena varix
- Enlarged lymph nodes or inguinal lymphadenitis
- Psoas abscess
- Enlarged psoas bursa
- Undescended or ectopic testis or retractile testis
- Lipoma of spermatic cord
- Hydrocele of femoral hernia sac
- Femoral aneurysm
- **Adenolymphocele** or **'hanging scrotum'** due to Onchocerceases can be confused with giant groin hernia in African patients[35].

In females
- Femoral hernia
- Hydrocele 'of canal of Nuck' (Figs. 9.57A & B). Hydrocele of canal of Nuck is the most common differential diagnosis of inguinal hernia in a female.

In males

Femoral hernia

- Zieman's technique – Impulse is felt on ring finger.
- Finger invagination test – Inguinal canal is empty.
- Position of neck of sac – Neck of hernia sac lies below the inguinal ligament and lateral to pubic tubercle.
- Ring occlusion test – Pressure on femoral canal, hernia does not come out.

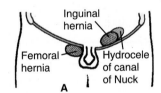

Fig. 9.57A. Differential diagnosis of inguinal hernia in females.

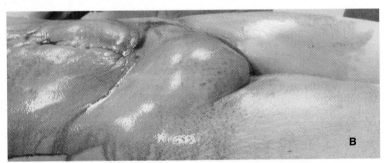

Fig. 9.57B. Large hydrocele of canal of Nuck, right side.

Saphena varix

- Saccular enlargement of the termination of long saphenous vein.
- Swelling disappears when the patient lies down.
- Impulse on coughing present, it is a fluid thrill.
- Schwartz's test is positive.
- Venous hum is sometimes heard.

Enlarged lymph nodes or inguinal lymphadenitis

- Primary site of infection should be searched from umbilicus to toes.

Psoas abscess (Fig. 9.58)

- It is a reducible painless swelling which gives impulse on coughing.
- Swelling is lateral to femoral artery.
- Iliac part of the abscess if present shows cross fluctuations across inguinal ligament.

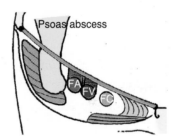

Fig. 9.58. Psoas abscess.

Enlarged psoas bursa

- It lies in front of hip joint and under psoas major muscle.
- Osteoarthritis of hip joint is present.
- Swelling diminishes when the hip is flexed.

Undescended or ectopic testis or retractile testis

- Scrotum of the same side is empty.
- Swelling in inguinal canal or around.
- Testicular sensations are present on handling the lump.

Lipoma of spermatic cord

- Edge of the lump slips under finger.

Hydrocele of femoral hernia sac

- Extremely rare condition, neck gets blocked with omentum or adhesions.
- Fluctuations present

Femoral aneurysm

- Expansile pulsation is diagnostic.

In Females

Femoral hernia

It looks like inguinal hernia if having expansile impulse on coughing.

Hydrocele of canal of Nuck (Figs. 9.57 A & B)

- It is named after Anton Nuck, 1650-1692, Professor of Anatomy and Medicine, Leiden, the Netherlands.
- The processus vaginalis that persists after birth is called "Canal of Nuck".
- Canal of Nuck extends upto labia majora from inguinal canal.
- Canal of Nuck may not disappear but gets blocked and produces a cyst called "Hydrocele of canal of Nuck".

Complications of a hernia

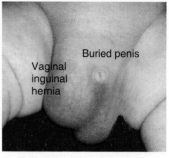

Fig. 9.59. Congenital, vaginal inguinal hernia, right side.

- Irreducibility
- Strangulation
- Inflammation
- Hydrocele of sac
- Obstruction
- Incarceration
- Torsion of sac

Negatives in direct inguinal hernia:

- Never congenital.
- Never in females.
- Does not descend into scrotum.
- Does not strangulate except Ogilvie hernia.

INGUINAL HERNIA IN INFANTS AND CHILDREN

- Congenital inguinal hernias in infants are 99% indirect, 0.5 to 1% are direct and less than 0.5% are femoral hernias. 50% of these hernias are present in first year of life, more common in first 6 months.
- Indirect inguinal hernia is less common in girls than boys (1 : 9).
- Repair of the congenital inguinal hernia is the most common operation in children.
- 3-5% infants are born with inguinal hernia.
- 80-90% inguinal hernias occur in boys.
- Inguinal hernias are found on the right side in 60% cases and on the left side in 30% and bilaterally in 10% cases (Fig. 9.59). The incidence of bilateral hernias is more in females (20-40%).
- Undescended testes or ectopic testes are associated with inguinal hernia in 90% cases.
- Incidence of incarceration is 12%, mostly occur within first 6 months of life, incidence increases in premature infants upto 30-40%.
- Any irreducible hernia needs urgent operation.
- 60% have patent processus vaginalis on other side of body also. 20% will develop indirect inguinal hernia. Laparoscopy avoids unnecessary groin exploration on the other side.
- The presence of a patent processus vaginalis is a necessary but not sufficient variable in developing a congenital indirect inguinal hernia. In other words, all congenital indirect inguinal hernias preceded by a patent processus vaginalis, but not all patent processus vaginalis go on to become inguinal hernias.[36]
- Incarceration occurs in 10% of inguinal hernias in childhood. In 45% girls with incarcerated inguinal hernias the contents of the sac consist of various combinations of adnexal structures.

These structures are usually a sliding component of sac.

- Hernia in children is often observed when child strains or cries. History alone may be sufficient as bulge cannot be elicited at will.
- Congenital indirect inguinal hernia is most common during first year of life, but it may not appear till middle or old age. The increased intra-abdominal pressure opens deep inguinal ring and allows the contents of abdomen to enter patent processus vaginalis.
- **Silk glove sign:** Coverings of hernia sac are felt as they slide over spermatic cord by rolling it under index finger over pubic tubercle.

Management

- **Time of operation:** Infant must be operated within first year as incidence of incarceration is maximum in this period. Infant of more than one year can have a planned operation and not an urgent operation.
- In a newborn baby, wait for three months, as strangulation is uncommon due to following reasons:
  - Wide neck
  - Almost no inguinal canal as superficial inguinal ring overlaps deep inguinal ring.
- Operate at the age of less than 5 years, do herniotomy only.
- Above 5 years of age:
  - Herniotomy
  - Deep inguinal ring narrowing
- 80% cases of incarcerated hernia in infants and children can be managed conservatively.
- The complications are 20 times greater after emergency repair of incarcerated hernia than after elective procedure.[12]
- Inguinal hernia in infants and children needs surgery due to high risk of incarceration.
- There is no role of laparoscopic hernia repair in infants and young children.[13]
- Irreducible or incarcerated hernia without strangulation should be reduced and operated within 48-72 hours, this avoids post-operative complications.
- Irreducible or incarcerated hernia with strangulation should be operated urgently.
- An infant with a direct inguinal hernia must be investigated for connective tissue disorders such as Ehler-Danlos syndrome.
- More than 50% patients of testicular feminising syndrome have an inguinal hernia. A female infant with bilateral inguinal hernia should be suspected for feminising syndrome.

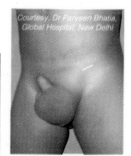

"Historically it was recommended that all boys under 2 years of age and all girls under 5 years of age undergo operative exploration of the contralateral inguinal canal in search of a clinically silent patent processus vaginalis. This approach has been replaced in large part by laparoscopic exploration. If a patent processus vaginalis is demonstrated, a second inguinal incision is made."[14]

Fig. 9.60. Incision in infants in congenital hernia.

Operation

Incision (Fig. 9.60)

3 cm long transverse incision, in inguinal skin crease.

Steps

- Scarpa's fascia is incised.
- Operation is further done by either of two methods:
  - Through the external inguinal ring (Mitchell Bank's technique)
  - Through incising external oblique facia / aponeurosis

  No added benefit is gained by opening the inguinal canal or dividing the external inguinal ring.
- Sac is found as a glistening structure.
- Sac is separated from vas deferens and cord structures by injecting 1-2 ml normal saline.
- Base of the sac is ligated with 3-0 polyglactin and the sac is excised 1/2 to 1 cm distal to the ligature.
- Wound is closed.

Mitchell Bank's operation consists of:

- High ligation of sac
- Removal of indirect sac

Laproscopic inguinal hernia repair

Classic open inguinal hernia repair is the gold standard repair but laparoscopic inguinal hernia repair is performed in many centers. There are two ways:

- **Intracorporeal legation**. Primary repair is done lateral to spermatic cord with interrupted sutures or 'Z' plasty or "flip-flop hernioplasty",[37] in which two folds of peritoneum are used to cover internal inguinal ring.
- **Laproscopic assisted extracorporeal closer**: A small stab wound is made over internal inguinal ring and a suture is passed through the abdominal wall behind the peritoneum. It is then directed around the internal inguinal ring and passed out the same stab wound and tied extracorporally under laparoscopic visualization.

Post-operative Complications in Infants and Children

Intraoperative complications

- Division of ilioinguinal nerve
- Division of vas deferens
- Haemorrhage

Post-operative complications

- Wound infection occurs in 1-2% case.
- Scrotal haematoma.
- 80% recurrence occurs in first year post-operative.
- Following are the common causes of recurrence:
  - Missed hernia sac.
  - Broken sutures and ligature at the neck of sac.
  - Failure to repair a large deep inguinal ring.
  - Injury to floor of inguinal canal so a direct inguinal hernia develops.
  - Severe infection to inguinal canal.
  - Hereditary connective tissue disorder.

MANAGEMENT OF INGUINAL HERNIA

"It will appear excess of daring to write at the present day of the radical treatment of hernias"
                                                                              — **Edoardo Bassini, 1890**

Before deciding to operate a case of inguinal hernia curable aggravating factors are treated i.e. chronic cough, prostatic enlargement, colonic tumour and ascites.

> Inguinal hernia patient should be operated to remove swelling and pain and to avoid strangulation (4-6% lifetime risk of strangulation). Most surgeons feel that herniorrhaphy becomes more difficult, longer the repair is delayed. At present, conventional wisdom is that all inguinal hernias should be repaired, however based on clinical judgement, one may elect not to advise repair in an elderly patient with asymptomatic, broad based direct hernia.[15]

Inguinal hernia is treated by operation.
The treatment of inguinal hernia can be divided into two categories:
* Conservative treatment
* Operative treatment

Conservative Treatment

No treatment

Following patients are not given any treatment:
* Short life expectancy due to malignancy or other life threatening sickness.
* Severe and debilitating general illness due to systemic disease.
* Those who refuse to surgical as well as non-surgical treatments.
* **"Watchful waiting"** is advised to elderly patients who have small uncomplicated asymptomatic hernia.

Truss (Figs. 9.61 & 9.62)

Truss may cure a hernia in a newborn baby. Except in a newborn, it does not cure a hernia. The truss is used to avoid protrusion of hernia from deep inguinal ring to inguinal canal and out of superficial inguinal ring.

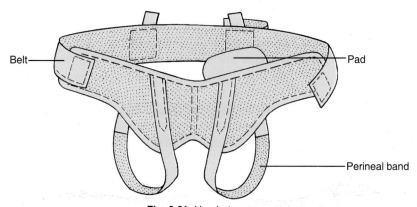

Belt

Pad

Perineal band

Fig. 9.61. Hernia truss.

Indications of truss

Use of truss should not be encouraged. It should be condemned for:
- Those who refuse for surgery. They must be explained that surgery is the best form of treatment as truss is not curative and is also associated with complications.
- Elderly patients who have risk of recurrence due to chronic bronchitis, BPH and chronic constipation.
- Patients with short life expectancy like:
  - Patients with cardiorespiratory disorders who have high risk of complications due to anaesthesia.
  - In infants and children, continuous use of truss for a period of two years may cure hernia.

Trusses can provide symptomatic relief of hernias and are used more commonly in Europe.[16] Sir Winston Churchill used truss for years. Correct measurement and fittings are required for the use of truss.

Conditions required for truss

- Patient must be intelligent
- Hernia should be reducible

Contraindications for use of truss

- Irreducible hernia
- Strenuous job
- Chronic bronchitis
- Hernia associated with huge hydrocele
- Hernia associated with undescended testis
- Patient with poor intelligence or moron

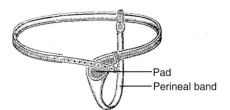

Fig. 9.62. Rat tail truss.

Complications and dangers of truss

Use of truss is not to be encouraged, it should be condemned due to its complications and adverse effects. A few complications and dangers of truss are mentioned below:
- It causes atrophy of muscles of inguinal area, which increases the chances of recurrence after surgery.
- It can cause strangulation or obstruction of hernia if not properly applied. Pad slips to the side of the hernia lump and presses it which may lead to strangulation.
- It can damage the contents of hernia sac if hernia is not properly reduced before a truss is applied.
- If the local area is not kept clean and dry, it will cause dermatitis and other skin problems leading to difficulty in healing after operation or even contraindication to operation and use of truss.
- Hernia sac may develop adhesions with inguinal canal which may cause problems during the operation.
- Atrophy of spermatic cord develops.
- Hernia repair becomes difficult as dissection is difficult due to atrophy and fibrosis.

What is the name of the commonly used truss?

- "Rat tail spring truss" (Fig. 9.61) with a perineal band.
- The perineal band prevents the slipping of truss.
- For very large hernias which cannot be reduced a "Bag truss" is used to support the hernia.

How measurements are taken for truss?

Measurements are taken from tip of greater trochanter to third piece of sacrum and to greater trochanter of the other side.

How to use truss?

- Lie down comfortably.
- Reduce the hernia.
- Put truss pad on hernia site and fix the belt.
- Use the truss throughout the day and remove it only when going to bed and put on truss again before getting out of bed.

Disadvantage of truss

It causes atrophy of inguinal muscles, so the truss is not advised for the young patients as it may cause recurrence if hernia repair is done.

Mechanism of action of truss

- The anterior wall of inguinal canal is pressed against the posterior wall of inguinal canal so the inguinal canal is blocked.
- It also closes the weak area of Hesselbach's triangle in direct inguinal hernia.
- It closes superficial and deep inguinal rings.
- Adhesions gradually develop and block the inguinal canal.

Operative Treatment

It is the treatment of choice.

Goals of hernia surgery:

- To eliminate peritoneal sac of hernia, especially in indirect inguinal hernia.
- To close fascial defect in posterior wall of inguinal canal.
- To avoid recurrence.

KEY POINTS

- *Surgery is the treatment of choice for inguinal hernia.*
- *Surgery can be open or laparoscopic.*

Guidelines for surgery in the groin hernia

• *NICE guidelines advise laparoscopic repair for recurrent and bilateral inguinal hernia and open mesh repair for primary unilateral inguinal hernia. Open mesh repair is the operation of choice for the primary unilateral inguinal hernia.[17,38]*
• *Most surgeons feel that all cases of inguinal hernia should be operated for the following reasons:*
  – *To prevent complication e.g. strangulation (4-6% lifetime risk of strangulation).*
  – *Because herniorrhaphy becomes more difficult.*
• *Asymptomatic small and easily reducible direct inguinal hernia should be left alone as there is almost no risk of strangulation.*
• *Symptomatic direct inguinal hernia and indirect inguinal hernia require repair as there is small risk of strangulation.*
• *Irreducible inguinal hernia should be operated urgently to avoid strangulation.*
• *All femoral hernias should be operated urgently.*

Operations for inguinal hernia

• Herniotomy – Excision of hernia sac.
• Herniorrhaphy – Repair of posterior wall of inguinal canal and repair of internal inguinal ring.
• Hernioplasty – Reinforcement of posterior wall of inguinal canal with implants or fascial flaps.

Comparison of open and laparoscopic inguinal hernia repairs

Open Inguinal Hernia Repair	Laparoscopic Inguinal Hernia Repair
1. Cost effective*	Costlier
2. Short learning curve	Long learning curve
3. Can be done under local anaesthesia	Can be done under general anaesthesia
4. No major complications	Serious, visceral and vascular injuries can be caused
5. Does not require a high level expert	Requires a high level expert
6. Procedure of choice for primary unilateral inguinal hernia	Good for recurrent and bilateral inguinal hernia
7. Much of post-operative discomfort and pain	Not much post-operative discomfort and pain
8. Return to work takes longer	Return to work takes shorter

* Laparoscopic hernia repair in UK has an additional NHS cost of £300 over open repair, similar figures are from other countries.[18]

Treatment strategy of recurrent inguinal hernia

Usually the laparoscopic hernia repair is advised for recurrent inguinal hernia, but if the previous surgery was a laparoscopic repair then open mesh repair is advised. If recurrence occurs after open repair then laparoscopic repair is selected. If it is a re-recurrence after laparoscopy and open mesh repair then patient should be referred to a highly specialised hernia centre. Recurrences are best managed by placing a second prosthesis through a different approach.[19]

Special Features of Direct Inguinal Hernia in Relation to Surgery

- Hernia sac may have no neck, so cannot be excised but only pushed in and some interrupted sutures are applied.
- Whole of posterior wall of inguinal canal may become weak.
- Direct hernia patient usually an elder individual with poor tissue repair, BPH and constipation, so stress on hernia repair may lead to recurrence.
- Recurrence in direct inguinal hernia is twice as common as in indirect inguinal hernia.

NOTE

Operations for recurrent inguinal hernia are often more difficult and have a higher potential for complications than a primary repair. A laparoscopic approach has the advantage that it allows the repair to be done through virgin territory[20] in a case of recurrence after open repair.

Inguinal Hernia Operation in Females (Fig. 9.63)

The round ligament of uterus replaces the spermatic cord in female. It is ligated and excised at deep inguinal ring and the deep inguinal ring and inguinal canal are closed.

- **Closure of inguinal canal:** Inguinal canal is closed after excision of round ligament of uterus.
  - Inguinal canal is closed by a few interrupted sutures. The suture takes bite of conjoint tendon then of fascia transversalis from posterior wall of inguinal canal and then of inguinal ligament.

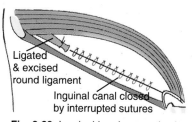

Fig. 9.63. Inguinal hernia operation in females.

- Following points are to be noted in females:
  - Round ligament is thinner than spermatic cord.
  - Round ligament is less vascular than spermatic cord.
  - Inguinal canal in females is smaller than males.
  - There is almost no cremaster muscle.
- A landmark study by Koch et al. based on Swedish Hernia Register (1992-2003) showed[39]
  - Their is higher proportion of emergency hernia repair in women than men
  - Women had higher risk of reoperation for recurrence than men.
  - Women who are originally diagnosed with an indirect or direct hernia at primary repair are likely to have a femoral hernia found at reoperation for a recurrence (41.6% versus a corresponding 4.6% of men).

STRANGULATED INGUINAL HERNIA (Fig. 9.64)

"Always explore in cases of persistent vomiting if a lump, however small, is found occupying one of the abdominal rings and its nature is uncertain."

— **Augustus Charles Bernays (1854-1907)**

"The danger is in delay, not in the operation."

— **Sir Astley Cooper**
Anatomist and Surgeon.
Guy's Hospital, London, England

Causes of Strangulation

• Narrow neck
• Rigid rim of neck

Strangulation is common in the following hernias:

• Femoral hernia
• Obturator hernia
• Indirect inguinal hernia

Constriction factors in strangulated inguinal hernia

• Neck of sac
• External inguinal ring in children
• Adhesions between contents and sac wall

Contents of sac in strangulated inguinal hernia (Figs. 9.65 A & B)

• Small intestine – Most common
• Omentum – Common
• Large intestine – Less common
• Ovary and fallopian tube in females – Occasionally

Incidence

• Strangulated inguinal hernia in infants occur more commonly in females, the incidence is 5 : 1 in female and male.
• In female infants, ovary or fallopian tube or both are commonly found in sac.
• Incidence of strangulation is 4% in inguinal hernia. It is 2.8% after 3 months of age and 4.8 % after 2 years of age.
• Treatment of choice of strangulated inguinal hernia is surgery but the patient has to be resuscitated first.

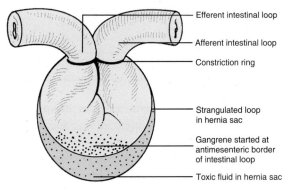

Efferent intestinal loop

Afferent intestinal loop

Constriction ring

Strangulated loop in hernia sac

Gangrene started at antimesenteric border of intestinal loop

Toxic fluid in hernia sac

Fig. 9.64. Strangulated hernia, diagrammatic representation.

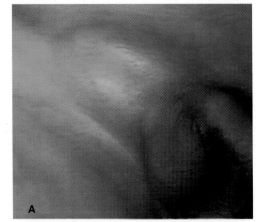

A

Fig. 9.65A. Strangulated right indirect inguinal hernia.

- In females, the commonest content in sac is ovary.
- The mortality in strangulated hernia increases with age: at 60 years it is 3%, at 70 years it is 6% and at 80 years it is 12%.

- *Muhammad Ali (Cassius Clay), the famous world boxing champion, used to say "I am the greatest" and "I float like a butterfly and sting like a bee".*
  He could not fight the famous "The second fight" with Sonny Liston on 16th November 1964 as he developed strangulated inguinal hernia three days before the fight and had to undergo an emergency operation. The fight was postponed for six months.

Pathology of strangulated hernia (Fig. 9.66)

Reducible hernia becomes irreducible, then obstructed and ultimately strangulated. Though all hernias do not strangulate. Narrow-neck hernia should be operated at early stage due to the danger of strangulation.

Reducible hernia
↓
Irreducible hernia
↓
Obstructed hernia
↓
Strangulated hernia

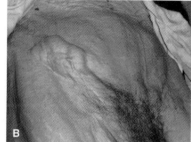

Fig. 9.65B. Strangulated recurrent right inguinal hernia (Holthouse's hernia).

First, acute intestinal obstruction develops. The intestine within the hernia sac starts dilating. Venous return is affected by occlusion of veins due to constriction and congestion. Ulcerations in mucosa and haemorrhage in the wall of intestine inside the hernia sac occur and intestine becomes congested and bright red. Serous fluid oozes in the sac. Venous stasis increases and arterial supply is impaired, if occlusion is not relieved. Ecchymoses appear in serosa of intestine. Blood oozes in the lumen of intestine and in sac. Intestine loses the shine and becomes flabby. Bacteria migrate from lumen of intestine to the sac. Mesentery in the sac becomes congested, haemorrhagic with thrombosed

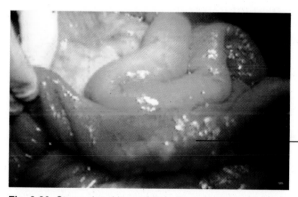

—Strangulated loop of ilium changing color with hotpacks to viability, resection was avoided

Fig. 9.66. Strangulated loop of ilium from strangulated hernia.

vessels. Gangrene changes the colour of intestine from purple to black to green due to decomposition of blood. If gangrene extends to intra-abdominal bowel then peritonitis develops.

Gangrene first appears at the following sites in intestine:
- Place of constriction.
- Antimesenetric border of intestine as it is farthest from blood vessels.

Distension of loop of intestine increases
↓
It causes venous obstruction and venous pressure increases
↓
Venous return further decreases
↓
Intestine becomes oedematous and purple coloured
↓
Arteries also pressurised and compromised
↓
Sac fluid becomes blood-stained and infected
↓
Intestine becomes grey, atonic, listless and friable
↓
Exudation occurs into the sac
↓
Bacterial transudation occurs
↓
Gangrene starts and intestine becomes greenish to black
↓
Perforation
↓
Peritonitis

Bacteria Present in Strangulated Hernia Sac

Common bacteria present in the fluid collected in the sac of strangulated hernia are:
- *E. coli*
- Anaerobic streptococci
- Anaerobes
- Klebsiella

Clinical Features of Strangulated Hernia

- Pain
- Nausea
- Vomiting
- Tense, tender, irreducible hernia

- The patient develops sudden pain.
- Pain continues till the patient is operated and perforation or paralytic ileus develops.

> **NOTE**
>
> - *Sudden disappearance of pain may be a bad sign due to perforation.*
> - *Sudden cessation of pain is due to:*
>   - *Perforation of intestine (Fig. 9.67)*
>   - *Paralytic ileus*
>   - *Spontaneous reduction of strangulation. It happens especially after injection of analgesics and muscle relaxants.*

- Sudden severe pain develops over a hernia which becomes generalised abdominal pain.
- Pain is of colicky nature.
- Sometimes the content is small bowel then pain may be only at umbilicus.
- Nausea and vomiting follow pain.
- Following features of obstruction develop:
  - Pain in abdomen
  - Vomiting
  - Distension of abdomen
  - Absolute constipation
- Hernia becomes
  - Tense
  - Tender
  - Irreducible
  - Absence of impulse on coughing
  - Increase in size of swelling occurs

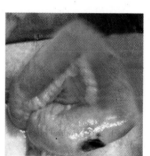

Fig. 9.67. Perforation of intestine, in a hernia sac.

- General condition of patient deteriorates. Features of septic shock develop.
  - Pulse, feeble and fast
  - Hypotension
  - Toxic look
  - Bowel sounds are absent
  - Cold and clammy skin with perspiration
- Highest incidence of strangulation occurs in first few months of life and young patient.
- Hernia can strangulate at any time.
- Development of irreducibility of a reducible hernia is a sign of impending strangulation and urgent surgery is a must.
- Vomiting becomes forceful and frequent.

> *Contents of hernia that are prone to get strangulated are:*
>
> - Small intestine
> - Omentum
> - Part of circumference of intestine
> - Ovary or fallopian tube in a female child
> - Colon rarely strangulates

Strangulated Richter's hernia (Fig. 9.68)

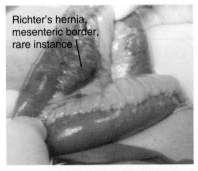

Richter's hernia, mesenteric border, rare instance

- A strangulated Richter's hernia may not be having features of obstruction due to partial blockage of lumen of intestine.
- Pain is a constant feature.
- The patient may be passing normal stool.
- There may not be nausea and vomiting.
- Absolute constipation is not present and instead there may be diarrhoea, clinical features may mimic acute gastroenteritis.
- Absolute constipation develops after which paralytic ileus develops.
- Intestinal obstruction is not present unless half of the circumference of the bowel is involved.

Fig. 9.68. Strangulated Richter's hernia.

Strangulated Richter's hernia occurs in the following hernias:

– Femoral hernia
– Obturator hernia

Strangulated Littre's hernia

Meckel's diverticulum is sometimes found strangulated in the sac of strangulated inguinal hernia. Strangulation of Meckel's diverticulum is not unusual. (Figs. 9.69 A & B).

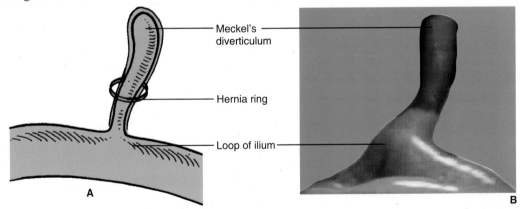

Meckel's diverticulum

Hernia ring

Loop of ilium

A

B

Fig. 9.69A. Littre's hernia, long Meckel's diverticulum.

Fig. 9.69B. Strangulated Littre's hernia, gangrenous Meckel's diverticulum.

Strangulated omentocele (Fig. 9.70)

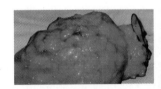

- The omentum can stand the compromise to blood supply for a much longer period than intestine.
- Pain is always present.
- Vomiting and absolute constipation are absent initially.
- Gangrene starts at the centre of entrapped portion of omentum or in most distal part and is usually delayed.

Fig. 9.70. Strangulated omentum.

- Infection in omentum leads to abscess formation.
- There is no feature of acute intestinal obstruction.

NOTE

Strangulated hernia is an extremely dangerous condition, Queen Caroline, wife of King George II of England died of a strangulated umbilical hernia in 1736 at age of 55.

Treatment of strangulated inguinal hernia

- I.V. Fluids
- Nasogastric aspiration
- I.V. antibiotics
- Catheterisation
- Urgent surgery

More patients died of fluid and electrolyte problems than of delaying an operation for a few hours in strangulated hernia. That is why, the first step in the treatment of strangulated hernia is to ressuscitate the patient.

- Admit the patient in hospital.
- Do not elevate the foot end of bed in strangulated hernia for fear of reduction of gangrenous bowel.
- Nasogastric tube suction.
- I.V. Fluids.
- Narcotic injections to reduce pain.
- Patient is prepared for urgent surgery.
  [**Conservative treatment** is indicated only if the patient is an infant. It includes:
  – Analgesia.
  – Gallow's traction (the judgement of Solomon's position).
  – There is no danger of rupture of intestine and reduction of gangrenous intestine.
  – Forcible reduction is discouraged.
- Taxis (forcible reduction) is contraindicated nowadays due to its complications which are:
  – Contusion of intestine.
  – Rupture of sac and reduction of contents intraperitoneally or extraperitoneally.
  – Reduction en masse, strangulated sac is reduced with strangulated bowel still intact (Fig. 9.71 A & B).
  – Reduction into a loculus of sac, sac ruptures at the neck and reduction happens in extraperitoneal space.

Important steps in strangulated hernia surgery

- Adequate incision
- Identify sac
- Aspirate the toxic fluid from the sac before dividing constriction
- Divide constricting ring protecting inferior epigastric vessels

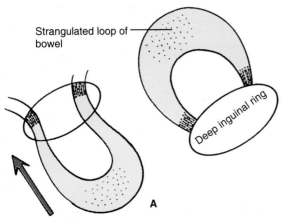
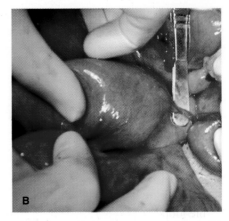

Strangulated loop of bowel

Deep inguinal ring

A

B

Fig. 9.71. Reduction en masse, taxis can reduce the hernia with strangulation intact, **B.** Laparotomy was done in this case to relieve strangulation.

- Check the viability of the contents
- Resection of gangrenous bowel if required
- Repair of hernia
- Broad spectrum antibiotics

Operation for Strangulated Inguinal Hernia

Anesthesia

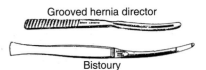

Grooved hernia director

Bistoury

Fig. 9.72. Hernia director and bistoury.

General anesthesia or spinal anesthesia are usually preferred over local anesthesia. Local anesthesia is given to save the life of the patient if his condition does not permit general anesthesia or spinal anesthesia.

General anesthesia is the best anesthesia for strangulated hernia as you may require to perform intestinal resection if gangrene of bowel loop is present.

Steps

- Same steps as in herniotomy operation till the sac is identified.
- **Fundus first method:** Fundus of sac is opened first or aspiration of toxic fluid is done before handling the constriction at the neck due to the following advantages:
  - Contamination of peritoneal cavity by toxic or infected fluid of the sac is avoided.
  - Strangulated loops of bowel will not slip inside peritoneal cavity without proper examination of intestine loop to rule out any gangrene.
- Constriction is divided after examining the contents of sac. The constriction is divided at upper and lateral side with the help of grooved hernia director or bistoury (long and narrow knife with one side sharp and other side blunt) (Fig. 9.72).
- This method of division of constriction ring has the following advantages:
  - Cutting the constriction on medial side may cause injury to inferior epigastric vessels.
  - Grooved hernia director prevents injury to intestinal loop.

Site of constriction ring (Fig. 9.73)

The constriction ring can be situated at any of the following sites:
• Superficial inguinal ring
• Deep inguinal ring
• Midway between superficial and deep inguinal rings
• Anywhere along the sac

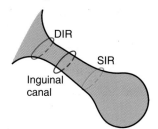

Fig. 9.73. Sites of constriction in strangulated indirect inguinal hernia.

Precautions

• Strangulated loop of intestine should not slip inside the peritoneal cavity.
• If the loop without proper examination by chance slips in the peritoneal cavity then try to take out the loop with Babcock's tissue forceps.
• Strangulation in Maydl's hernia may involve only the loop inside peritoneal cavity and not the loop inside the hernia sac and the gangrene can be missed if whole loop is not taken out and examined.
    Now the decision is made for viability of the strangulated loop.

The signs of non-viability of the bowel loop are:

• The loop of intestine is green and black.
• Bowel loop is flaccid and shineless.
• No peristalsis is seen in the loop of intestine.
• No pulsation is found in arteries of mesentery.

What to do if there is doubt about viability of intestinal loop?

• Wrap the loops of bowel with hot and moist packs.
• Request anaesthetist to give 100% oxygen for at least 10 minutes and then see the loops of bowel for viability.
• Observe the following features:
    – Pink color appears and discoloration disappears.
    – Peristalsis returns.
    – Pulsations in the blood vessels of mesentery appear.

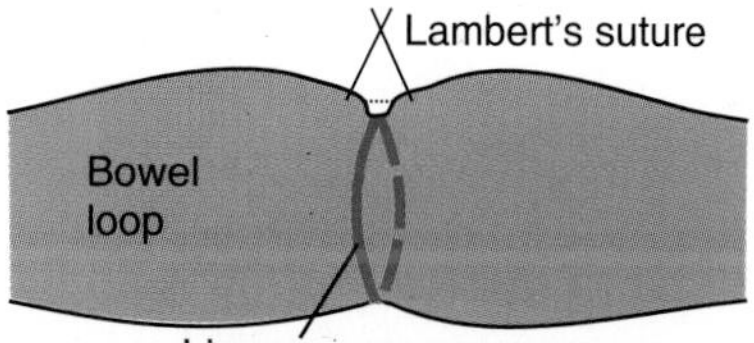

Fig. 9.74. Lambert's suture for linear gangrenous area.

In case the strangulated loop is found viable then

• The bowel loop is returned back to the peritoneal cavity.
• Proceed further for herniotomy and herniorrhaphy.
• Hernioplasty is not advised due to high chance of post-operative wound infection.

In case the strangulated bowel loop is not found normal and

• If a linear area at constriction site in bowel loop is found gangrenous then it can be invaginated with Lambert's sutures (Fig. 9.74).
• If the whole loop of bowel is found gangrenous, and
    – When the general condition of patient is satisfactory then perform resection of the loop of the bowel and perform end-to-end anestomosis.

– When the general condition does not permit as informed by anesthetist then exteriorize the bowel loop. As soon as the general condition of the patient improves resection of the bowel can be performed.
– When non-viable bowel is a large bowel then exteriorization of bowel with Paul-Mikulicz's resection is performed.
– When the omentum is strangulated then transfix it and excise the gangrenous portion.

Mucosa is more vulnerable than the seromuscularis to the effects of ischaemia and if the outer layers survive then mucosa may slough out and leave an annular stricture. It is called "Intestinal stenosis of Garre".[21]

Strangulated Richter's hernia (Figs. 9.75 A & B)

If the gangrene is localised to a small area and not involving the whole circumference then the gangrenous area of the loop of intestine is buried inside the lumen of the bowel and few interrupted sutures are applied.

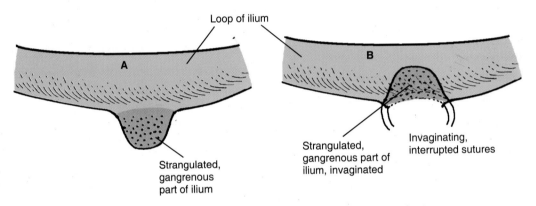

Fig. 9.75A. Strangulated Richter's hernia, **B.** Invaginating interrupted sutures.

NOTE

Mortality from strangulated hernia
Mortality is related to duration of the strangulation and the age of the patient. A longer duration leads to a greater degree of tissue oedema, ischaemia and risk of outright necrosis.[26]

KEY POINT

If on exploration the bowel is found to be pink on release, arterial pulsations in mesentery present and peristalsis is there, then replace the bowel in abdominal cavity. If the bowel is purple, green or dark without pulsations and persistalsis, then resect the bowel.

SLIDING HERNIA (HERNIA-EN-GLISSADE)

"Sliding hernia occurs due to slipping of posterior parietal peritoneum on underlying retroperitoneal structures."

The posterior wall of the sac is formed by not only posterior parietal peritoneum but also by retroperitoneal structures.

On Right Side (Fig. 9.76 A)

* Caecum forms posterior wall of hernia with peritoneum. Appendix may also be there.

On Left Side (Fig. 9.76 B)

* Sigmoid colon and its mesentery form the posterior wall of hernia with peritoneum.
* Urinary bladder can be one of the contents of sliding hernia on both right and left side.
* Left side hernia may also contain small bowel in 1 : 2000 cases.

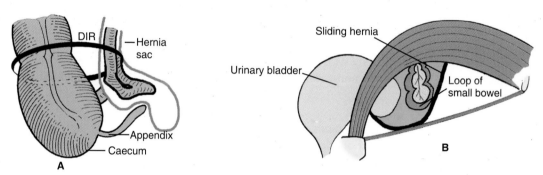

Fig. 9.76A. Sliding hernia, right side, **B.** Sliding hernia, left side.

KEY POINT

If caecum and appendix are the contents of a hernia sac. It cannot be a sliding hernia.

Incidence

* One in 2000 cases is inguinal hernia.
* One in 8000 cases is sac-less sliding hernia.

Aetiology

* It occurs due to slipping of posterior parietal peritoneum over retroperitoneal tissues. It starts as indirect hernia and then becomes sliding hernia.

Causative Factors

* Abnormal attachment of posterior peritoneum to underlying retroperitoneal tissues
* Caecal mesentery
* Congenital abnormality in sigmoid colon attachment

Accessory Factors

The following factors accentuate the conditions favouring development of sliding hernia:
- Obesity
- Lax and flabby abdominal musculature

Complications

- Irreducibility
- Strangulation

Clinical Features

- It is usually big indirect inguinal hernia.
- It occurs usually after 40 years of age and its incidence increases with age.
- It exclusively occurs in males.
- It is more common on left side, 5 out of 6 cases are on left side.
- Bilateral cases are rare.
- There is no specific diagnostic feature of sliding hernia.
- It is suspected in big scrotal hernia.
- If large intestine is present along with small intestine then the large intestine (caecum or sigmoid colon) is usually found to be non-strangulated and the small intestine loops are found to be strangulated.
- It may be sac-less hernia
- It may occur with both direct and indirect hernia.
- It reappears slowly after reduction.
- It is a large global scrotal hernia.
- It does not get reduced totally.
- Its sac is thick.
- It strangulates easily.

Treatment

It is treated by operation.
   The conservative treatment has no role.
- The internal inguinal ring becomes wider due to big hernia.
- The sac of hernia is anterior and medial to the spermatic cord.
- It is better not to open the sac if it is diagnosed preoperatively.
- Do not dissect and try to separate the viscus from posterior wall of the sac.
- Extra big sac can be excised, otherwise reduce the sac totally.
- Close the sac.
- Reduce the hernia.
- Further repair is like any indirect inguinal hernia repair.

La Roque repair

The mesentery of sigmoid colon is reefed up and shortened and the entire sigmoid colon is replaced within the adbominal cavity.[27,28]

> **KEY POINT**
>
> *In sliding inguinal hernia do not try to separate the viscus from posterior wall of the sac.*

BILATERAL INGUINAL HERNIA (FIG. 9.77)

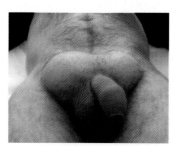

- Bilateral inguinal hernia incidence is 10% in infants and 12% in adults.
- Bilateral inguinal hernia occurs more in female infants than male infants.
- In every case of bilateral inguinal hernia, metabolic collagen defect must be investigated before hernia repair is attempted.
- Laparoscopic method of hernia reapir is preferred in bilateral inguinal hernia than open method as it is economical and less painful.

Fig. 9.77. Bilateral inguinal hernia.

GIANT INGUINAL HERNIA (FIG. 9.78)

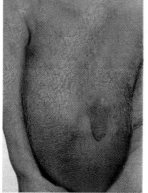

- Giant inguinal hernia is an indirect inguinal hernia reaching upto the middle of the thigh or lower. Giant inguinal hernias are usually of long standing period, may be present for decades. Giant inguinal hernia contains small bowel and omentum. Giant inguinal hernia should not be operated by inexperienced or a learning surgeon.

REFERENCES

Fig. 9.78. Giant inguinal hernia.

1. **Burkitt HG.**, (2001). Essential surgery, 3rd edition, p. 349.
2. **Russell RCG** *et al.*, (2000). Bailey and Love's short practice of surgery, 23rd edition, p. 1146.
3. **Burkitt HG.**, (2001). Essential surgery, 3rd edition, p. 348.
4. **Carey LC.**, (1967). Acute appendicitis occurring in humans : a report of 10 cases, *Surgery*, 61: 236–8.
5. **Rains JH** *et al.*, (1971). Bailey and Love's short practice of surgery, 15th edition, p. 1065.
6. **Russell RCG.** *et al.*, (2000). Bailey and Love's short practice of Surgery, 23rd edition, p. 1149.
7. **Smith GD, Crosby DL, Lewis PA.**, (1996). Inguinal hernia and single strenuous event. *Ann. R. Coll. Surg. Eng.*, 78: 367.
8. **Cameron AE.**, (1994). Accuracy of clinical diagnosis of direct and indirect inguinal hernia. *Br. J. Surg.*, 81: 250.
9. **Kark A, Kurzen M, Waters KJ.**, (1994). Accuracy of clinical diagnosis of direct and indirect inguinal hernia. *Br. J. Surg.*, 81: 1081.
10. **Bradley M, Morgan D, Pentlow B, Roe A.**, (2003). The groin hernia–an ultrasound diagnosis? *Ann. R. Coll. Surg. Engl.*, 85: 178–180.
11. **Della S V, Groebli Y.**, (2000). Diagnosis of non-hernia groin masses. *Ann. Chir.*, 125: 179–183.
12. **Rowe MI, Clatworthy HW Jr.**, (1970). Incarcerated and strangulated hernias and children. *Arch. Surg.*, 101: 136–43.

13. **Bennett DH.**, (2005). Core topics in general and emergency surgery, 3rd edition, p. 57.

14. **Funfer MM** *et al.*, (1996). Laparoscopic exploration of the contralateral groin in children: an improved technique. *J. Laparoscopic surg.*, 1: 51.

15. **Kurzer M & Allen EK.**, (2005). Inguinal hernia repair: an update, Recent advances in surgery 28, Irving Taylor & Colin Johnson, pp. 75–85.

16. **Cheek CM, Williams MH, Farndon JR.**, (1995). Trusses in the management of hernia today. *Br. J. Surg.*, 82: 1611–13.

17. **National Institute for Clinical Excellence.** (2001). Guidance on the use of laparoscopic surgery for inguinal hernia. Technology Appraisal Guidance No. 18. London: NICE.

18. **Wantz GE.**, (1997). Laparoscopic herniorrhaphy, *J. Am. Coll. Surg.*, 184: 521–522.

19. **Townsend CM** *et al.*, (2004). The sabiston textbook of surgery, **2,** 17th edition, p. 1217.

20. **Burkitt HG.**, (2001). Essential surgery, 3rd edition, p. 353.

21. **Kirk RM.**, (2000). General surgical operations, 4th edition, p. 131.

22. **Gilbert AI.**, (2007). Generation of the plug and patch repair: Its development and lesson from history, Mastery of surgery, 5th edition, Lippincott Williams & Wilkins, pp. 1942.

23. **Kang SK, Burnett CA, Freund E,** *et al.*, (1999). Hernia: is it a work-related condition? *Am. J. Ind. Med.* 36: 638.

24. **Javid PJ, Brooks DC.**, (2007). Maingot's abdominal operations, 11th edition, McGraw-Hill, p. 107.

25. **McIntosh A, Hutchinson A, Roberts A,** *et al.*, (2000). Evidence-based management of groin hernia in primary care—a systematic review. *Fam. Pract.* 17: 442.

26. **Javid PJ, Brooks DC.**, (2007). Maingot's abdominal operations, 11th edition, McGraw-Hill, p. 120.

27. **Fischer JE.**, (2007). Surgery of hernia, Mastery of surgery, 5th edition, 1857.

28. **La Roque GP.**, (1919). *Surg. Gynaecol. Obstet.*, 29: 207.

29. **Badoe EA.**, (1973). *Afr. J. Med. Sci.*, 4: 51–58.

30. **Rains JH** *et al.*, (1971). Bailey and Love's short practice of surgery, 15th edition, p. 1249.

31. **Rains JH** *et al.*, (1971). Bailey and Love's short practice of surgery, 15th edition, p. 1245.

32. **Amyand C.**, (1736). Of an inguinal rupture, with a pin in the appendix caeci, encrusted with stone. *Phil. Trans. Royal Soc.*, 39: 329.

33. **Bhatia P** *et al.*, (2008). Lap management of Amyand's hernia; Global News Letter, **8,** p. 2.

34. **D'Alia C, Schiavo W, Tonante MG, Taranto A, Gagliano F, Bonanno, L.**, (2003). Amyand's hernia: Case report and review of literature. Hernia, 7: 89–91.

35. **King M, Bewes P, Cairns J, Thomtor J.** *et al.*, (2005). Hernias, primary surgery, non-trauma, **1,** Oxford Publications, p. 206.

36. **Itani K.M.F., Hawn M.T.** (2008). Biology of hernia formation, *Surg. Clin. N. Am.* **88,** 1. p. 28.

37. **Yip K.F., Tam P.K., Li, M.K.** (2004). Laparoscopic flip flop hernioplasty an innovative technique for pediatric hernia surgery, *Surg. Endosc*, 18(7): 1126–29.

38. **Woods B.** *et al.*, (2008). Open repair of inguinal hernias. An evidence based review, *Surg. Clin. N. Am.*; 88, 153.

39. **Koch A.**, *et al.*, (2005). Prospective evaluation of 6895 groin hernia repairs in women. *Br. J. Surg.*; 92:1553–8.

10 Femoral Hernia

"Most errors in clinical medicine are made by making a cursory incomplete examination than due to lack of knowledge and skill".
— **Henry Cohen**

Femoral hernia is more common in females due to wider pelvis. It is specially more common in multiparous elderly women due to stretching of pelvic ligaments during pregnancy.
- It accounts for 17% of all groin hernias (excluding incisional hernia).
- It is the third most common hernia after inguinal and incisional hernias.
- It accounts for 20% of hernias in females and 5% of hernias in adult males (Fig. 10.1).
- 70% of femoral hernias occur in females.
- Female to male ratio is 2 : 1.
- Female patients are elderly but male patients are of 30-45 years.
- Femoral hernia is never congenital. No evidence of a congenital sac has ever been found.[1]
- Pregnancy is the most important causative factor. Increased abdominal pressure by repeated pregnancy is one of the reasons of femoral hernia.
- It cannot be controlled by a truss.
- 25% of femoral hernias become incarcerated or strangulated.
- It is prone to get strangulated due to its narrow neck.
- In 40% of cases, first of all strangulation occurs.
- Operation should be performed as early as possible due to risk of strangulation.

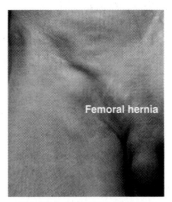
Fig. 10.1. Femoral hernia in a male, rare instance.

FEMORAL RING

It is an oval opening of 1.25 cm diameter. It is larger in females than in males. It is closed by thickened extraperitoneal tissue from inside which is called "femoral septum". It is pierced by few lymphatics.

FEMORAL SHEATH (Fig. 10.2)

Femoral sheath envelops femoral vessels. The sheath rests upon pectinius and adductor longus muscles medially and posas major and iliacus muscles laterally. Femoral canal lies in front of pectinius muscle. It has three compartments:
- Medial compartment – contains femoral canal.
- Intermediate compartment – contains femoral vein.
- Lateral compartment – contains femoral artery.

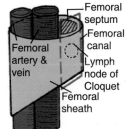
Fig. 10.2. Femoral sheath.

SAPHENOUS OPENING (Fig. 10.3)

It is also called "fossa ovalis". It is an opening in fascia lata situated 4 cm below and lateral to pubic tubercle. The upper and lateral margins of saphenous opening are thickened and sharp and are known as "falciform process". Once the femoral hernia comes out of saphenous opening, it is turned upwards by falciform process. The saphenous opening is covered by loose areolar tissue called "cribriform fascia".

Long saphenous vein and lymphatics pass through saphenous opening.

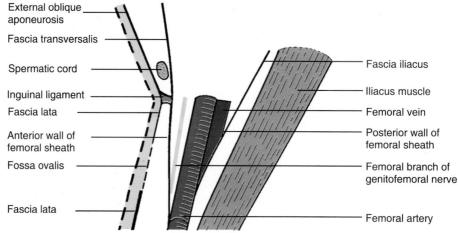

Fig. 10.3. Saphenous opening and femoral sheath.

Hey's Ligament (Fig. 10.4)

It is named after William Hey, English surgeon (1736 – 1819).

The lateral margin of saphenous opening is also called Hey's Ligament.

COURSE OF FEMORAL HERNIA (Figs. 10.5 A & B)

It passes out through femoral ring then passes through femoral canal and

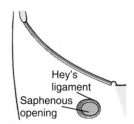

Fig. 10.4. Hey's ligament.

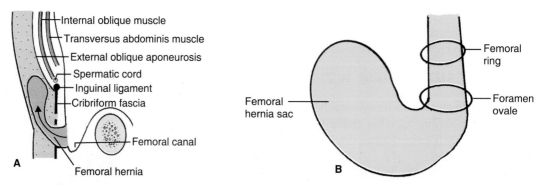

Fig. 10.5A. Course of femoral hernia diagrammatic representation, **B.** Retort-shaped course.

comes out in thigh through saphenous opening. It then turns up in subcutaneous tissue in thigh and may reach above inguinal ligament.

Sites of Constriction in Strangulated Femoral Hernia (Figs. 10.6 A-D)

Constriction occurs at the following sites:
• Lacunar ligament
• Neck of sac

In 40% of cases, obstructing agent is not Gimbernat's (Lacunar) ligament but the narrow neck of the femoral sac itself.[2]

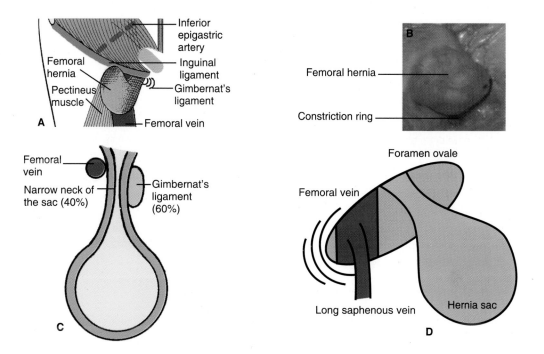

Fig. 10.6. Sites of constriction in strangulated femoral hernia, **A.** Gimbermat's ligament, diagrammatic representation, **B.** Open view, **C.** Neck of the sac and **D.** Foramen ovale.

CAUSES OF FEMORAL HERNIA

The main causes of femoral hernia are:
• Width of femoral ring.
• Size and shape of femoral ring.
• Increased intra-abdominal pressure.
• If insertion of iliopubic tract is narrow (less than normal 1-2 cm) or is medially displaced then width of femoral ring increases and a femoral hernia can develop.

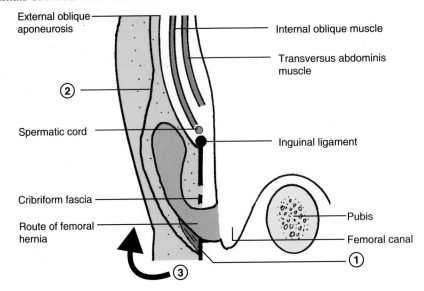

Fig. 10.7. Factors responsible for upward direction of femoral hernia sac after coming out of saphenous opening.
1. Falciform process. 2. Attachment of fascia of scarpa to fascia lata below saphenous opening. It does not allow it to move down but it has to go up. 3. Repeated flexion movements of thigh push the hernia up.

- Occurrence of femoral hernia increases after inguinal herniorrhaphy (both open and laparoscopic). It is due to the following factors:
  - A femoral hernia was missed in previous surgery.
  - Normal femoral plug sometimes is indistinguishable from femoral hernia and its manipulation during laparoscopic inguinal herniorrhaphy causes a true femoral hernia.
  - A new femoral hernia develops.

Theories of Aetiology of Femoral Hernia

True cause of femoral hernia is not known.

Following theories are forwarded by researchers:

Congenital preformed peritoneal sac theory

Many authors supported this theory in early twentieth century that there is a preformed sac by birth.[3,4] Keith has declined this theory.[5]

Acquired theory

This theory states that femoral hernia occurs due to acquired factors.
- Keith rejected congenital theory in 1923. "There is never a congenital preformed femoral hernia sac passing through the femoral ring". Increased intra-abdominal pressure is the main reason.[5]
- McVay demonstrated that width of femoral ring is the main aetiological factor.[6]

Coverings of Femoral Hernia (Fig. 10.8)

• Skin
• Superficial fascia (Camper's fascia and Scarpa's fascia)
• Cribriform fascia
• Anterior layer of femoral sheath
• Fatty contents of femoral canal
• Femoral septum
• Peritoneum

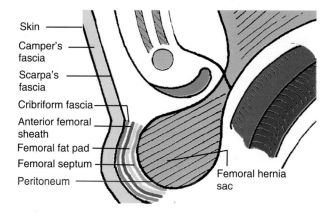

Skin
Camper's fascia
Scarpa's fascia
Cribriform fascia
Anterior femoral sheath
Femoral fat pad
Femoral septum
Peritoneum
Femoral hernia sac

Fig. 10.8. Coverings of femoral hernia.

Classification of femoral hernia

I Typical femoral hernia
II Atypical femoral hernia
  • External femoral hernia or Hesselbach's hernia
  • Prevascular hernia or Teale's hernia or Narath's hernia
  • Retrovascular or Serafine's hernia
  • Lacunar ligament femoral hernia or De Laugier hernia
  • Cloquet hernia or Pectineal hernia or Callisen's hernia

Femoral hernias are divided in two groups:

Typical Femoral Hernia

It is a hernia which protrudes through fascia transversalis and then passes through femoral ring and then via femoral canal it travels down and comes out through cribriform fascia in thigh.

Atypical Femoral Hernia (Fig. 10.9)

These hernias take pathways other than femoral canal.

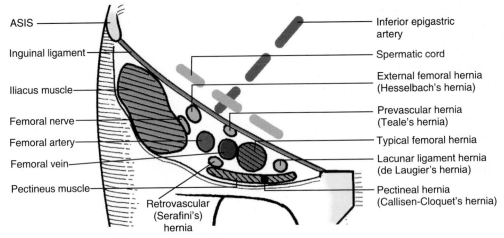

ASIS

Inguinal ligament

Iliacus muscle

Femoral nerve

Femoral artery

Femoral vein

Pectineus muscle

Retrovascular
(Serafini's)
hernia

Inferior epigastric
artery

Spermatic cord

External femoral hernia
(Hesselbach's hernia)

Prevascular hernia
(Teale's hernia)

Typical femoral hernia

Lacunar ligament hernia
(de Laugier's hernia)

Pectineal hernia
(Callisen-Cloquet's hernia)

Fig. 10.9. Typical and atypical femoral hernias.

Hesselbach's femoral hernia or external femoral hernia

This hernia occurs outside the femoral canal, under inguinal ligament in front of femoral nerve and external iliac artery.

Prevascular hernia or Narath's or Teale's femoral nerve

It is named after Albert Narath (1864-1924), Professor of Surgery, Heidelberg, Germany.
- Hernia occurs in front of the femoral vessels due to lateral displacement of psoas muscle in patients with congenital dislocation of hip.
- It is a hidden hernia.
- It has expansile cough impulse.
- It usually reduces.
- It is wide-necked, so there are less chances of strangulation.
- Repair is difficult due to its proximity to femoral vessels.

De Laugier's or Lacunar ligament femoral hernia

It is named after Stanislas Laugier, 1799-1872, Surgeon, Hotel Diu, Paris, France.
- It occurs through a gap in lacunar ligament (Gimbernat's ligament).
- It is more medial than classical or typical femoral hernia.
- It always occurs when strangulation occurs.

Pectineal or Cloquet's femoral hernia

It was first reported by Cloquet.
- It occurs behind the fascia covering pectineus muscle. It passes behind femoral vessels.
- It may coexist with a usual femoral hernia.
- It is prone to strangulate like femoral hernia.

Retrovascular or Serafini's femoral hernia

This hernia protrudes in thigh behind femoral vessels

CLINICAL PATHOLOGY

Due to rise of intra-abdominal pressure, the abdominal viscus or peritoneum with extraperitoenal fat is pushed through femoral ring to femoral canal. The hernia goes down from septum crurale then through femoral canal and then through cribriform fascia, finally it turns up and comes out as a swelling below the inguinal ligament. Sometimes it even goes above the inguinal ligament. The full course of femoral hernia takes the shape of a retort.

The strangulation occurs commonly in femoral hernia due to:
• Narrow neck of sac at femoral ring.
• Tortuous narrow path of hernia sac.
• Tough and unyielding boundaries of femoral ring.

Clinical Features of Femoral Hernia (Fig. 10.10)

The ratio of femoral hernia to all groin hernias is 2% to 8%.[7]

Femoral hernia is never congenital.

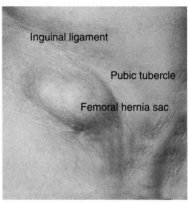

Fig. 10.10. Large femoral hernia.

Age

• Most common between 40-70 years. The peak distribution occurs in the 50's.[8]
• It is rare before 40 years of age and uncommon in children.
• It occurs in one percent of children with groin hernias.[14]

Sex

Inguinal hernia is the commonest hernia in females.
• Femoral hernia is more common in females than males, 4-5 times more common in females.
• Femoral hernia is common in multiparous females.

Side

• Right side is twice affected than left side.
• In 20% of the cases, it is bilateral.

The reason of higher incidence of femoral hernia on right side is not known.[9]
In this context, the following hypotheses have been made:
• Presence of sigmoid colon on left side offers internal support.
• Usually, right side is the dominant side of the body for most people hence tension on abdominal wall is more on right side.

Symptoms

Commonly a femoral hernia is symptomless.
• Small femoral hernia remains unnoticed till stragulation occurs.
• Pain usually does not occur. It occurs only due to the following reasons:
  – Strangulation
  – Omentum gets adherent and causes dragging pain

- A globular swelling may be present below and lateral to pubic tubercle. It becomes prominent on standing and straining and disappears on lying down.
- When it gets strangulated then symptoms of obstruction develop with pain at the hernia site spreading to whole abdomen.
- Richter's hernia is common in femoral hernia.

> - Femoral hernias are over diagnosed because of the presence of a prominent femoral fat pad, a so called "Femoral pseudo hernia".[10]

Signs

- The patient is examined in the standing position. Feel the lump and its neck, carefully determine the exact site of neck in relation to pubic tubercle and inguinal ligament.
- Painless swelling below inguinal ligament and below and lateral to pubic tubercle is felt.

Position (Fig. 10.11)

It is seen below the inguinal ligament and lateral to pubic tubercle.

In obese patients, the pubic tubercle is difficult to palpate so the tendon of adductor longus is palpated upward which leads to pubic tubercle. In obese persons, small femoral hernia may be overlooked unless carefully examined.

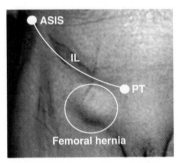

Fig. 10.11. Femoral hernia below inguinal ligament and below and lateral to pubic tubercle.

Femoral hernia may descend downwards, laterally or medially, it may go up and above the inguinal ligament, but usually seen as a lump behind the groin crease.

Size and shape

It is a globular swelling, usually small and takes the shape of a retort if goes above inguinal ligament.

Colour

Skin over hernia is of normal colour unless it is obstructed or strangulated, then it becomes red.

Temperature

Usually, the temperature is normal. It is hot if the hernia is inflamed or strangulated.

Tenderness

It is non-tender, but any attempt to forcibly reduce it will cause pain. Strangulation causes tenderness.

Reducibility

Complete reduction is difficult due to adhesions with peritoneal sac and narrow neck.

Expansile cough impulse

Due to irreducibility, most of the femoral hernias do not show expansile cough impulse.

Site

Site of occurrence is the most important sign in femoral hernia (femoral hernia is below inguinal ligament and below and lateral to pubic tubercle) as reducibility and expansile cough impulse—the two diagnostic signs of hernia—may be absent.

Consistency and composition

• It is firm and dull on percussion.

TYPES OF FEMORAL HERNIA

Femoral hernias are classified into two types according to the descent of its contents:
1. **Incomplete femoral hernia (Fig. 10.11)**
   Intestine reaches only to saphenous opening.
2. **Complete femoral hernia (Fig. 10.12)**
   Intestine passes out through the saphenous opening.
• The contents are omentum and extraperitoneal fat.
• Rarely a part of intestine or urinary bladder can be found in it.
• Rarely a femoral hernia has a big sac.
• Intermittent groin bulge or a tender groin mass is felt.
• Occult femoral hernia is always considered in small bowel obstruction specially if you are not dealing with adhesions due to previous abdominal surgery.
• It is usually missed as the cause for intestinal obstruction in elderly females.
• 10% of femoral hernias are misdiagnosed as inguinal hernia.
• The following two classical signs of a hernia are less prominent in femoral hernia:
   – Impulse on coughing
   – Reducibility
• This is due to:
   – Adherence of femoral hernia contents.
   – Narrowing of the neck of the sac of hernia.
• Cough impulse is rarely found as it is usually an irreducible hernia.
• It may be present as a tender lump if gets strangulated or incarcerated.

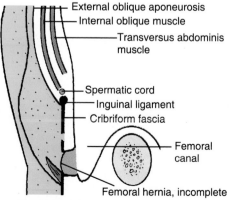

Fig. 10.11. Incomplete femoral hernia.

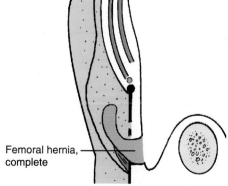

Fig. 10.12. Complete femoral hernia.

- Strangulated femoral hernia is easily missed unless the femoral region is carefully examined for a lump like a big grape.
- Femoral hernias are rare in native Africans.[11] It is postulated that chronic foot infection leads to repeated inflammation of groin lymph nodes and that the consequent fibrosis of the femoral canal prevents herniation.[12]

Strangulated Femoral Hernia

- The femoral hernia strangulates frequently.
- Gangrene develops early due to narrow and tough femoral ring.
- Obstructing agent is neck of the sac in 40% of the cases.
- Richter's hernia commonly occurs in this hernia.
- Early operation is the treatment of choice due to fear of strangulation.
- Truss is contraindicated.
- High operation of McEvedy is the preferred procedure.

How to Differentiate from Inguinal Hernia?

- Neck of femoral hernia sac lies below the inguinal ligament and lateral to pubic tubercle. In inguinal hernia, the neck lies above the inguinal ligament and medial to pubic tubercle.
- **Zieman's test:** Impulse is felt on coughing by ring finger.
- **Finger invagination test:** The inguinal canal is found empty.
- **Ring occlusion test:** When the hernia is reduced and pressure is exerted on femoral canal, hernia does not appear on coughing.

Femoral hernia is more common in females. It is due to:

- Femoral ring is larger in females due to wider female pelvis.
- Inguinal ligament forms a large angle with superior ramus of pubis.
- Femoral vessels are thinner in females so femoral canal become bigger as it gets more space in femoral sheath.
- Lacuna musculorum is thinner in females, so femoral canal is wider.

Differential Diagnosis of Femoral Hernia

- Usually a small irreducible soft mass is palpated. It shows that incarceration of the hernia sac is present.

Differential diagnosis of femoral hernia

- Inguinal hernia
- Enlarged inguinal lymph nodes
- Femoral artery aneurysm
- Rupture of adductor longus muscle
- Undescended and ectopic testis

- Saphena varix
- Lipoma in femoral triangle
- Psoas abscess
- An enlarged psoas bursa
- Hydrocele of a femoral hernia sac

Inguinal hernia *(Fig. 10.13)*

- It is more common than femoral hernia.
- Its sac is usually bigger than femoral hernia.
- Its neck of sac is above and medial to pubic tubercle while neck of femoral hernia is below and lateral to pubic tubercle.

Saphena varix

"Usually the saphena varix feels softer than a femoral hernia" –**Robert Milnes Walker**

- It is a saccular expansion of termination of long saphenous vein.
- It is associated with other varicose veins.

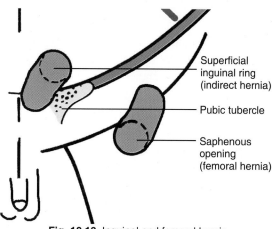

Fig. 10.13. Inguinal and femoral hernia.

- Swelling disappears completely on lying down while in femoral hernia it does not.
- Impulse on coughing is present in both but saphena varix has fluid thrill on coughing.

Schwartz's test

Tapping of the long saphenous vein below will transmit the impulse in saphena varix and will be felt by the fingers of the other hand.

- A venous hum sometimes can be heard on auscultating over saphena varix.
- Fluid thrill is called **Cruveilhier's Sign**. Fluid thrill is present when patient coughs and a tremor is felt by palpating fingers as if a water jet is entering.

Enlarged inguinal lymph nodes

- It may be associated with other enlarged lymph nodes.
- Solitary Cloquet's lymph node is difficult to differentiate from femoral hernia.
- Focus of infection should be searched from umbilicus to toe, terminal part of anal canal, vagina and urethra.

Lipoma in femoral triangle *(Fig. 10.14)*

- Due to the mobility of its edge below the finger it can be diagnosed clinically.

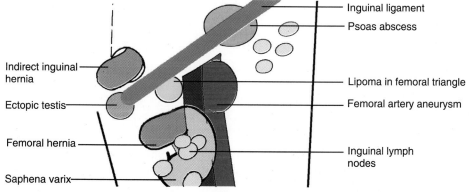

Fig. 10.14. Differential diagnosis of femoral hernia.

Femoral artery aneurysm

It is a pulsatile lump.

Psoas abscess (Fig. 10.15)

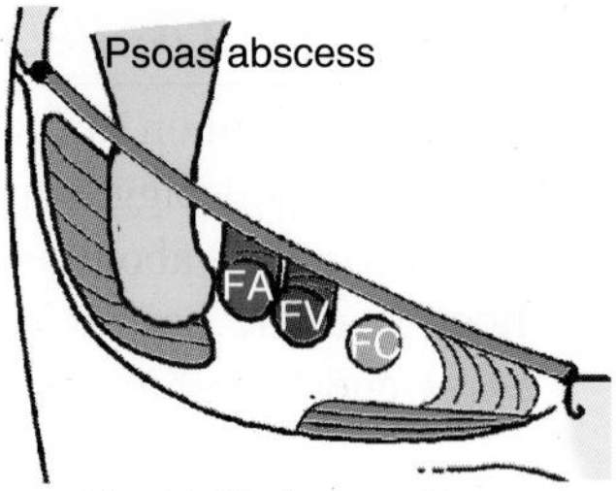

Fig. 10.15. Psoas abscess.

- Fluctuations are present.
- X-ray of spine will confirm the diagnosis.
- It is a cold abscess which descends down from Pott's spine.
- It is a reducible swelling and gives impulse on coughing.
- Swelling is lateral to femoral vessels.
- Cross-fluctuations across inguinal ligament are present if it has an iliac part also.
- Examination and X-ray of spine demonstrates spinal disease.

Rupture of adductor longus muscle

- Haemotoma in adductor longus muscle occurs in sportsmen specially in footballers.
- Swelling is more medial and bigger than femoral hernia.

Enlarged psoas bursa

- It lies in front of hip joint under psoas major muscle.
- It often communicates with hip joint.
- In osteoarthritis of hip joint, it becomes tense and enlarged and a cystic swelling appears below the inguinal ligament.
- The swelling diminishes in size when hip is flexed.

Undescended and ectopic testis (Fig. 10.16)

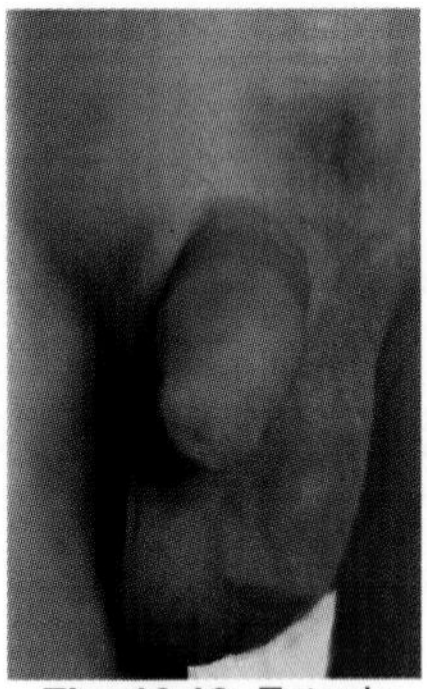

- Same side scrotum is empty.
- Swelling is typical in shape and has testicular sensation.
- Commonest site of ectopic testis is just above and lateral to superficial inguinal ring and superficial to external oblique aponeurosis in pouch of Denis Browne.
- Undescended testis is smaller than other side testis but ectopic testis is well developed.

Fig. 10.16. Ectopic testis.

Hydrocele of a femoral hernia sac

- It is an extremely rare condition.
- It occurs due to blockage or adhesions of neck of sac with omentum.

MANAGEMENT OF FEMORAL HERNIA

Conservative treatment—Contraindicated

Taxis should not be attempted in a femoral hernia as it may cause damage to the bowel.
    Conservative treatment is contraindicated due to the following reasons:
- Risk of strangulation is high.
- Truss cannot be applied properly as it gets displaced in movement due to flexion of the thigh.

Operative Treatment

It is the treatment of choice and should be performed at the earliest.

Herniorrhaphy is the operation of choice. It has the following approaches (Fig. 10.17):

(1) High approach operation or McEvedy's operation

- It is approached through an incision above the inguinal ligament and inguinal canal.
- It is the best operation for strangulated femoral hernia.
- It is a better procedure than low operation.
- It gives better access than low operation.
- It is more time consuming than low operation.

Advantages of high approach

- It can deal with cases of obstructed hernia or strangulated hernia.
- It can perform resection of bowel in strangulated hernia.
- Abnormal obturator artery can be seen and dealt with.

(2) Middle approach operation or inguinal approach or Lotheissen's operation

- It is approached through an incision near the inguinal ligament.
- It is through the inguinal canal.

Advantages of middle approach

- Sac can be excised flush with parietal peritoneum.
- The occult indirect inguinal hernia can also be identified.

(3) Low approach operation or Lockwood operation

Advantages of low approach

- It is approached below the inguinal ligament.
- It deals with hernia site directly.
- It is less time consuming.

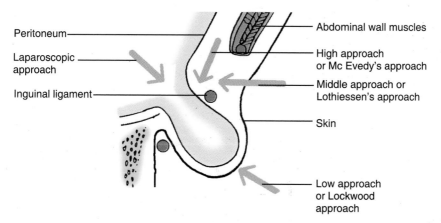

Fig. 10.17. Different approaches of femoral hernia operation.

Disadvantages of low approach

• Neck of the hernia sac cannot be approached properly so recurrence can occur as femoral ring repair cannot be done well.

Laparoscopic repair of femoral hernia

• Iliopubic tract is approximated with the Cooper's ligament by polypropylene sutures.
• A small piece of mesh is introduced in the femoral canal and fixed.

Henry's approach

A.K. Henry developed the lower middle approach for repair of bilateral femoral hernias. Henry's approach, via, a Pfannestiel incision, is of historical interest only.[13]

KEY POINT

In an obese lady with acute intestinal obstruction, incarcerated or strangulated femoral hernia must be specifically searched for.

REFERENCES

1. **Burkitt HG.**, Essential surgery, 3rd edition, 2001, p. 354.
2. **Souttar HS, Bailey & Love's.**, (1971). Short practice of surgery, 15th edition, p. 1069.
3. **Murray RW.**, (1910). Is the sac of a femoral hernia of congenital or acquired origin? *Am. Surg.*, 52: 668.
4. **Russell RH.**, (1923-1924). Femoral hernia and the saccular theory. *Brit. J. Surg.*, 11: 148.
5. **Keith A.**, (1923-1924). On the origin and nature of hernias. *Br. J. Surg.*, 11: 455–475.
6. **McVay CB, Savage LE.**, (1961). Etiology of femoral hernia. *Ann. Surg.*, 154 (Supl.): 25.
7. **Glassow F.**, (1985). Femoral hernia; A review of 2105 repairs in a 17-year period. *Am. J. Surg.*, 150: 353–356.
8. **Hachisuka T.**, (2003). Femoral hernia repair, *Surg. Clin. North Am.*, 83, 1189–1205.
9. **Waddington RT.**, (1971). Femoral hernia : a recent appraisal, *Brit. J. Surg.*, 58: 920–922.
10. **Bendavid R.**, (2002). Femoral pseudohernias. Hernia, 6: 141.
11. **Cole GJ.**, (1964). *Trans. R. Soc. Trop. Med. Hyg.*, 58: 441–447.
12. **Wosornu L.**, (1974). *Trop. Doct.*, 4: 59-63.
13. **Kirk RM.**, (2000). General surgical operations, 4th edition, p. 127.
14. **Brandt ML.**, (2008). Paediatric hernias, *Surg. Clin. N. Am.*, 88, 37.

11

Umbilical & Paraumbilical Hernias

"What one knows, he sees and what one looks for, he is more likely to see. Chance favours only the prepared mind."
— **Louis Pasteur**

One lakh procedures for umbilical, epigastric's Spigelian, and flank hernia repairs are performed in United States annually.[1]

Umbilical hernias (Figs. 11.1 A-C) develop at umbilical ring and may be present at the time of birth or later. Umbilical hernias are present in approximately 10% of all newborns and are more common in premature infants. A defect less than 1 cm in size closes in 95% spontaneously.[2] A defect greater than 1.5 cm in diameter seldom closes spontaneously.

The infantile umbilical hernia is a result of an abnormally large or weak umbilical ring in an otherwise normal abdominal wall.[14]

First known record of surgical repair of umbilical hernia was mentioned in the first century AD, done by Celsus.[3]

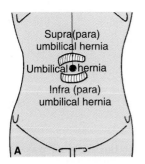 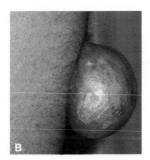 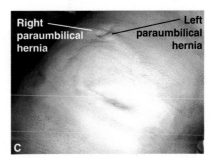

Fig. 11.1A. Umbilical and paraumbilical hernias, **B.** Huge umbilical hernia, **C.** Two paraumbilical hernias.

Following types of umbilical hernias are known:
- Umbilical hernia at birth or exomphalos or omphalocele. It is present at the time of birth.
- Umbilical hernia of infants and children.
- Umbilical hernia of adults.

- Umbilical hernia is due to failure of part or whole midgut to return to cealom during early fetal life.
- Gastroschisis is a congenital fissure of anterior abdominal wall not involving the site of insertion of the umbilical cord. Usually, accompanied by protrusion of the small intestine and part of large intestine.

COMPARISON BETWEEN GASTROSCHISIS AND EXOMPHALOS OR OMPHALOCELE

OMPHALOCELE	GASTROSCHISIS
1. Covered defect of umbilical ring.	1. Uncovered defect of anterior abdominal wall lateral to umbilicus.
2. Peritoneal sac is present.	2. Peritoneal sac is not present.
3. In 50% cases, there are associated abnormalities in males.	3. In 10-15%, cases there are associated abnormalities in males.
4. Liver is eviscerated.	4. No evisceration of liver.
5. Mortality is 37%.	5. Mortality is 90%.
6. Surgical closure is the treatment.	6. Surgical closure is the treatment.

EXOMPHALOS OR OMPHALOCELE OR UMBILICAL HERNIA AT BIRTH (FIGS. 11.2 A & B)

- It is a type of congenital umbilical hernia. In exmphalos, the part of midgut fails to return to coelomic cavity.
- The basic defect is failure of fusion of anterior abdominal wall.
- Exomphalos is also called "omphalocele". It is a developmental anomaly.

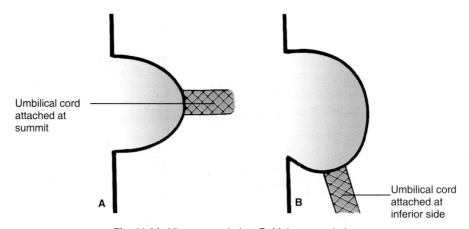

Umbilical cord attached at summit

Umbilical cord attached at inferior side

Fig. 11.2A. Minor exomphalos, **B.** Major exomphalos.

- Exomphalos is of two types:
  - Exomphalos minor
  - Exomphalos major
- Exomphalos minor – small fascial defect – less than 4 cm.
- Exomphalos major – large fascial defect – more than 4 cm.

Small Defect or Foetal Omphalocele

It develops after eight weeks of gestation when the gut fails to return to the abdominal cavity, then a defect develops in abdominal wall.

At the time of birth small defects may not be clinically appreciated, even single loop of small intestine will be missed in diagnosis and a hurried ligation of umbilical cord can damage the small bowel and may lead to umbilicoenteric fistula. The umbilical cord is attached to the sac on its summit.

Large Defects or Embryonic Omphalocele

It develops before eight weeks of gestation due to the failure of abdominal wall closure. In large defects, the abdominal organs like liver, stomach, intestine, pancreas, spleen and even urinary bladder can protrude and they may be visible through semiluscent membrane. In 50% of such patients, multiple anomalies are present such as congenital heart defects, Trisomy 21 and renal abnormalities. The Beckwith-Wiedemann syndrome (exomphalos, gigantism, macroglossia, visceromegaly and renal dysplasia) is one of the better known syndromes.[4] Surprisingly, the intestine lies freely in sac without adhesions and on the other hand, liver is seen with dense adhesions with sac. While performing a repair, the adhesions are to be kept in mind. The umbilical cord is attached to the sac on inferior side (Fig. 11.3).

> The sac of exomphalos is very thin and semitransparent. It consists of three layers:
> * Outer layer – Amniotic membrane
> * Middle layer – Wharton's jelly
> * Inner layer – Peritoneum

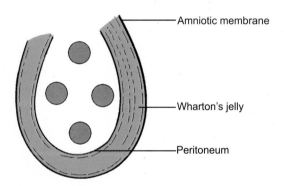

Fig. 11.3. Three layers of sac of exomphalos.

* Normally, intestine returns to abdominal cavity at 10th week of gestation. If it fails then umbilical hernia develops.
* It is rare to have umbilical hernia at the time of birth.
* It is due to intrauterine epithelization of exomphalos.
* It occurs 1 in 4000 births.
* It is diagnosed either in utero before birth or at the time of birth. Ultrasound can detect abdominal wall defect and umbilical hernia as early as at 15th week of gestation.
* Big omphalocele can cause problem during delivery. Caesarean delivery is preferred to vaginal delivery as vaginal delivery can cause rupture or dystocea (abnormal or difficult labour).

- These cases must be treated at specialized centres. If the ultrasound has diagnosed the hernia in prenatal period, then the mother should be shifted to specialized centre for delivery.

Treatment

When the defect is less than 4 cm, it is termed "Hernia of the umbilical cord". When the defect is greater than 10 cm, it is termed "Giant omphalocele".[5]

Small defects

- Sometimes a twist to the cord may reduce the contents of the sac into the peritoneal cavity and is retained by a strapping applied to it. Strapping is left for 15 days.
- Primary closure is easy as there is not much disproportion between volume of abdominal cavity and volume of the contents of hernia sac.

Large defects

These large defects are difficult to close as the thin membrane ruptures during repair. The operation is performed as emergency measure otherwise it may burst.

Techniques to deal with the large defects are as follows:
- **Non-operative treatment** – Painting of hernia sac with drying antiseptic solution gradually causes it to heal and later it develops into a ventral hernia which can later be easily operated.
- **Operative treatment**
  - **Skin flap closure:** Skin flaps are created on both sides of the swelling. These relaxing incisions are applied on both sides to bring the flaps to midline to cover the hernia.
  - **Staged closure:** First skin flap closure is done. Later on muscle approximation over the sac is done.
  - **Primary closure:** It is done in small hernia.

UMBILICAL HERNIA OF INFANTS AND CHILDREN

Cause

- It occurs due to the failure of round ligament (obliterated umbilical vein) to cross the umbilical ring (Fig. 11.4).

> - Absence of Richet's fascia, which is named after Louis Alfred Richet (1816-1891), Professor of Clinical Surgery, Faculty of Paris, France. Richet's fascia is a fold of extraperitoneal fascia enveloping the obliterated umbilical vein.

- Orda states that all defects result from the incomplete closure of the early natural umbilical defect and the absence of umbilical fascia.[6]

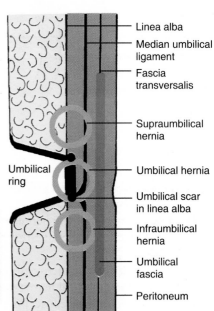

Fig. 11.4. Anatomy of umbilicus and hernias.

Incidence

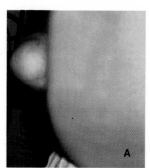

- Common in both sexes. It is more common in males than females, the ratio is 2 : 1.
- Usually symptoms are absent.
- Size increases if the infant cries and assumes the shape of a cone.
- Strangulation or obstruction is rare before three years of age.
  - It occurs 1 in 5 birth.
  - 90% hernias disappear by the age of two years.
  - If at the age of three months the umbilical fascial defect is more than 1.5 cm, then it will not disappear.

Fig. 11.5A. Umbilical hernia in a child.

  - A very rare complication is reported in Nigerian children, "spontaneous rupture". It occurs in the first year of life, precipitated by raised intra-abdominal pressure due to excessive crying. This needs urgent surgical intervention due to partial evisceration.[12]

Age

Weakness at umbilicus may be present at birth, but hernia may not be noticed for few months.

> **Ethnic group**
>
> Congenital umbilical hernias are more common in Negroes.
> It is eight times higher in black and Asian infants than white infants in USA although no genetic pattern is confirmed.[12]

Symptoms

Rarely, any symptom is observed.
    No intestinal obstruction due to wide neck.

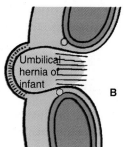

Fig. 11.5B. Umbilical hernia in an infant, diagrammatic represention.

Signs (Figs. 11.5 A - C)

Position

Centre of umbilicus.

Shape and size

Hemispherical, small or big.

Composition

Congenital umbilical hernia usually contains bowel hence, compressible and resonant on percussion.

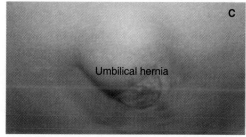

Fig. 11.5AC. Umbilical hernia in an infant.

Expansile cough impulse

It is present.

Treatment

- There is no age for surgery but it should be done before the child goes to school.
- **Below two years of age:** Only conservative treatment is done. It requires reassurance and strapping. 90% of cases are closed spontaneously within 12 to 18 months. Strapping is done with a pad or a big coin or a round piece of metal (Figs. 11.6 A & B). This is applied continuously and the sac gets obliterated by adhesions.
- **Above two years of age:** Herniorrhaphy is the treatment of choice.

Operations

- Simple apposition of fascial edges.
- Mayo's repair, there is no evidence that Mayo's operation is better than simple apposition of the fascial edges.

Simple apposition of fascial edges operation

- Umbilicus should be preserved to avoid psychological problem.
- Curved incision is made below the umbilicus.
- Neck of sac is incised.
- Contents of sac are pushed in the peritoneal canal.
- Neck of sac is ligated and sac is excised.
- Gap in linea alba is closed with non-absorbable sutures.
- Skin is closed.

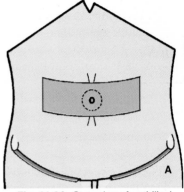

Fig. 11.6A. Strapping of umbilical hernia in infant.

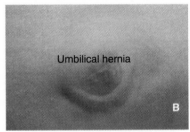

Fig. 11.6B. Reduction in size of umbilical hernia after use of strapping for nine months.

UMBILICAL HERNIA OF ADULT

"It is the protrusion of abdominal viscera or part of a viscus through a weak umbilicus." It is a hernia through a weak umbilical scar. Usually, it follows a neonatal umbilical sepsis but not due to persistence of infantile hernia (Fig. 11.7).

Pathology

It is due to protrusion through umbilical canal. The persistent raised intra-abdominal pressure results in umbilical cicatrix and umbilical hernia develops.

Boundaries of Umbilical Canal

- Anterior boundary – Linea alba.
- Posterior boundary – Umbilical fascia.
- Lateral side – Medial edges of rectus sheath.

Aetiology

The persistent raised intra-abdominal pressure results in umbilical hernia. It occurs in the following conditions:

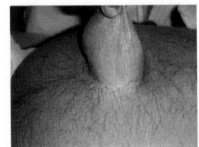

Fig. 11.7. True umbilical hernia in adult.

- Acute abdominal distension
- Ascites
- Peritoneal dialysis

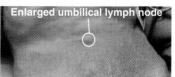

Sister Joseph nodule (Fig. 11.8)

It can mimic irreducible umbilical hernia
Sister (? Mary) Joseph, was a brilliant surgical assistant to
William J Mayo, who used to predict maliganancy by finding
a nodule at the umbilicus. In 1928, William J Mayo lectured
on this nodule but did not mention the name of Sister Joseph.
It was Hamilton Bailey, who in 1949 named this entity as
"Sister Joseph nodule."[10 & 11]

Fig. 11.8. Sister Joseph nodule, in a case of carcinoma of stomach.

Clinical Features

- True umbilical hernia in an adult is uncommon, most of these hernias are paraumbilical hernias.
- 90% of adult umbilical hernias occur in females.
- They have tendency to get incarcerated and strangulated, as neck of the hernia sac is usually quite narrow as compared to the size of the herniated mass. Dense fibrous hernia ring at the neck causes strangulation.[7]
- Almost all patients are obese and multiparous.[8]
- It is always painful as sagging of hernia causes traction on intestines, stomach and transverse colon. As hernia enlarges, it further sags down and pain increases.
- It is usually irreducible due to omental adherence to sac wall (Fig. 11.9).
- Pain occurs due to recurrent subacute intestinal obstruction.

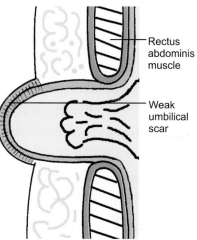

Fig. 11.9. Umbilical hernia in an adult containing omentum, diagrammatic representation.

Management

Surgery is the treatment of choice.

In small hernia (less than 2 cm) (Fig. 11.10A)

- Subumbilical incision and edge to edge suturing (primary tissue repair).

In larger hernia (more than 2 cm and less than 4 cm) (Fig. 11.10B)

- Mayo's repair.

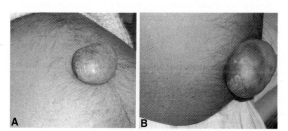

Fig. 11.10. True umbilical hernia in an adult, **A.** Small and **B.** Big.

In hernia more than 4 cm

- Prosthetic mesh hernioplasty gives the best results. It avoids recurrence in most of the cases of various size— small, medium and big size.

PARAUMBILICAL HERNIA (FIG. 11.11)

In umbilical hernia, the bulge occurs under the umbilicus but in paraumbilical hernia, the bulge occurs either above or below the umbilicus.

Paraumbilical hernia does not protrude through umbilicus. It protrudes in the midline through the linea alba above or below the umbilicus, hence called paraumbilical hernia.

Paraumbilical hernia is an acquired hernia due to disruption of fibres of linea alba.[9]

"It is a protrusion of abdominal contents through a defect in linea alba just above or below the umbilicus". It is of two types:

- **Supraumbilical hernia** – It occurs above the umbilicus. It is more common than infraumbilical hernia.
- **Infraumbilical hernia** – It occurs below the umbilicus.

Aetiological Factors

- Obesity
- Weak and flabby musculature of anterior abdominal wall due to:
  - Lack of abdominal wall exercise.
  - Presence of excessive fat.
- Repeated pregnancies.

Single Decussation Theory

Umbilical hernia is more common among individuals who have only a single midline aponeurotic decussation as compared with the normal triple decussation.[9]

Clinical Features

Special features of paraumbilical hernia
• Usually occurs in obese middle-aged females. • Size can be very big and associated with pain. • Strangulation may occur. • Surgery is a must.

- It is round or oval in shape.
- It can become very big (Fig. 11.12).
- If big, it sags down.

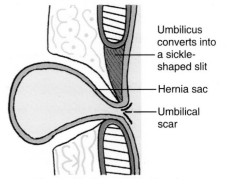

Umbilicus converts into a sickle-shaped slit

Hernia sac

Umbilical scar

Fig. 11.11. Paraumbilical hernia.

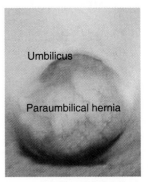

Umbilicus

Paraumbilical hernia

Fig. 11.12. Big paraumbilical hernia.

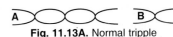

Fig. 11.13A. Normal tripple aponeurotic decussation, **B.** Abnormal single decussation.

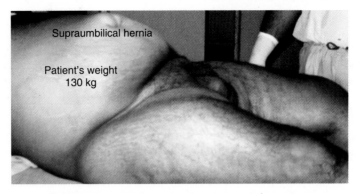

Fig. 11.14. Big paraumbilical hernia in an obese patient.

- Its neck is sometimes very narrow and causes strangulation.
- Usually it contains omentum or small intestine or both. Sometimes it may contain transverse colon also.
- Adhesions are common as a rule in long standing cases. Adhesions are usually between the contents and fundus. Sac becomes loculated due to multiple adhesions and thus, the paraumbilical hernia is usually not reducible (Fig. 11.14).
- Females are five times more affected than males.
- It is common between 35-50 years of age.
- It is common in obese female patients.
- Lump is dull on percussion due to omentum but is resonant if it contains intestine.
- Small paraumbilical hernia is painless but sometimes it is accompanied by some discomfort.
- Large hernia has dragging pain due to its weight.
- If it is irreducible due to adhesions of omentum with sac, then pain appears. Pain increases on prolonged standing and strenuous exercise.
- Gastrointestinal tract symptoms are common due to traction of small intestine, stomach, transverse colon and omentum.
- Subacute or partial intestinal obstruction causes recurrent intestinal colic.
- The adhesions are mainly between contents and the fundus. Neck of the sac usually remains free.
- Intertrigo and necrosis of skin may occur in large dependent hernia.
- Trophic ulcers develop due to friction.
- Expansile impulse on coughing is present if hernia is reducible but if it is not reducible, then it is not present.
- If hernia can be reduced, then edge of the defect in linea alba is easily palpable.

Treatment

The operation is the treatment of choice as hernia becomes irreducible and strangulated as time passes:
- Mayo's operation
- Mesh repair

> **NOTE**
>
> *Usually adhesions are present between the sac and contents. These adhesions are at the fundus of sac mainly and not at the neck, so the principle of the operation is "Neck first and fundus later" so as to avoid going through adhesions.*

> **KEY POINT**
>
> *Now there is a scientific evidence that collagen derangement is an aetiological factor in development of hernia.*

REFERENCES

1. **DuBay DA, Franz MG.**, (2003). Acute wound healing: the biology of acute wound failure. *Surg. Clinic. North Am.*, 83: 463–481.
2. **Brunicardi F.C.** *et al.*, (2005). Schwartz's principles of surgery, 8th edition, p. 132.
3. **Javid PJ, Brooks DC.**, (2007). Maingot's abdominal operations, 11th edition, McGraw-Hill, p. 122.
4. **Musehaweek U.**, (2003). Umbilical and epigastric hernia repair; *Surg. Clin. North Am.*, 83: 1208.
5. **Lawrence WW** *et al.*, (2003). Current surgical diagnosis and treatment, 11th edition, p. 1340.
6. **Townsend CM.**, (2004). Sabiston textbook of surgery, **2,** 17th edition, p. 1177.
7. **Orda R, Nathan N.**, (1973). Surgical anatomy of the umbilical structures. *Int. Surg.*, 58: 454.
8. **Brown SP.**, (2005). Core topics in general and emergency surgery, 23rd edition, Elsevier, p. 60.
9. **Askar DM.**, (1984). Aponeurotic hernias: Recent observation upon paraumbilical and epigastric hernias. *Surg. Clin. North Am.*, 64, 2: 315–333.
10. **Schwartz IS.**, (1987). Sister (? Mary) Joseph Nodule, *N. Eng. J. Med.*, 316: 1348–9.
11. **Bailey H.**, (1949). Demonstration of physical signs in clinical surgery, 11th edition Baltimore, William & Wilkins, 1227.
12. **Cuschieri A.** *et al.*, (2002). Essential surgical practice, 4th edition, Arnold, p. 173.
13. **Radhakrishnan J.**, (1995). Umbilical hernia, In Nyhus LM, Condon RE (Eds). Hernia, 4th edition, Philadelphia, J.B. Lippincott.
14. **Salameh JR.,** (2008). Primary and unusual abdominal wall hernias, *Surg. Clin. N. Am.*; 88, 45.

12

Epigastric Hernia

"The operation is a silent confession of the surgeon's inadequacy."

— John Hunter, (1728-1793)

- "Epigastric hernia is a protrusion of extraperitoneal fat through the linea alba between umbilicus and xiphisternum."
- Epigastric hernia was first described by Villeneuve in 1285.[1]
- Usually, it contains extraperitoneal fat and hence is also known as "fatty hernia of linea alba" (Fig. 12.1 & 12.2).
- When the development of hernia starts, it contains only extraperitoneal fat but as it grows it pulls a pouch of peritoneum which is empty or contains a portion of omentum. It does not contain a viscus as the neck of the sac is very narrow.

AETIOLOGY

Epigastric hernia was earlier regarded as a congenital defect[2] but now regarded as an acquired lesion. Although epigastric hernias have been described in infants.[8]

Two hypotheses are considered as far as development of epigastric hernia is concerned:

- **Decussation hypothesis of Askar[3]**
  - Epigastric hernia occurs where single midline pattern of decussation occurs instead triple decussation. Kornekov et al. found that thickness and density of fibres is more imprtant than decussation for development of hernia.[3]
- **Vascular lacunae hypothesis by Lang and colleague[4]**
  - Epigastric hernia occurs from the weak spot in linea alba where vessels pierce it. Increased abdominal tension forces preperitoneal fat derive from falciform ligament along the blood vessels inlarging the fascial defect and causing epigastric hernia.[2]
- A sudden strain while lifting weight can tear interlacing fibres of linea alba and can cause epigastric hernia. It is therefore common in young manual workers.
- Epigastric hernia occurs due to disruption in functional anatomy of abdominal wall. The aponeurotic sheets of anterior abdominal wall have fibres which are directed obliquely. The change of shape of these fibres occurs in various dimensions during abdominal distension as in respiration. The linea alba moves in length and breadth during abdominal distension so tearing of fibres occur resulting in epigastric hernia.

CLINICAL FEATURES

- The incidence of epigastric hernia varies from 0.5-10%.
  - It is more common in males. The male to female ratio is 4 : 1. It is rare in infants and children.

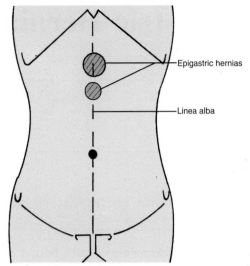

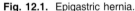

Fig. 12.1. Epigastric hernia.

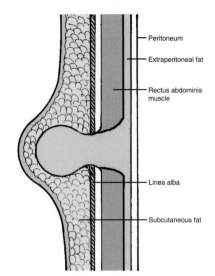

Fig. 12.2. Protrusion of preperitoneal fat through linea alba.

- Mostly seen in manual workers of 30-45 years age.
- It is symptomless hernia in 75% of cases.
- Usually felt better than seen.
- It is commonly diagnosed in routine health checkups.
- Epigastric hernia occurs most commonly above the level of umbilicus, probably due to excessive strain on the abdominal wall aponeurosis[5] (Fig. 12.3).
- Symptoms if present are:
  - Vague upper abdominal pain.
  - Nausea.
  - Epigastric tenderness.
    a) Pain increases on lying down and on exertion.
    b) Palpation reveals a midline mass.
- Pain is more when patient lies down due to traction of hernial contents.
- Incarceration of fat and omentum is common.
- Incarceration and strangulation of viscera is rare.
- The epigastric hernia protrudes through linea alba and its fibres form the hernia ring.
- Rectus sheath of one or both sides may form the lateral boundaries of epigastric hernia ring.
- If the defect is more than 1.5 cm, then the lateral boundaries of hernia ring are formed by rectus sheaths and also medial edges of rectus muscles, one or both.[6]

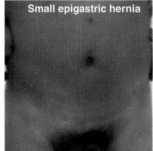

Fig. 12.3. Small epigastric hernia, midline, above umbilicus.

Epigastric hernia presents in one of the three presentations:

- **Symptomless**
  - It is discovered on routine examination.

- **Painful swelling**
  - Tight clothes may cause pain.
  - Pain is situated locally.
  - There is increase of pain during physical activity.
  - Hernia is tender to touch.
  - Pain is usually because of partial strangulation of fat nodule.
- **Referred dyspepsia**
  - Features of peptic ulcer are present but ulcer must be excluded as a patient of epigastric hernia may also get peptic ulcer as anybody else.

NOTE

- *Epigastric hernia neck is too small to contain bowel.*
- *Clinical features sometimes simulate Acid Peptic Disease (APD).*
- *Pain is due to strangulation.*
- *If painful then surgery is must.*

Differential Diagnosis

Most of the complaints of the epigastric hernia patient are similar to those of PUD. They must be investigated for PUD as most of the epigastric hernias are asymtpomatic.

Investigations

In obese patients, the lump is difficult to palpate so ultrasound or CT scan of abdomen is required.

TREATMENT

- **Asymptomatic epigastric hernia**
  - No treatment, only reassurance is required.
- **Symptomatic epigastric hernia**
  - Operation is the treatment of choice.
  - If the gap is less than 2 cm, then simple repair of linea alba with non-absorbable suture is done.
  - If the gap is more than 2 cm, then vertical Mayo's repair is done.
  - If the gap is more than 4 cm, then polypropylene mesh hernioplasty is done.
- **When exploration of sac is done**
  - If the omentum is found healthy, then it is pushed back in abdomen.
  - If the omentum found strangulated, then it is excised.
- Arroyo and co-workers in Spain showed recurrence rate after primary suture to be 11% and after using a tension free mesh repair to be only 1%.[7]

Post-operative Complications of Epigastric Hernia

- Haematoma
- Infection

- Recurrence between 7-9%
  - In 50% of cases there is no recurrence but a persistent second hernia is present.

> **KEY POINT**
>
> *Epigastric hernia usually contains exatraperitoneal fat or a nodule of omentum in sac but there is no viscus as its neck is too small to permit any viscus.*

REFERENCES

1. **Javid PJ, Brooks DC**., (2007). Maingot's abdominal operations, 11th edition, McGraw-Hill, p. 123.
2. **Moschowitz AV**., (1914). The pathogenesis and treatment of herniae of the linea alba, *Surg. Gynical. Obstetric.*, 18: 504.
3. **Askar OM**., (1978). A new concept of the aetiology and surgical repair of paraumbilical and epigastric hernias. *Am. R. Coll. Surg. Engl.*, 60: 40–42.
4. **Lang B, Lau H, Lee F**., (2002). Epigastric hernia and its etiology. Hernia, 6(3).
5. **Muschoweek U**., (2003). Umbilical and epigastric hernia repair, *Surg. Clin. North Am.*, 83: 1207.
6. **Arroyo A, Garcia P, Perez F,** *et al.*, (2001). Randomized clinical trial comparing suture and mesh repair of umbilical hernia in adults, *Br. J. Surg.*, 88(10): 1321–1323.
7. **Skandalakis JE, Skandalakis LJ, Colborn GL, Androvlakins J,** *et al.*, (2007). Mastery of surgery, 5th edition, Lippincott Williams & Wilkins, p. 1959.
8. **Salameh JR**., (2008). Primary and unusual abdominal wall hernias. *Surg. Clin. N. Am.*, 88, 47.

13

Incisional Hernia

"Abdominal closure: if it looks all right, it is too tight. If it looks too loose, It's all right."
— **Matt Oliver**

In adults, incisional hernia accounts for 80% or more of ventral hernias.[1]

Incisional hernia is a very common problem encountered by a surgeon. In the United States, each year approximately 2 million laparotomies are performed, resulting in a reported incisional hernia rate of between 2% and 11%.[2] 90,000, incisional hernia repairs are performed each year in the United States.[3]

"Herniation at the site of previous surgery or injury is called incisional hernia" (Figs. 13.1 A & B)

• Incisional hernia is also known as "post-operative hernia" or "ventral hernia".
• It usually follows a laparotomy wound as deeper layers of the wound give way during early post-operative period.
• Incisional hernia occurs in 14% of abdominal operations.
• Recurrent rates after incisional ventral hernia repair have been reported to 10-50%.[4]

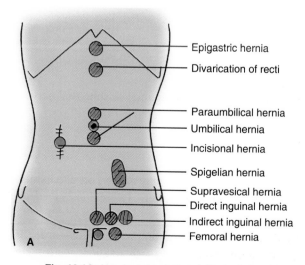
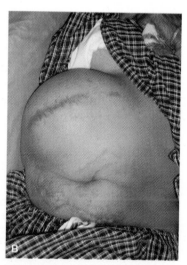

Epigastric hernia
Divarication of recti

Paraumbilical hernia
Umbilical hernia
Incisional hernia

Spigelian hernia
Supravesical hernia
Direct inguinal hernia
Indirect inguinal hernia
Femoral hernia

Fig. 13.1A. Hernias of anterior abdominal wall, **B.** Huge post-cholecystectomy incisional hernia (Incisional hernia can develop at the site of any previous hernia operation).

AETIOLOGY AND RISK FACTORS

Commonly stated risk factors for incision hernia include age and gender. Many studies have found that age more than 65-70 years predisposes patients to wound dehiscence and is common in men.

The risk factors can be divided in three groups:

(I) Defects with the Patient

- Age
- Obesity
- Peritonitis
- Poor general condition
- Repeated pregnancy
- Smoking
  - Sorenson supported what Raymond Read first had described many years ago, that smoking is a significant independent risk factor (fourfold increase) for development of incisional hernia.[5]
- Diabetes
- Other causes are malignancy, jaundice, steroids and anaemia with hypoproteinemia.

(II) Defects with Operation Technique (Fig. 13.2)

- Emergency surgery
- Bowel surgery
- Wound infection—It is the most common cause.
- Wound dehiscence
- Poor operation technique
- Absorbable sutures i.e. catgut
- Continuous sutures
- Tight suturing
- Deeper layers of incision are not repaired well.
- Injury to motor nerves in the following operations:
  - Kocher's incision for cholecystectomy 8th, 9th and 10th intercostal nerves can get damaged.
  - Battle's pararectal incision for appendicectomy.
  - Mc. Burney's incision for appendicectomy, it can damage ilioinguinal or subcostal nerve.
- Midline infraumbilical incision. It is the most common site of incisional hernia.
- Vertical incision
- Drainage tube through incision
- Intraoperative blood loss more than 1 litre
- Failure to close fascia at trocar site, the size if more than 10 mm may cause port site hernia.
- The other important aspect in repair of recurrent hernias is that repetition of a previously inadequate technique which frequently fails.[6]

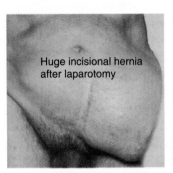

Huge incisional hernia after laparotomy

Fig. 13.2. Post-operative incisional hernia.

- Mechanisms of recurrence of ventral hernia described in the literature, in decreasing order of frequency, are infection, lateral detachment of mesh, inadequate mesh fixation, inadequate mesh overlap, missed hernias, increased intra-abdominal pressure and trauma.[7]

(III) Post-operative Causes (Fig. 13.3)

- Post-operative abdominal distension
- Post-operative peritonitis
- Early removal of sutures (controversial factor)
- Steroids in post-operative period
- Post-operative straining e.g. vomiting, sneezing and coughing
- Post-operative vigorous ventilation and pulmonary complications

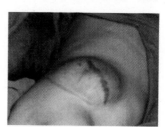

Fig. 13.3. Right post nephrolithotomy incisional hernia.

Obesity

Fat splits the muscle fibres by acting as screw-driver and thus makes the muscles weak. So the incisional hernia is common in obese persons. Obesity has never been shown to cause a wound healing effect. However, increased mechanical forces are likely to contribute to abdominal wall wound failure. Class II data show an increased incidence of incisional hernia formation in obese patients.[8] Ultrasound and computer tomography help to evaluate obesity and can be very helpful in predicting incision hernia development.

Suture material

- Absorbable suture material, such as use of chronic catgut for closure of laparotomy wound, leads to incisional hernia and even burst abdomen, as it cannot withstand high pressure.
- Even mild infection can cause early dissolution of catgut.
- So always use non-absorbable sutures for closing the abdomen wound such as monofilament polypropylene or ethilon.

Continuous suture (Fig. 13.4)

Usually the length of suture material looks sufficient before starting a continuous suture, at the end when we put the knots, usually tension is built up due to insufficient length of suture.
- Sometimes suture is taken from the edge of the wound and tension cuts it.
- Relaxed incision under anaesthesia is smaller than without anaesthesia and is a reason for tight suture.
- The length of the suture material should be at least four times of incision size.
- Hodgson did a meta-analysis of 2000 incisional hernia cases and found that if the fascia is closed with non-absorable continuous suture at initial laparotomy, incidence of incisional hernia is the lowest.[5]
- When flank incision cuts the intercostal nerves that are trophic to abdominal muscles then muscle

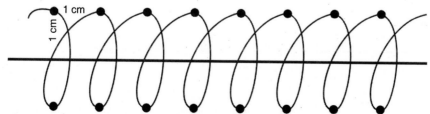

Fig. 13.4. Length of suture should be four times of incision length and distance between sutures and the edge of the wound should be atleast 1 cm.

becomes weak, thin and fibrotic, and loses its tone and bulges out. It is called denervated flank bulge (DNFB). It is not a true hernia. DNFB cannot be repaired.[9]

Retention suture

Use of internal retention sutures has been reported to reduce inguinal hernia recurrence rate to 3%.[24]

Tension on suture line

Tight suture cuts the tissue and throttles the tissue causing death of the tissue (necrosis) and the tissue becomes weak and later hernia occurs through this area.

The incisional hernia rate is lower if SL : WL (SL = suture length, WL = wound length) ratio is 4 or more, suturing with lower ratio is associated with threefold increase in the rate of incisional hernia.[10] Abdominal wall incision may lengthen by 30% when it is loaded or if the abdomen becomes distended post-operative.[11] Clinical studies of acute wound failure respond through principles in achieving low wound dehiscence rates, wide tissue bites, short stitch intervals and non-strangulating tension on suture. A 1 cm stitch interval with 1 cm tissue bite achieves the 4 : 1 SL : WL ratio.[12]

Incisional hernia develops when suture line fails, suture line too loose or suture pulls through this develops before the laparotoy wound scar is mechanically capable of with standing the distraction forces. The provisional matrix (PM) is composed of immature and weak matrix glycoproteins and collagen isoforms. In addition, the scar-to-wound interface is not developed.[13]

Midline incision

Midline incisions are more prone to incisional hernia.

The increasing use of non-absorbable sutures as polypropylene is reducing the incidence of incisional hernia in midline incision. So use non-absorbable sutures in midline incisions.

Wound bursting strength in Cadavers is twice as great for transverse as midline incisions when sutures are placed 1 cm from wound edge.

Vertical incision

Vertical incisions are also more prone for incisional hernia than transverse incisions. So wherever possible vertical incisions should be avoided and transverse incisions are preferred. Vertical incisions should be closed with non-absorbable sutures.

Drainage tube

A drainage tube must always be introduced through a separate stab wound and not through the main incision as it has more chances of developing incisional hernia.

Wound infection

Infection in deep layers of wound causes burst abdomen and incisional hernia. Wound infection is commonly cited as the most significant independent prognostic factor for incisional hernia.

Straining

Straining like coughing, vomiting, sneezing if violent in post-operative period can disrupt the deeper layers of the wound and predispose the wound for incisional hernia. The patient should be treated for these factors in post-operative period. It is better if these are avoided by preventing measures as post-operative steam inhalation and incentive spirometry.[14]

Post-operative distension of abdomen

It is a common condition after laparotomy specially if paralytic ileus develops.

The post-operative distension puts strain on sutures specially in early post-operative period. It predisposes to incisional hernia.

Peritonitis

Peritonitis is always associated with infection. Peritonitis may be preoperative or post-operative, both lead wound infection and may lead to burst abdomen and incisional hernia.

Poor general condition of the patient

Poor nutritional status of the patient leads to poor healing of the wound which predisposes to incisional hernia.

Steroids

Steroids usually delay the healing and thus predispose to incisional hernia.

TYPES OF INCISIONAL HERNIA (Fig. 13.4)

These are of two types:
- Type I – Situated in upper abdomen or in midline in lower abdomen.
- Type II – Situated in lateral part of lower abdomen

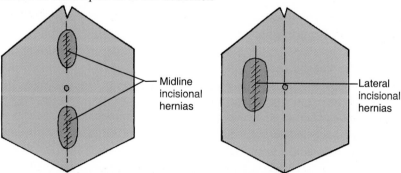

Fig. 13.4. Incisional hernia, Type I and II.

Type-I Incisional Hernia

- Wide gap in musculature
- Margin of defect smooth and regular
- Reducible hernia
- Hernia reduces spontaneously as patient lies down
- Not multiloculated sac
- No risk of strangulation
- Can be treated with simple abdominal corset

Type-II Incisional Hernia

- Small gap
- Irregular
- Irreducible hernia
- Does not reduce spontaneously
- Multiloculated sac
- Risk of strangulation
- Surgery is must

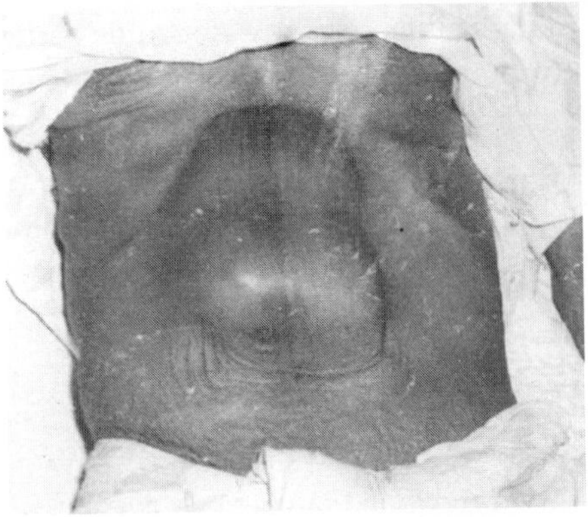

Pathology

Fig. 13.5. Huge incisional hernia.

- Incisional hernia usually starts in early post-operative period as asymptomatic process. It starts as partial disruption of deeper layers of laparotomy wound.
- Infection causes disruption of the sutures so muscles are separated leading to weak scar formation which leads to incisional hernia due to increased intra-abdominal pressure.
- Lateral abdominal muscles retract and become fibrotic which further enlarges the hernia defect and the hernia.

CLINICAL FEATURES OF INCISIONAL HERNIA (Fig. 13.5)

The first sign of an incisional ventral hernia is usually an asymptomatic bulge noticed by the patient. Hernia becomes more obvious with the position.[15]

- It is common in obese elderly females.
- History of trauma or operation and wound infection may be present.
- It usually occurs through lower abdominal incision.
- It may develop from a small weak spot of incision scar.
- It may develop from any part of scar but development of incisional hernia at lower end of scar is more common.
- It may involve the whole scar.
- Incisional hernia smaller than 4 cm is a small hernia and more than 4 cm is a large hernia. Large incisional hernias have more recurrence rate.[28]
- Usually, the incisional hernia is wide-necked so it is asymptomatic.
- Recurrent pain in incisional hernia is quite common and it is due to:
  - Adhesions between contents and sac.
  - Strangulation occurs either in narrow-necked hernia or in any loculus of large hernia.
- On examination, a scar is found.
- A reducible swelling with expansile impulse on coughing is present.
- Swelling is present through scar.
- Strangulation is not common in incisional hernia.
- Defect in abdominal wall is palpable.

Differential Diagnosis

Clinical detection of incisional hernia in an obese individual or in patients who had multiple abdominal surgeries can be difficult on physical examination. CT scan, ultrasonography and contrast gastro-intestinal series can be used to evaluate these patients.[16,17,26,27]

The differential diagnosis of incisional hernia are as follows:
- Tumour
- Cold abscess
- Haematoma
- Foreign body granuloma

NOTE

- *Incisional hernia starts as partial disruption of deeper layers of laparotomy wound in post-operative period.*
- *It occurs more commonly through lower abdominal scars than upper abdominal scars.*
- *It rarely strangulates.*
- *An adhesion between sac and contents is almost always present.*
- *It is dangerous to reduce large incisional hernia due to fear of respiratory embarrassment.*
- *More than half of all incisional hernias present within the first 2 years after the primary operation, but a significant percentage of incisional hernias occur many years after the primary operation.[18]*

Planning and Preoperative Preparation for Operation

- Weight reduction in obese patients is utmost important. It is essential before surgery because return of hernia contents in abdomen can lead to respiratory embarrassment, paralytic ileus due to compression of intestinal loops and recurrence.
- Breathing exercises are taught two weeks before the operation to improve respiratory reserve.
- Patient is advised to take six small meals instead three big meals to avoid post-prandal distension.
- Constipation has to be avoided. Start mild laxative one week before the surgery to avoid straining in post-operative period.

The goals of hernia repair

The goals of hernia repair should be as follows
- Prevention of visceral eventration
- Incorporation of the remaining abdominal wall in the repair
- Provision of dynamic muscular support.
- Restoration of abdominal wall continuity in a tension-free manner

TREATMENT

Preventive Measures

- In obese persons weight should be reduced before the surgery.
- Chronic bronchitis should be treated before the surgery.
- During laparotomy one should be careful about operative techniques. The closure of abdomen should be done with care. The deeper layers must be sutured properly.
- It is important to prevent post-operative wound infection.
- Post-operative steam inhalation and incentive spirometry should be used to avoid chest infection.

Palliative Treatment

Conservative treatment for incisional hernia is through the use of hernia belt or truss, the use of which is not encouraged.

Abdominal belt sometimes gives relief. It is only indicated in reducible type-I incisional hernia – If the belt is used continuously for a long time without allowing it to come out then it may help by causing adhesions.

Curative Treatment

Surgery is the curative treatment.

> ### *Loss of Domain*
>
> The giant ventral hernia with loss of abdominal domain can be a challenging problem.
> In large incisional hernia some abdominal contents permanently stay in incisional hernia sac outside the abdominal cavity as they have lost the "domain" inside the abdominal cavity. The musculature of abdominal wall also shrinks or retracts due to loss of some of its contents in incisional hernia sac. So any attempt to reduce the contents of hernia sac back to the abdominal cavity causes Abdominal Compartment Syndrome presented as cardiorespiratory embarrassment.

ABDOMINAL COMPARTMENT SYNDROME (ACS) (Figs. 13.6 A & B)

The effects of raised intra-abdominal pressure leads to "abdominal compartment syndrome". The normal intra-abdominal pressure is 0-5 mm Hg. If the abdominal pressure is raised above 5 mm Hg it causes adverse effects.

ACS is the complex of adverse physiological consequences that occurs as a result of an acute rise in intra-abdominal pressure (usually > 20 mm of Hg).

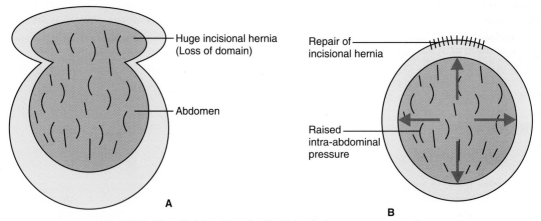

Fig. 13.6A. Huge incisional hernia, **B.** Abdominal compartment syndrome.

Common Causes of ACS

- Iatrogenic – Tension pneumothorax in laparoscopy.
- Abdominal wall – Incisional hernia repair for large hernia.
- Intra-abdominal – Intra-abdominal trauma, acute intestinal obstruction and neoplasm.

Treatment

All cases of incisional hernia require surgery at some stage. Routine indications for operation are:
• Type II incisional hernia.
• Irreducible type I hernia.
• Type I hernia when conservative treatment fails.
    Incisional hernia operations are carried out in two stages:

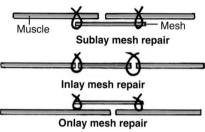

Fig. 13.7. Repair of incisional hernia defect, diagrammatic representation.

First stage

• Excision of unhealthy skin and redundant peritoneum.
• Adhesiolysis – Removal of adhesions.
• Return of the contents of hernia to peritoneal cavity.
    – Encircling elliptical incision is made enclosing the unhealthy skin.
    – Skin is separated from sac, which is thinned out to peritoneum.
    – Sac is opened at neck.
    – Adhesions are removed, if omentum is adherent part of it then it may be excised.
    – Contents are returned to peritoneal cavity.

Second stage

Repair of the defect.

Suture repair or Mayo repair or Tension-free anatomical approximation
Only small hernias less than 3 cm size should be treated with it and Mayo's repair.
    Various layers of abdominal wall are approximated separately with non-absorbable sutures after incision of the scar. To reduce the tension one can give releasing incisions in anterior rectus sheath in lateral part in midline incisionl hernia.

Open mesh repair (In more than the 3 cm size defect) (Figs. 13.7-13.10)
• Sublay repair
• Inlay repair
• Onlay repair

    Studies have shown that suture repair of incisional hernias has 45-90% recurrence rate.

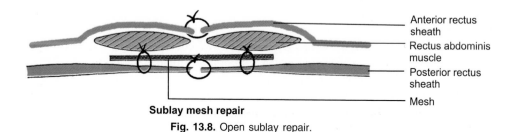

Sublay mesh repair

Fig. 13.8. Open sublay repair.

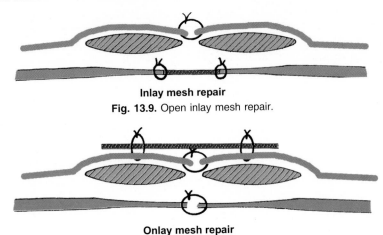

Inlay mesh repair

Fig. 13.9. Open inlay mesh repair.

Onlay mesh repair

Fig.13.10. Open onlay mesh repair.

Laparoscopic repair

Laparoscopic approach in incisional hernia repair gives better visualization than open method in multiple fascial defects. Complete visualization of fascia underlying the previous incision allows the identification of smaller "Swiss-cheese" defects that could be missed in an open approach.

Other techniques where loss of domain develops

- Ramirez technique (component separation technique)
- Relaxing technique
- Pneomoperitoneum technique
- Tissue expanders
- Keel operation
- Cattell's operation
- Nuttal's operation
- Darning (fascial suture or skin ribbon hernioplasty)
- Rives-Stoppa-Wantz retrorectus repair

Open onlay mesh repair technique

- Old scar and redundant skin is excised.
- Sac is carefully dissected.
- Sac is opened and adhesions are released.
- Sac is excised.
    A mesh is placed to cover the defect and overlaps by 5 cm on all sides. It is a tension-free repair.
    The mesh is fixed with underlying fascia with non-absorbable sutures.
    The disadvantges of this repair are:
- Repair is under tension.
- Extensive subcutaneous dissection causes seroma formation.
- Mesh infection develops if the wound is infected

Open inlay mesh repair technique

The mesh is sutured with the edges of defect in fascia. The mesh will be in contact with the viscera so the mesh is chosen correctly such as polypropylene and polygalactin composite (Vipro) mesh.[16]

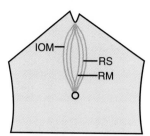

Fig. 13.11. Ramirez technique (component separation technique)

Open sublay mesh repair technique

The peritoneum and posterior rectus sheath are closed and then the mesh is placed over them and sutured with it with non-absorbable sutures.

- **Ramirez technique[19,29] (component separation technique) (Fig. 13.11)**
  - This method includes release and medial advancement of anterior rectus sheath, rectus muscle and internal oblique to close the defect.
  - The need of mesh application is eliminated.
  - Relaxing incisions are placed on external oblique aponeurosis.
  It can cover the defect of 20 cm by advancing structures on both sides of midline by 10 cm.
- **Relaxing technique (Fig. 13.12)**
  - Multiple small incisions are given on both sides of fascia.
  - Incisions should not interfere with blood supply.
  - This technique is specially helpful in large incisional hernias.
- **Pneumoperitoneum technique**
  - Pneumoperitoneum is created with carbon dioxide by introducing a Tenckoff catheter intraperitoneally as in laparoscopic surgery and repeated insufflation to increase abdominal domain is reported.[20]
  - It improves the cardiorespiratory adaptation.
  - It increases the volume of peritoneal cavity.
- The technique of serial preoperative therapeutic pneumoperitoneum offers one approach to the problem of peritoneal volume loss.[21]
- There is renewed interest in serial abdominal pneumoperitoneum and other techniques for the development of autologous tissue sources to repair these difficult wounds.
- **Tissue expanding techniques (Fig. 13.12)**
  - The expanders are placed under skin or in submuscular plane to create space.
  - It is kept for a few minutes before proper surgery.
  - Tissue expanders and relaxing incisions, in stages are described to approach this challenging problem.[22,23]
- **Keel operation (Fig. 13.13)**
  - Hernia sac is not opened and pushed back inside the abdomen. Suturing is done with

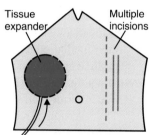

Fig. 13.12. Relaxing incisions and tissue expander.

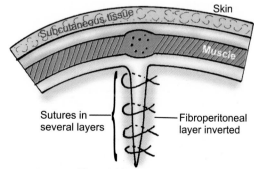

Fig. 13.13. Keel operation.

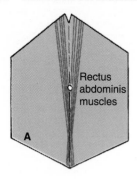

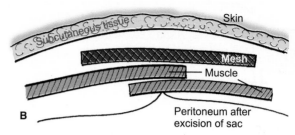

Fig. 13.14A. Nuttal's operation, **B.** Modified Nuttal's operation.

non-absorbable suture in a few layers so it protrudes inside peritoneal cavity, like Keel of a ship, it is called "Keel Operation".

- **Cattell's operation**
  - The sac is dissected out and is opened. Contents are reduced. Peritoneum is repaired. Different layers are sutured layer-by-layer in midline with non-absorbable sutures. Two lateral incisions are made in aponeurosis on either side half inch away from midline, then medial edges are sutured over previous line of sutures in midline and lateral margin are sutured over it in the midline.

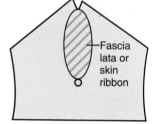

Fig. 13.15. Darning with fascial lata or skin ribbon.

- **Nuttal's operation (Fig. 13.14A)**
  - The anterior rectus sheath is incised on either side of the defect. The insertion of rectus abdominis muscle is detached from pubic symphysis and reattached on opposite pubic tubercle with 1-0 polypropylene.
    Overlapped rectus abdominis muscles are sutured together without tension.
  - Anterior rectus sheath is now closed again.
- **Modified Nuttal's operation (Fig. 13.14B)**
  - Nuttal's operation can be reinforced with mesh also.
  - The polypropylene mesh covering the size of the defect can be placed over the repaired fascial layer.

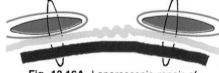

Fig. 13.16A. Laparoscopic repair of incisional hernia.

- **Darning repair by facial sutures or skin ribbon hernioplasty (Fig. 13.15)**
  - If the hernia gap cannot be closed without tension then darning is done with skin ribbon or fascial sutures.
- **Rives-Stoppa-Wantz technique**
  - Rives describes in 1973 a procedure where a big mesh is placed between rectus muscle and posterior rectus sheath. Recurrence rate was 6.7%. Wantz learned this technique from Rives.
- **Laparoscopic repair (Figs. 13.16 A-D)**
  - Park[18] *et al.* found that laparoscopic repair is having following advantages over open repair:

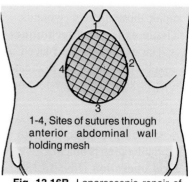

1-4, Sites of sutures through anterior abdominal wall holding mesh

Fig. 13.16B. Laparoscopic repair of incisional hernia, mesh application.

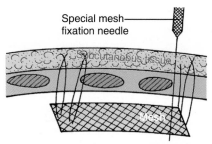

Fig. 13.16C. Laparoscopic repair of incisional hernia, mesh application, method of fixation of mesh.

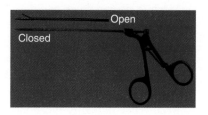

Fig. 13.16D. Shoeman's needle.

– Hospital stay was shorter in laparoscopic repair.
– Post-operative complications were lower in laparoscopic repair.
– The operative time was longer in laparoscopic repair (95 minutes versus 75 minutes) which was the only disadvantage.

Contraindications of laparoscopic repair of incisional hernia

Some of the following contraindications were absolute contraindications earlier but now with better experience they are becoming relative contraindications:
• Extensive previous abdominal surgery.
• Multiple recurrent incisional hernias.
• Big incisional hernia with loss of domain.
• Hernia with incarcerated bowel.
• If other bowel surgery is also required.

Position – Supine

Pneumoperitoneum

It is created with Veress needle.

Ports

• One 10 mm port for camera (camera port)—above or below the hernia.
• Two 5 mm ports (working ports)—one on each side of hernia.
• Palmar's point: Sometimes it is difficult to find safe area to introduce veress needle to create pneumoperitoneum due to big incisional hernia. Three safe points are:
  – **Palmar's point:** Left subcostal midclavicular point at lateral edge of rectus abdominis muscle[30].
  – Right subcostal midclavicular point.
  – Below xiphisternum in epigastrium.

Steps

• Adhesions are divided. While releasing, adhesions remain near anterior abdominal wall rather than bowel. It avoids injury to bowel.
• Size of defect is measured.

- Mesh is shaped so as to cover 5 cm more than the defect on all directions.
- Mesh is folded and introduced through 10 mm port, Inside the peritoneal cavity, mesh is unfolded.
- The mesh is held to abdominal wall with four sutures at four corners which are passed through abdominal wall through four small stab wounds with special needle (Shoeman's needle).
- Now the mesh is fixed with tacks or metal clips.
- Stab incisions are closed conveniently.
- Recurrence rate after incisional ventral hernia repair is reported to range from 10% to 50%.
- Pre operative pneumoperitoneum is required for tension free repair of recurrent ventral hernia. Intraperitonial polypropylene mesh can cause adhesive and erosion in abdominal viscera [31-35].

NOTE

Complications of prosthetic mesh repair in incisional hernia are as follows:
- *Infection of the mesh.*
- *Sinuses and fistulae formation.*
- *Mesh displacement and erosion in surrounding structures, appeared to be technique-specific.[36]*
- *Exposed mesh with wound infection.*

PPM mesh coated with ePTFE prevents adhesions with abdominal viscera.[25]

KEY POINT

The length of the suture material should be at least four times of incision size to avoid tension on suture line in incisional hernia repair.

REFERENCES

1. **Larson GM.** (2000). Ventral hernia repair by laparoscopic approach, *S. Cl. N. Am.*, **80**, 4, 1329.
2. **Read Re, Yoder G.**, (1989). Recent trends in the management of incisional herniation, *Arch. Surg.*, 124: 485–488.
3. **Franz MG.**, (2007). Complications in surgery, Lippincott Williams & Wilkins, p. 523.
4. **Langer S, Christiansen J.**, (1985). Long-term results after incisional hernia repair. *Acta Chir. Scand*, 151: 217–219.
5. **Voeller G.**, (2007). Ventral abdominal hernia, Mastery of surgery, 5th edition, p. 1951.
6. **Cobb WS,** *et al.*, (2005). Laparoscopic repair of incisional hernias, *S. Cl. N. Am.*, 85: 91–103.
7. **Awad ZT, Puri V, Le Blanc K, Fitzgibbons RJ, Iqbal A,** *et al.*, (2005). Mechanisms of ventral hernia recurrences after mesh repair and a new classification, *J. Am. Coll. Surg.*, 201:132–140.
8. **Mannien MJ, Lavonius M, Perhoniemi VJ.**, (1990). Results of incisional hernia repair: a retrospective study of 172 unselected hernioplasties. *Eur. J. Surg.*, 157: 29–31.
9. **Voeller G.**, (2007). Ventral abdominal hernia, Mastery of surgery, 5th edition, pp. 1955–56.
10. **Pollock AV, Evans M.**, (1989). Early prediction of late incisional hernias. *BJS.*, 76: 953–954.
11. **Jenkins TPN.**, (1976). The burst abdominal bowed: A mechanical approach, *BJS.*, 63: 873.
12. **Carlson MA.**, (2001). Acute wound failure, wound healing. *Surg. Clin. N. Am.*, 77(3):607–35.
13. **Bucknall TE, Cox PJ, Ellis H.**, (1982). Burst abdomen an incisional hernia: A prospective study of 1129 major laparotomies, *BMJ*, 284: 931–933.

14. **Irvin TT, Stoddard CJ, Greaney MG.**, (1977). Abdominal wound healing: A prospective clinical study *BMJ*, **2**, 351–352.
15. **Keith W. Millikan.**, (2003). Incisional hernia repair, *Surg. Clin. North Am.*, 83: 1227.
16. **Admirer AA, Dolich MO, Sisley AC, Samimi KJ.**, (2002). Massive ventral hernias: Role of tissue expansion in abdominal wall restoration following abdominal compartment syndrome, *Am. Surg.*, 68: 491–496.
17. **Bebawi MA, Moqtaberi F, Vijay V.**, (1997). Giant incisional hernias stages repair using pneumoperitoneum and expanded polytetra fluoethylene, *Am. Surg.*, 63: 375–381.
18. **Park A, Birch DW, Loverics P.** *et al.*, (1998). Laparoscopic and open incisional hernia repair: A comparison study, *Surgery*, 124: 816–822.
19. **Ramirez OM, Grotto JA.**, (2001). Closure of chronic abdominal wall defects: the components separation technique. In: Bendavid R, Ed. Abdominal wall hernia; Springer, Verlag, 487.
20. **Caldirone MW, Romano M, Bozza F,** *et al.*, (1990). Progressive pneumoperitoneum in management of giant incisional hernias, *Br. J. Surg.*, 77: 306–308.
21. **Raynor RW, Del Geurico LRM.**, (1989). The place for pneumoperitoneum in repair of massive hernia, *World J. Surg.*, 13: 581–585.
22. **Franz GM.**, (2007). Complications in surgery, Lippincott Williams & Wilkins, 541.
23. **Stoppa RE.**, (1989). Treatment of complicated groin and incisional hernias; *WJS.*, 13: 545-54.
24. **Sitzmann JV, McFadden DW.**, (1989). The internal retention repair of massive ventral hernia. *Am. Surg.*, 55: 719–723.
25. **Cameron AEP, Gray RCF, Talbot RW** *et al.*, (1980). Adbominal wound closure: A trial of polypropylene and dexon for *J. Surg.*, 67: 487–491.
26. **Deitch EA, Engel JM.**, (1980). Ultrasonic diagnosis of surgical diseases of the anterior abdominal wall, *Surg. Gynecol. Obstet.*, 151: 484–486.
27. **Rubio PA, Del Castillo H, Alvarez BA.**, (1988). Ventral hernia in a massively obese patient diagnosed by computerized tomography, *South Med. J.*, 1307–1308.
28. **Anthony J, Berger PC, Kem LT,** *et al.*, (2000). Factors affecting recurrence following incisional herniorhaphy, *World J. Surg.*, 24: 95–100.
29. **Ewart CJ, Lankford AB, Gamboa MG.**, (2003). Successful closure of abdominal wall hernias using the component separation technique. *Ann. Plast. Surg.*, 50: 269–273.
30. **Chang FH** *et al.*, (1994). *J. Am. Assoc. Gynaecol. Laparosc.*, 1: 57.
31. **Itani K.M.F., Hawn M.T.** (2008). Biology of hernia formation, *Surg. Clin. N. Am.* **88,** p. 9.
32. **Mayagoitia J.C., Suarez D., Arenas J.C.,** *et al.* (2006). Preoperative progressive pneumoperitoneum in patients with abdominal-wall hernias. *Hernia* 10(3): 213–7.
33. **Novitsky Y.W., Harrell A.G., Cristiano J.A.,** *et al.* (2007). Comparative evaluation of adhesion formation, strength of ingrowth, and textile properties of prosthetic meshes after long-term intra-abdominal implantation in a rabbit. *J. Surg. Res.* 140(1): 6–11.
34. **Robinson T.N., Clarke J.H., Schoen J.,** *et al.* (2005). Major mesh-related complications following hernia repair: events reported to the Food and Drug Administration. Surg. Endosc. 19(12): 1556–60.
35. **Perrone J.M., Soper N.J., Eagon J.C.,** *et al.* (2005) Perioperative outcomes and complications of laparoscopic ventral hernia repair. *Surgery*; 138(4): 708–16.
36. **Bachman S.,** *et al.*, (2008). Prosthetic material in ventral hernia repair: How do I choose? *Surg. Clin. N. Am.*; 88, 103.

14

Divarication of Recti (Diastasis Recti)

"The most important part of the stethoscope is the part between the ears —
Your brain
—John Apley

- Divarication of recti is the separation of two rectus abdominis muscles with bulging of abdominal contents through the gap.
- On raising legs, the bulge is clearly visible.
- On relaxing, fingers can be inserted in the gap.
- Strangulation does not occur.

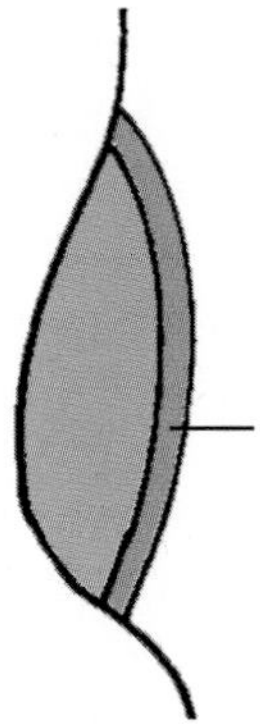

CLINICAL FEATURES (Figs. 14.1 A & B)

- Common in elderly multiparae.
- Sometimes seen in babies and young children.
- Fingers can be insinuated through the gap between two recti.[1]
- Bulge is visible on raising both legs straight up.
- Bulge is noticed during coughing and straining.
- No chance of obstruction or strangulation.

CAUSES

- Multiple pregnancies.
- Repeated midline abdominal operations.
- After chronic distention of abdomen which is due to other causes.

Fig. 14.1A. Divarication of recti, side view.

Rectus abdominis muscle

Anatomical basis of divarication of recti

The rectus muscles are two vertical long muscles originating from lower ribs near midline on each side of midline and are inserted to the pubic symphysis. At origin, these muscles are separated by a gap but at insertion they are very close. So when they contract they are separated by a larger distance from each other in upper abdomen. This separation during contraction is further helped by contraction of two muscles of both sides. These are:
- Internal oblique muscles
- Transverses abdominis muscles

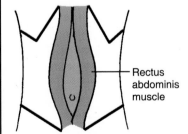

Rectus abdominis muscle

Fig. 14.1. Divarication of recti, front view.

The gap which is created during contraction of muscles is further increased if linea alba is weak. This causes protrusion of abdominal contents through this wide gap.

TREATMENT

- No treatment is required in babies and children as it disappears with their growth and development.
- Abdominal binder or belt is sufficient in adults.
- Operation is not required usually as it does not cause strangulation.

KEY POINT

Divarication of recti does not require any treatment except an abdominal binder.

REFERENCE

RCG Russell *et al.,* (2004). Bailey & Love's short practice of surgery, 24th edition, p. 1292.

15

Spigelian Hernia (SH)

"The two unforgivable sins of surgery, the first great error in surgery is to operate unnecessarily; the second, to undertake an operation for which the surgeon is not sufficiently skilled technically."
— **Max Thorek, (1880-1960)**

Adriaan Van Spieghel Der, 1576-1625, Professor of Anatomy and Surgery, Padua, Italy. He was born in Brussels and educated in Padua.

Spiegel described the following structures:
- Spigelian hernia (Fig. 15.1)
- Spigelian fascia (Fig. 15.2)
- Spigelian line
- Caudate lobe of liver

It is also called "spontaneous lateral ventral hernia" or "Hernia of the semilunar line".

In 1764, Klenklosch recognized the spontaneous nature of these hernias and called them "Hernia of the spigelian line."[1]

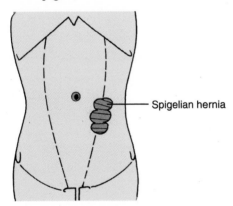

Fig. 15.1. Left Spigelian hernia.

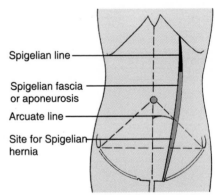

Fig. 15.2. Spigelian fascia aponeurosis and belt.

Spigelian hernia is the protrusion of preperitoneal fat or a peritoneal sac containing or not containing an intra-abdominal organ, across a congenital or acquired defect in Spigelian line.[2]

SPIGELIAN FASCIA (ZONE) OR APONEUROSIS

It is composed by aponeurosis of the following three muscles:
- External oblique muscle

- Internal oblique muscle
- Transversus abdominis muscle

Actually, it is the true aponeurosis of transeversus abdominis muscle lateral to lateral border of rectus muscle.

It is mainly formed by fusion of internal oblique and transversus abdominis aponeurosis between rectus abdominis muscle and transversus abdominis muscles.

It is between lateral margin of rectus muscle and Spigelian line (semilunar line), from eight costal cartilage to pubic tubercle.

- The spigelian zone is 0.3 to 3.7 cm wide.

"S" Belt or Spigelian Hernia Belt

It is a hernia prone area between Monro's line and inter ASIS line in Spigelian aponeurosis. At the junction of semilunar and semicircular lines, Spigelian fascia is the widest and is the weakest and therefore, Spigelian hernia occurs maximum in this area.

ANATOMICAL EXPLANATION OF AETIOLOGY OF SPIGELIAN HERNIA (Fig. 15.3)

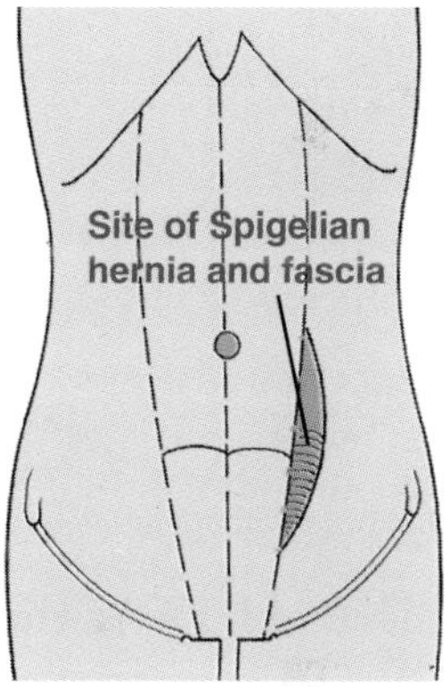

Above the arcuate line aponeurosis, fibres run at right angle and form a strong barrier but below the arcuate line aponeurotic fibres run parallel and so this area becomes a weak area. It is a triangular area which is also pierced by inferior epigastric vessels contributing to more weakness.

This triangular area is the commonest site of Spigelian hernia (Fig. 15.4). Its boundaries are:

- Above – Arcuate line
- Below – Inferior epigastric vessels
- Laterally – Linea semilunaris

Hernia occurs near the junction of linea semicircularis and linea semilunaris.

The hernia ring is formed by aponeurosis of internal oblique and transversus abdominis muscles.[3]

Fig. 15.3. Anatomical explanation of aetiology of Spigelian hernia.

Theories of Aetiology

Spigelian hernia can be congenital or acquired.[4] Following theories have been put forward:

- Perforating vessels may weaken the area in Spigelian fascia and a small lipoma or fat enters here which gradually leads to hernia formation.

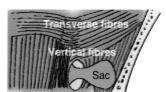

Fig. 15.4. Site of Spigelian hernia.

- Preperitoneal fat may enter and separate internal oblique and transversus abdominis muscles and thus creating a weak area through which Spigelian hernia develops[5] (Fig. 15.5).
- Factors causing raised intra-abdominal pressure, i.e., obesity, multiple pregnancies and COPD facilitate development of Spigelian hernia.
- Rapid loss of weight sometimes causes Spigelian hernia.

Semilunar Line, Spigelian Line or Linea Spigeli

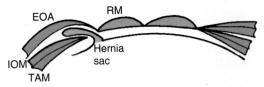

Fig. 15.5. Spigelian hernia protruding between external oblique aponeurosis and internal oblique muscle.

- This line is not clearly seen during surgery.
- Spigelian line is a semilunar line visible on anterior abdominal wall which marks the transition from muscular to aponeurotic area in transversus abdominis. It extends from costal margin to pubic tubercle. It is convex laterally and concave medially. The lateral border of rectus is also marked similarly but Spigelian line is different from it. The Spigelian aponeurosis is the aponeurosis between these two lines. The Spigelian aponeurosis is the widest between umbilicus and interspinal level. More than 90% of Spigelian hernia occurs in this Spigelian hernia belt.

Spigelian hernia passes through transversus abdominis and internal oblique aponeurosis. The external oblique aponeurosis remains intact and is pushed out with skin (Figs. 15.6 A-C).

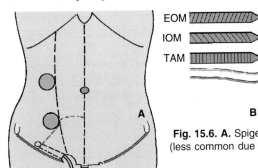

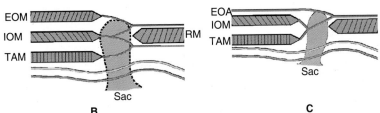

Fig. 15.6. A. Spigelian hernia, above and below umbilicus, **B.** Above umbilicus (less common due to more resistance), **C.** Below umbilicus (more common due to less resistance).

CLINICAL FEATURES (Figs. 15.7 A-D)

Spigelian hernia constitutes 0.12% of all abdominal wall hernias[8]. It is common between 50-60 years of age in both males and females and equally on both right and left sides.

- Spigelian hernia is diagnosed when the patient stands and strains, a bulge appears in the lower abdominal wall which is reduced with a gurgling sound when pressure is applied. In patients with a reducible hernia, the most common features are pain and a lateral bulge on standing. Pain is intermittent and nonspecific.[9]
- Swelling is not big, a slight swelling is seen lateral to rectus muscle at the level of arcuate line.
- Contents and sac are usually under external oblique muscle so hernia ring is not felt.
- Hernia usually protrudes intraparietally so it becomes difficult to diagnose and so it is included in differential diagnosis of obscure abdominal pain.
- Preoperative diagnosis is difficult and only 50% of cases are diagnosed pre-operatively.[1,2]
- 14% patients present with strangulation.

TREATMENT

Conservative

Abdominal support by a belt is needed.

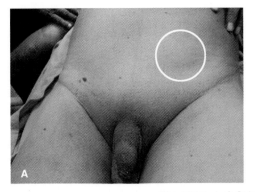
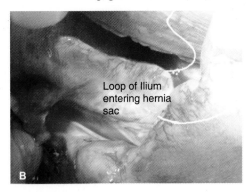

Fig. 15.7A. Left Spigelian hernia, **B.** On operation.

Surgery for Spigelian hernia

- Incision is applied over the swelling.
  - Sac is identified, opened, contents are reduced, sac is ligated and excised.
  - Repair transversus abdominis, internal and external oblique muscles.
- "Prefix mesh plug" can be used to block opening of hernia.

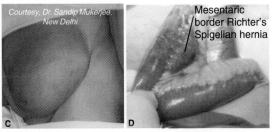

Fig. 15.7C. Huge left Spigelian hernia, **D.** Mesenteric border Richter's Spigelian hernia.

NOTE

Spigelian hernia is a rare occurrence.[6] Mr. Ng found that 10 clinicians of more than 25 years practice in Hong Kong have not seen even one case of Spigelian hernia.[7]

KEY POINT

Spigelian hernia is an interparietal hernia at arcuate line in Spigelian aponeurosis.

REFERENCES

1. **Opson RO, Davis WC.,** (1968). Spigelian hernia: rare or obscure? *Am. J. Surg.,* 116: 842–846.
2. **Read RC.,** (1960). Observations on the aetiology of spigelian hernia: *Ann. Surg.,* 152: 1004–09.
3. **Skandalakis JE, Skandalakis LJ, Colborn GL, Androvlakins J,** *et al.,* (2007). Mastery of surgery, 5th edition, Lippincott Williams & Wilkins, p. 1861.
4. **Weiss J, Lernan OZ, Nissan S.,** (1974). Spigelian hernia, *Ann. Surg.,* 180: 836–839.
5. **Spangen L.,** (1989). Spigelian hernia, *World J. Surg.,* 13: 573–580.
6. **Fischer JE** *et al.,* (2007). Editor's comment, Mastery of surgery, 5th edition, Lippincott Williams & Wilkins, p. 1886.
7. **Ng WT.,** (2004). *Br. J. Surg.,* 91: 640.
8. **Howlihan TJ.,** (1976). A review of spigelian hernia, *Am. J. Surg.,* 131: 734–735.
9. **Salameh J.R.** (2008). Primary and unusual abdominal wall hernias *Surg. Clin. N. Am.* **88,** 1 p. 50.

16

Internal Hernias

"It is less dangerous to leap from the Clifton suspension Bridge than to suffer from acute intestinal obstruction and decline operation."
— **Frederick Treves, 1835-1923**

Internal herniation in the absence of adhesions is uncommon and a preoperative diagnosis is unusual.[1]

AETIOLOGY

- **Congenital causes (Figs. 16.1 - 16.5)**
  - Hernia through foramen of Winslow.
  - Due to malrotation of the gut e.g. paraduodenal hernia.
  - Due to abnormal opening in mesentery e.g.,
    a) Trans-mesenteric hernia
    b) Trans-transverse mesocolon hernia
    c) Trans-sigmoid mesocolon hernia
  - Due to abnormal holes in ligament e.g.,
    a) Trans-gastrocolic ligament hernia
    b) Trans-gastrohepatic ligament hernia
    c) Trans-omental hernia
    d) Trans-broad ligament hernia

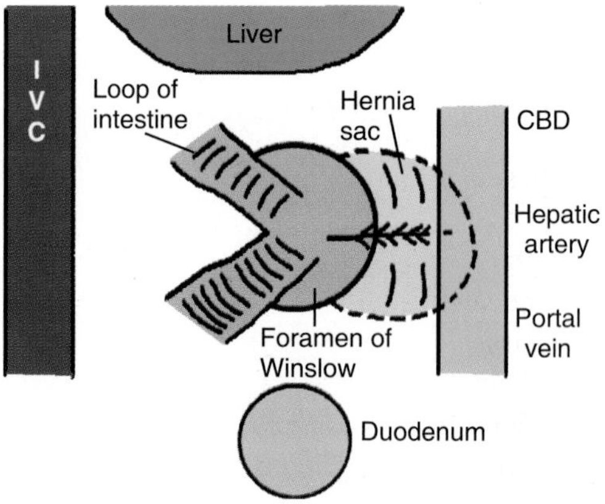

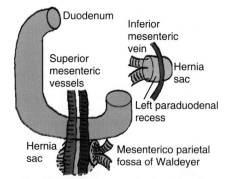

Fig. 16.1. Hernia through foramen of Winslow.

- **Acquired (Fig. 16.6)**
  - Hernia through adhesions of previous operation.
  - Hernia through defects in mesentery caused by previous operation if it was not approximated in whole length after resection and anastomosis e.g., retroanastomotic hernia which occurs after gastrojejunostomy.
  - Hernia through colostomy and ileostomy sites.
  - **Para-transplantation hernia:** Its a rare complication of kidney or liver transplantation. 'Entrapment of bowel or omentum occurs through a defect in peritoneum covering the transplanted kidney or around Roux-en-y loop in liver transplantation.' Volvulus of small intestine is a fatal complication.[7]

Pathology

The internal hernias are of two types:

Fig. 16.2. Common paraduodenal hernias.

- True hernia.
- Internal prolapse
- **True hernia**

  It has a sac. Orifice involved may be
  - Normal orifice: Foramen of Winslow.
  - Paranormal orifice: Peritoneal fossae i.e. paraduodenal, ileocaecal, paracolic, intersigmoid and supravesical.
- **Internal prolapse**

  It has no sac. They may occur through:
  - Abnormal orifice in omentum or mesentery: Transeomental hernia and transemesocolonic hernia.
  - Anomalous orifice: Congenital defects in ligament or in mesentery.
  - Surgical defects or surgically altered anatomy i.e. anastamosis and stomas.
  - Commonest true internal hernia is a paraduodenal hernia.[2]

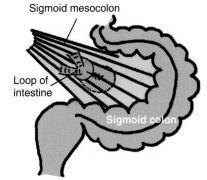

Fig. 16.3. Transmesenteric hernia, through sigmoid mesocolon.

CLINICAL FEATURES

- These are more common in males.
- No external hernia or bulge.
- Signs of intestinal obstruction may be present.
- Ninety percent cases of internal hernia present with acute intestinal obstruction like:
  - Pain
  - Vomiting
  - Distension
  - Absolute constipation (obstipation)

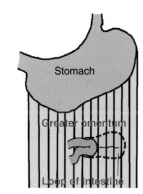

Fig. 16.4. Transomental hernia.

Investigations

- X-ray abdomen – Shows distended loops of intestine.
- CECT abdomen.
- Diagnostic laparoscopy.
- Exploratory laparotomy.

Differential Diagnosis

- Adhesions due to previous surgery account for 60% of all small bowel obstruction, including adhesions at prosthetic tissue interface.[8]
- Incarcerated or strangulated hernia, e.g., inguinal and femoral hernias.
- Neoplasm – Primary neoplasm of small bowel causing obstruction.
- Intussusception of small bowel.

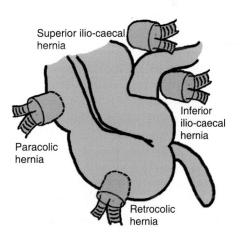

Fig. 16.5. Paracaecal hernias.

- Volvulus of small bowel.
- Stricture of small bowel.
- Gallstones causing small bowel obstruction.

TREATMENT

Diagnosis is frequently delayed.[3] In these patients the use of dilute barium or water soluble contrast small bowel studies are often helpful.[4-5]

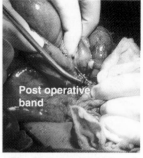

Fig. 16.6. Acquired internal hernia.

> **NOTE**
>
> *The essence of the treatment is early intervention which is the only means to prevent gangrene of bowel.*

- Operation should be performed at the earliest to avoid strangulation.
- Hernia is reduced and bowel is assessed for viability after giving 100% oxygen and moist packs application. If gangrene has developed then resection is done.
- Defects are closed with non-absorbable sutures.
- Some Iatrogenic retroanastomotic hernia, according to Markowitz AM, are the result of formation of internal hernia ring after construction of gastrojejunostomy.[6] In strangulated hernia, the incision should be placed on the ring where blood vessels, nerves, and viscera are prevented from injury.

> **KEY POINTS**
>
> - *Internal hernias are intra-abdominal hernia.*
> - *5% cases of all intestinal obstruction are caused by internal hernia.*
> - *80% of internal hernia have strangulation or gangrene.*

REFERENCES

1. **Russell RCG,** *et al.,* (2004). Bailey & Love's short practice of surgery, 24th edition, p. 1193.
2. **Cuschieri A,** *et al.,* (2002). Essential surgical practice, 4th edition, p. 168.
3. **Brown SP.,** (2005). Acute conditions of the small bowel and appendix, Core topics in general and emergency surgery, 3rd edition, pp. 170–171.
4. **Chen SC,** *et al.,* (1999). Water soluble contrast study predicts the need for early surgery in adhesion small bowel obstruction, *Br. J. Surg.,* 1986: 1692–8.
5. **Brochwocz MJ,** *et al.,* (2003). Small bowel obstruction: The water soluble follow-through revisited. *Clin. Radiol.,* 50: 393–7.
6. **Markowitz AM.,** (1964). Retroanastomotic hernia: In: Nyhus LM, Harkins HN, Eds., Hernia. Philadelphia: JB Lippincott, 607.
7. **Kiryakides GK, Simmons RL, Bules J,** *et al.,* "Paratransplant hernia", three patients with a new variant of internal hernia, *Am. J. Surg.,* 136: 629–30.
8. **Earle DB.,** *et al.,* (2008), Prosthetic-material in inguinal hernia repair: How do I choose? *Surg. Clin. N. Am,* 88, 188.

17 Recurrent Inguinal Hernia

"The surgeon's best hernia repair is the one with which they have had the greatest experience"
— **Crawford & Philips**

"Experience reveals that, despite the advances made in the field of hernia surgery where prostheses and laparoscopy have made significant contributions, the need to know anatomy and to be able to perform a pure tissue repair has become indispensable and imperative. Recurrences are still and often the result of inadequate dissection, failure to recognize a hernia, repair under tension, or an inappropriate use of a prosthesis."
— **Robert Bendavid 2007**

Recurrence of inguinal hernia occurs in about 1–5% of patients, but the rate is higher when surgical technique is poor.

* Rate of recurrence 2-8% (Fig. 17.1).
* Ideally it should be less than 1%.
* Recurrence usually occurs within one year of operation.

GENERAL CAUSES OF RECURRENCE

* Chronic cough
* Obesity
* Weak muscle tone
* Straining while passing urine as in BPH
* Straining while passing stool as in habitual constipation
* Smoking
  - It causes collagen deficiency and makes tissues weak and prone for recurrence.

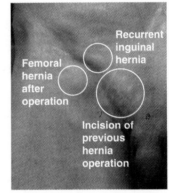

Fig. 17.1. Recurrent inguinal and femoral hernias.

> - "Recently molecular biological investigations have proven the theory of distrubed composition of extracellular matrix in patients with recurrent hernia. In particular, there is a decreased ratio of collagen type I and III".[1]

Intraoperative causes

* Absorbable sutures.
* Tension on suture line – It causes devitalization of tissue which gets replaced by fibrous tissue. The fibrous tissue is weak and causes recurrence.
* Improper ligation of sac.
  - Low ligation of sac (at fundus or body) causes recurrence.
* When the inventor of a new technique for hernia repair, such as Shouldice, operates, the recurrence

rate is low. But when the same procedure is done by others at non-specialized centres, the recurrence rate increases, more than 20% from Shouldice's method.

- Imperfect haemostasis leads to haematoma which causes infection. This infection further leads to weak scar which may result in recurrence.
- The other important aspect especially in the repair of recurrent hernias is that repetition of previously inadequate technique frequently fails.[2]

Post-operative causes

- Wound infection is the commonest cause of recurrence.
- Lifting of heavy weight within three months of operation.
- Persistent straining in post-operative period is due to:
  - Cough
  - BPH / urethral stricture
  - Straining at defaecation

False recurrence

Sometimes the recurrence is not a true recurrence. It is due to:
- A new hernia – After the operation of indirect inguinal hernia a new direct hernia develops.
- An old hernia – One hernia was overlooked at the time of first operation when two hernias were present.

The following type of hernias are more prone for recurrence:

- Very large hernia
- Large direct inguinal hernia
- Sliding hernia
  - Most important cause of early recurrence is faulty technique.
  - Most important cause of late recurrence is tissue failure.
  - Majority of incisional hernias start in post-operative period due to partial disruption of deep layers of the wound.
  - Large reported series shows reccurence rate <1%[3] with TEP. Another series[4] showed recurrence rate of 3.2% IPOM, 0.8% TAPP and 0% TEP.
  - The reported recurrence rate following primary inguinal hernia repair is around 1%, while the recurrence rate following the repair of multiple recurrent hernias is 12%. A prospective randomized, controlled, trial of incisional hernia repair established a 0% recurrence with the use of an alloplastic mesh implant and a 54% recurrence rate following a primary repair using in situ.

69.2% direct inguinal hernia recurrence occurs in medial position of floor of inguinal canal.[4]

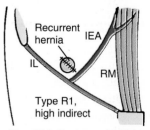

Fig. 17.2. Recurrent inguinal hernia type R1.

CLASSIFICATION OF RECURRENT HERNIA

Giampiero Campanelli[5] *et al.* gave a simple anatomo-clinical classification and have classified the recurrent inguinal hernia into following grades:[6] (Figs. 17.2-17.4)

- **Type R1**
  - First recurrence
  - High 'Indirect'
  - Reducible
  - Less than 2 cm size of defect in thin person
- **Type R2**
  - First recurrence
  - Low 'Direct'
  - Reducible
  - Less than 2 cm size of defect in thin person
- **Type R3**
  - Re-recurrence
  - Involves whole wall
  - Non-reducible more than 2 cm size of defect in overweight patient

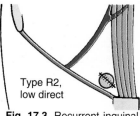

Fig. 17.3. Recurrent inguinal hernia type R2.

- Recurrence rate after repair of inguinal hernia increases with increased length of follow-up period,[7] 50 percent in 1st operative year, 75 percent at 2 years and 90 percent at 3 years.[15]
- Recurrence rates also increase when dedicated, expert post-operative examinations are used for assessment.[8]
- Inguinal hernia recurrence rates are 1% to 11% when general surgeons use these techniques outside the dedicated centers.[9]

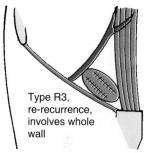

Fig. 17.4. Recurrent inguinal hernia type R3.

TREATMENT OF RECURRENT HERNIA

The interval between the first and the second operation should be at least 6 months to allow optimum recovery of the tissues to be used again for repair.[10]

If the previous repairs were open anterior then the recurrence should be dealt with either laparoscopically or using an open preperitoneal technique.[11]

- First time recurrence without infection is repaired by Lichtenstein repair.
- Subsequent recurrence and first time recurrence after Lichtenstein repair is dealt with Laparoscopic repair.

A recent multicentre randomized trial showed that the recurrence rate after repair of recurrent hernia, even by an experienced surgeon was 3-6% in laparoscopic group and 17.2% using an open anterior technique.[12]

- Polypropylene mesh hernioplasty is the operation of choice.
- The recurrence after operating a recurrent hernia is more common with open hernia repair than laparoscopic hernia because the approach in open repair hernia is through the unhealthy tissue, i.e., scar tissue and in laparoscopic repair it is through healthy tissue, i.e., virgin route.
- Treatment of the precipitant factors is important.
- Kuntz operation prevents the recurrence completely. It is recommended in elderly patients with multiple recurrences.
- In every case of recurrence and specially in re-recurrence, a cause must be diagnosed so that the further recurrence after operation is avoided.

> **NOTE**
>
> *Recurrence after laparoscopic inguinal hernia repair probably is more with technical error than other factors. To produce the best quality, repair requires advanced laparoscopic skills and routine and strict adherence to the standardized principles of the preperitoneal technique.[13]*

> **KEY POINT**
>
> *Recurrence is related to experience of surgeon, technical failure, tissue failure and infection.*

REFERENCES

1. **Jansen PL, Mertens Pr P, Klinge U, Schumpelic KV.,** (2004). The biology of hernia formation, 136: 1–4.
2. **Klinge U, Conze J., Krones CJ, Schumpelick V:** (2005). Incisional hernias: Open techniques, *World J. Surg.,* 29: 1066–72.
3. **Klaiber C,** *et al.,* (1999) Totallly endoscopic preperitoneal prothesis in recurrent inguinal hernia. *In*: Schumpelick V, Kingsnorth AW (Eds), Incisional Hernia, Berlin; Springer-Verlag, p. 424–430.
4. **MacFadyen BV Jr, Arregui ME, Corbitt JD, Jr.** *et al.,* (1993). Complication of laparoscopic herniorrhaphy. *Surg. Endosc.,* 7: 155–9.
5. **Campanelli G, Pettinari D, Cavalli M, Avesani EC.,** (2006). Inguinal hernia recurrence; Classification and Approach, *Journal of Minimal Access Surgery,* **2,** p. 147.
6. **Campanelli G, Cavagnoli R, Buratti MS, Clofri U, Casirani R.,** (2004). The preperitoneal prosthetic approach for the repair of Recurrent Inguinal Hernia, Wantz technique; New procedures in open hernia surgery, p. 85.
7. **Franz GM.,** (2007). Complications in Surgery, Lippincott Williams & Wilkins, 530.
8. **Franz GM.,** (2007). Complications in Surgery, Lippincott Williams & Wilkins, 533.
9. **Rutledge RH.,** (1993) The Cooper ligament repair: *Surg. Clin. North Am.,* 73(3): 471–485.
10. **Welsh DRJ, Alexander MAJ.,** (1993). The shouldice repair: *Surg. Clin. North Am.,* 73(3): 451–469.
11. **Kurzer M, Belshaw PA, Kark AE.,** (2002). Prospective study of open preperitoneal mesh repair for recurrent inguinal hernia. *Br. J. Surg.,* 89: 90–93.
12. **Neumayer L, Giobbie, Hurder A, Jonasson O,** *et al.,* (2004). Open mesh versus laparoscopic mesh repair of inguinal hernia. *N. Engl. J. Med.,* 350: 1819–1827.
13. **Kukleta JF.,** (2006). Causes of recurrence in laparoscopic inguinal hernia repair, *Journal of Minimal Access Surgery,* **2,** p. 190.
14. **Obney N, Chanck.,** (1984). Repair of multiple time recurrent inguinal hernias with reference to common causes of recurrence, *Contemp. Surg.,* 25: 24.
15. **Shell DH.,** *et al.,* (2008). Open repair of ventral incisional hernias. *Surg. Clin. N. Am.;* 88, 63.

18

Rare Hernias

"In study of some apparently new problems we often make progress by reading the work of the great men of the past."
— **Charles H. Mayo, (1865-1939)**

"It is important to know about rare hernias also as any strangulated hernia may prove fatal whether common or rare."
— **Author**

Following rare hernias are seen in surgical practice (Figs. 18.1A & B)

INTERSTITIAL HERNIA

It is defined as a hernia in which the sac emerges between the anterior abdominal muscles.[1]

Hesselbach demonstrates in 1814 an interstitial hernia in an autopsy, the sac was between internal and external oblique.

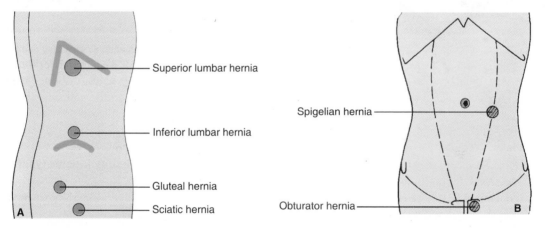

Fig. 18.1A. Rare hernias on side and back of abdomin, **B.** Rare hernia on anterior abdominal wall.

Aetiology

The aetiology of interstitial hernia is explained by the following two theories[2]:
- **Congenital theory**
  - All interstitial hernias are due to a congenital defect.[2]
- **Mechanical theory**
  - There is an area of weakness in the muscles of inguinal area.[2]

Classification

Interstitial hernias are classified into the following three groups by Field[3] in 1921:

- **Preperitoneal or intraparietal** – The sac lies between peritoneum and fascia transversalis.
- **Interparietal** – The sac lies between internal oblique muscle and external oblique aponeurosis.
- **Extraparietal** – The sac lies outside the external oblique aponeurosis in subcutaneous tissue.

The inguino-interstitial group is further divided into following four types:
- **Type I** – The sac is located between fascia transversalis and transverse abdominal muscle.
- **Type II** – The sac located between transverse abdominis and internal oblique.
- **Type III** – The sac located between internal and external oblique muscles.
- **Type IV** – The sac located between external oblique aponeurosis and Scarpa's fascia.
  - The hernia sac lies in between different muscle layers of abdominal wall.
  - The hernial sac is usually incomplete.

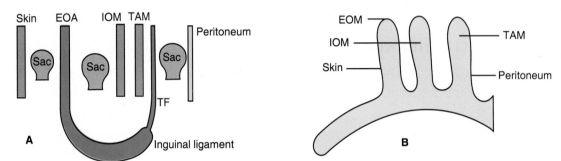

Fig. 18.2A. Interstitial hernia, very rare between internal oblique muscle and transversus abdominis muscle due to formation of conjoint tendon, **B.** Protrusion of peritoneal sac between different layers of abdominis muscles.

Clinical Features

- Most of the patients are males.
- Mostly present as intestinal obstruction due to incarceration or strangulation.
- Delay in operation is due to delay in diagnosis which may lead to high mortality in some types of interstitial hernia (preperitoneal).
- It occurs in 0.08% cases.
- Plain X-ray of abdomen reveals intestinal obstruction.
- MRI is helpful in diagnosis of interstitial hernia.
- Ninety percent of interstitial hernia is presented with intestinal obstruction and undescended testis.

Treatment

Exploratory laparotomy is done, then prolene mesh is applied but if the wound is contaminated then mesh is not used. If recurrence occurs, then elective prosthetic repair is done.

OGILVIE HERNIA (Figs. 18.3 A & B)

It is named after Sir William Heneage Ogilvie, 1887-1971, English surgeon. He also gave "Ogilvie Syndrome", false or pseudocolonic obstruction.
- It is a type of direct inguinal hernia.

- It is also called funicular direct inguinal or prevesical hernia.
- There is a congenital defect in conjoint tendon.
- A strangulation is the common feature of this hernia.
- If it contains urinary bladder then history of swelling becoming less prominent after micturition is present.

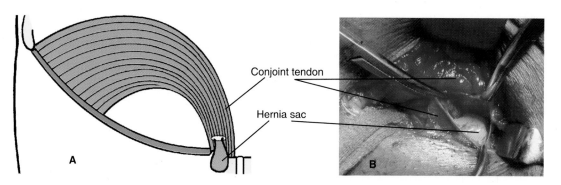

Fig. 18.3A. Right Ogilvie hernia, diagrammatic representation, **B.** On exploration.

LUMBAR HERNIA

Posterior abdominal wall is having the following boundaries:

- Lateral–A line straight up from ASIS touching ribs.
- Medial–5 lumbar vertebrae.
- Superior–Lower ribs.
- Inferior–Iliac crest.

Hernia in lumbar region of abdomen is called lumbar hernia.

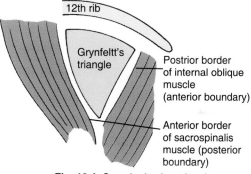

Fig. 18.4. Superior lumbar triangle.

- 5% of lumbar hernia occur outside lumbar triangles and 95% occur inside lumbar triangles.
- Incarceration and strangulation occur in about 10% cases.[4]

Lumbar hernia is of the following types:

- Superior lumbar hernia (SLH) – It is a primary hernia (Fig. 18.4).
- Inferior lumbar hernia (ILH) – It is a primary hernia.
- Primary lumbar hernia – It is rare, only few hundred cases have been so far reported.
- Secondary lumbar hernia or acquired lumbar hernia or incisional lumbar hernia – It occurs after open renal surgery.

Superior Lumbar Hernia (SLH)

"SLH is the protrusion of abdominal contents through superior lumbar triangle." Rarer than inferior lumbar hernia.

Superior lumbar triangle (Grynfelt's or Lesgaft's triangle) has the following boundaries:
- Superior boundary – 12th rib.
- Medial boundary – Sacrospinalis muscle.
- Lateral boundary – Posterior border of internal oblique muscle.

Inferior Lumbar Hernia (ILH) or Petit's Triangle

"It is the protrusion of abdominal contents through inferior lumbar triangle more common than superior lumbar hernia."

Hernias in the inferior lumbar triangle are most often small and occur in young athletic women.[5]

Inferior lumbar triangle or Triangle of Petit is named after Jean Louis Petit, 1674-1750, Director of the Academie de Chirurgia, Paris, France. It has the following boundaries:
- **Lower boundaries** – Iliac crest.
- **Medial boundaries** – Anterior border of latissimus dorsi muscle.
- **Lateral boundaries** – Posterior border of external oblique muscle.

Clinical Features of Lumbar Hernia

Primary lumbar hernia are rare, only few hundred cases so far have been reported. Superior lumbar hernia is also called Grynfeltt's hernia and is less common than inferior lumbar hernia.
- Soft reducible swelling in the region of superior or inferior lumbar triangle.
- Expansile impulse on coughing is present.
- Phantom hernia – It is a hernia in lumbar region due to paralysis of lumbar muscles due to polio.
- Inferior lumbar hernia is usually a small swelling. Incarceration appears in 10% cases.
- Recurrence rate is very low.

Differential Diagnosis

Lipoma

- Lipoma sometimes simulates hernia as fat feels like liquid at body temperature.
- Moves over underlying contracted muscles.
- It is non-reducible.
- There is no impulse on coughing.

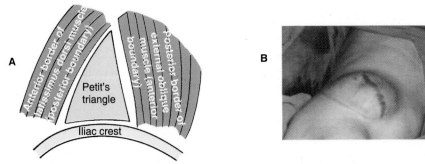

Fig. 18.5A. Inferior lumbar triangle, **B.** Right secondary inferior lumbar hernia.

Cold abscess

- A paravertebral abscess may point in any lumbar triangle.
- It is a cystic swelling.
- Fluctuation is present.
- Impulse on coughing may be present.
- X-ray of thoracic and lumbar spine is diagnostic.

Treatment

- Excision of sac and herniorrhaphy is the treatment of choice.
- Phantom hernia – It is operated like an incisional hernia.
- Recurrence is very low.
- It can also be repaired by laparoscopic techniques either intraperitoneal or retroperitoneal route.[6]

OBTURATOR HERNIA (Fig. 18.8)

To understand obturator hernia one must understand the basic anatomy of the following structures:
- Obturator area
- Obturator foramen (Fig. 18.6)
- Obturator canal
- Obturator membrane

- **Obturator area** is bounded by the following structures:
  - **Above:** Superior ramus of pubic bone.
  - **Below:** Ischiopubic ramus and adductor magnus.
  - **Medial:** Pubic arch and abductor muscles.
  - **Lateral:** Hip joint and upper part of femur.
- **Obturator foramen:**
  - It is a big hole in the hip bone.
  - It is formed by ischium and pelvic bones.
  - It is covered by obturator membrane.
- **Obturator canal:**
  - It is approximately 3 cm long.
  - It connects pelvic cavity to outside.
  - It is the site of protrusion of obturator hernia.
  - It has the following boundaries:
    a) **Superior and lateral boundaries:** Obturator groove of pelvis bone.
    b) **Inferior boundary:** Upper free edges of: (i) Obturator membrane; (ii) Obturator externus muscle; (iii) Obturator internus muscle.
  - It is 2-3 cm long and passes through the following structures:
    a) Obturator artery   b) Obturator vein   c) Obturator nerve
     In strangulated obturator hernia incision is made at lower margin of hernia ring to avoid injury to obturator vessels and nerve.
- **Obturator membrane:** It is a membrane which covers the whole obturator foramen except the obturator groove.[7]

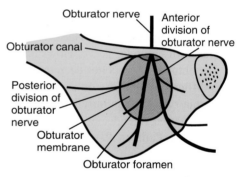

Fig. 18.6. Obturator foramen, membrane, canal and nerve.

Clinical Features

- It is the most lethal hernia of abdominal wall, mortality rate is 13% to 14%.[8]
- It is an extremely rare hernia.
- It is six times more common in females.
- It is common in females of more than 60 years of age.
- It is common in females who have recently lost considerable weight due to loss of fat. So it is common in thin built elderly females.
- It is more common in females than in males because obturator foramen is wider in females.

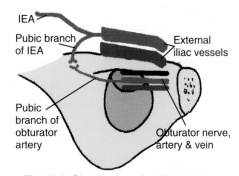

Fig. 18.7. Obturator canal and structures passing through it.

- It is difficult to diagnose as no swelling is present.
- Strangulation is common in obturator hernia.
- It is diagnosed on laparotomy only which is done for acute intestinal obstruction.
- To make hernia visible, position the lower limb in the following positions to make the hernia prominent
  - Flexion, Abduction, External rotation
- It is found beneath pectineus muscle.
- Patient limps with semi-flexed leg as movement causes pain.
- The Hannington-Kiff sign is a specific sign in obturator hernia. It is an absent adductor reflex in thigh.[9]
- Pain is referred to knee on the same side due to the articular branch of obturator nerve (Howship-Romberg Sign).
- The obturator hernia lies deep to the pectineus muscle and is difficult to diagnose on examination.
- Hernia swelling can only be palpated by rectal or vaginal examination. A tender swelling is felt at the site of obturator foramen. Pain on P/V and P/R examination indicates strangulation.
- Richter's hernia is common in obturator hernia.
- Fullness in femoral triangle on one side is suggestive of obturator hernia.
- Small bowel is the commonest organ involved in obturator hernia.

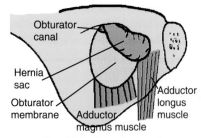

Fig. 18.8. Obturator hernia.

Important features of obturator hernia

- Six times more common in females.
- Strangulation is common.
- Hernia can be only palpated by P / V and P / R examination.
- Common in females above 60 years of age.
- Richter's hernia is common.

Treatment

If obturator hernia is diagnosed then early operation is performed as it gets strangulated. The operation has the following two approaches:

- **Abdominal approach**

When the diagnosis is known preoperatively, posterior preperitoneal approach, either laparoscopic or open through lower paramedian or midline or Pfannen steil incision is preferred.[14]

It is the best approach. Dilate the obturator foramen by big artery forceps and reduce the hernia sac. Take care of obturator vessel as they can get damaged. If case is undiagnosed, laparotomy is done.

- **Femoral approach**
  - Vertical incision is made medial to femoral vessels.
  - Retract the adductor longus muscle and divide or separate pectineus muscle to expose obturator externus muscle.
  - Usually the hernia sac is found protruding at upper border of obturator externus muscle.
  - Herniorrhphy is performed by repairing the defect in obturator foramen.
- Retropubic approach (Cheatle Hernia approach) may also be used in certain cases.
- Obturator hernia can also be dealt with an approach through urinary bladder wall.
- Obturator hernia can be operated by laparoscopic method,[10] extra or transperitoneally.
- It is better to place a PPM preperitoneally covering obturator foramen & femoral and inguinal areas.[15]

GLUTEAL HERNIA (Fig. 18.9)

- It is a rare hernia, occurs through greater sciatic foramen, either above or below the pyriformis muscle, as a bulge in gluteal region.

Differential Diagnosis

Following conditions simulate gluteal hernia:
- Lipoma
- Cold abscess
- Fibrosarcoma under gluteus maximus muscle
- Gluteal aneurysm

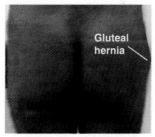

Fig. 18.9. Right Gluteal hernia.

Treatment

All such swellings must be explored by operation. Sac is excised. Contents are reduced. Defect is repaired by non-absorbable sutures. A proper repair reduces the chances of recurrence.

SCIATIC HERNIA (Fig. 18.10)

"It is the rarest hernia of abdominal wall.
It occurs through lesser sciatic foramen."

- It is the protrusion of peritoneal contents through greater or lesser sciatic foramen.
- It lies under gluteus maximus muscle.
- It is divided into three types by pyriformis muscle:
  - Supra-pyriformis hernia

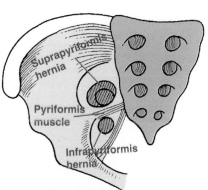

Fig. 18.10. Sciatic hernia.

- Infra-pyriformis hernia
- Sub-pyriformis hernia

Clinical Features

- A globular swelling appears which distorts the contour of the gluteal area.
- It is painless and non-tender.
- Loops of bowel in the hernia sac produce gurgling sound.

Differential Diagnosis

Following conditions simulate sciatic hernia:
- Cold abscess
- Lipoma
- Gluteal aneurysm
- Fibrosarcoma under gluteal maximus muscle

Treatment

All such swellings must be explored by operation. Sac is excised. Contents are reduced. Defect is repaired by non-absorbable sutures.

PERINEAL OR MERY'S HERNIA (Figs. 18.11 & 18.12)

Perineal hernia was first reported by Scarpa in 1821.

"Perineal hernia is a herniation of the abdominal contents through the pelvic floor." It is a rare hernia.

- Perineum a diamond-shaped area. It has the following boundaries:
  - **Anterior**
    a) Pubic symphysis
    b) Arcuate ligament
  - **Posterior**
    a) Coccyx
  - **Anterolateral**
    a) Ischiopubic rami
    b) Ischial tuberosities
  - **Posterolateral**
    a) Sacrotuberous ligament
- Perineum is divided into the following two regions by a transverse line between two ischial tuberosities:
  - **Anterior region:** Urogenital triangle
  - **Posterior region:** Anal triangle
- Anterior perineal hernia occurs through urogenital triangle or anterior to superficial transverse perineal muscle. It is exclusively found in females.

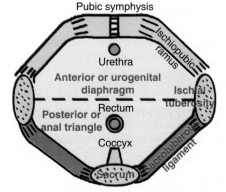

Fig. 18.11. Perineum.

- Posterior perineal hernia occurs through anal triangle or posterior to superficial transverse perineal muscle.

- Protrusion occurs through pelvic floor.
- Usually the sac is wide-necked.
- Obstruction is rare.
- Cystocele and rectocele are not perineal hernia.

Types of Perineal Hernia

- **Anterolateral or Pudendal hernia** – Hernia occurs in labia majora.
- **Posterolateral or Ischiorectal hernia** – Hernia protrudes in ischio-rectal fossa through
  - Levator ani.
  - **Hiatus of Schwalbe** (an opening to ischiorectal fossa through a gap between origin of levator ani and obturator fascia).
- **Median hernia** – sliding hernia – complete rectal prolapse.
  - **Post-operative perineal hernia:** It occurs through perineal post-operative scar after perineal prostatectomy, abdominal perineal resection of rectum or pelvic exenteration.[11]

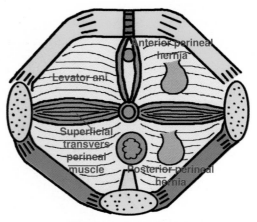

Fig. 18.12. Perineal hernias.

Perineal hernia is five times more common in females due to the following reasons:

- Broader pelvis
- Pregnancy and childbirth:
  a) Changes in pelvis occur due to prolonged pressure.
  b) Obstetric trauma.

Treatment

Repair is usually done by an abdominal approach.

Incision is made directly over the swelling. The sac is opened and the contents of the sac are reduced. The sac gets adhered with the surrounding structures and the adhesions are cleared. Sac is excised. Repair is done by muscle apposition or prosthetic mesh repair.

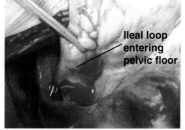

Fig. 18.13. Anterior perineal hernias.

SUPRAVESICAL HERNIA (Fig. 18.14)

- "It is a hernia in which the sac protrudes through the supravesical fossa."
- Sir Astley Cooper recognized the hernia in 1804. The term supravesical hernia was proposed by Warvi and Orr.[12]

- **External supravesical hernia**
  It is the protrusion of peritoneal viscera through supravesical fossa. It is medial to direct inguinal hernia site.
- **Internal supravesical hernia**
  The protrusion of abdominal viscera occurs through supravesical fossa and it is confined to the vicinity of urinary bladder. It is of three types:

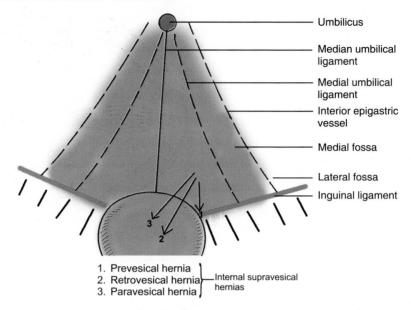

1. Prevesical hernia ⎫
2. Retrovesical hernia ⎬ Internal supravesical
3. Paravesical hernia ⎭ hernias

Fig. 18.14. Supravesical hernias, laparoscopic view.

- Anterior or prevesical hernia.
  a) Retropubic hernia
  b) Invaginating hernia
- Posterior or retrovesical hernia
- Lateral or paravesical hernia

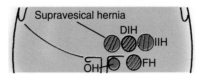

Fig. 18.15. Supravesical hernia, anterior view.

SOME RARE HERNIAS

Barth's Hernia

Hernia of loops of intestine between the serosa of the abdominal wall and that of a persistent vitelline duct.

Cooper's Hernia

A femoral hernia with additional tracts into the scrotum or towards the labium majus, and towards the obturator foramen.

Diverticular Hernia

Littre's hernia.

Dry Hernia

A hernia in which the sac and its contents are intimately adherent to each other.

Encysted Hernia

Scrotal and oblique inguinal hernia in which the intestine enveloped in its own proper sac, passes into the tunica vaginalis testis and has three coverings of peritoneum. It is also called Hey's hernia.

Fat Hernia

Hernial protrusion of properitoneal fat through the abdominal wall. It is also called hernia adiposa.

Hesselbach's Hernia

Hernia of a loop of intestine through the cribriform fascia.

Holthouse's Hernia (Fig. 18.16)

An inguinal hernia that has turned outward into the groin.

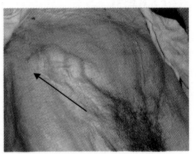

Fig. 18.16. Holthouse's hernia.

Inguinoproperitoneal Hernia

Hernia that is partly inguinal and partly properitoneal. It is also called Kronlein's hernia.

Hernia-en-bissac

It is also called properitoneal or Kronlein's hernia. It has a double sac. One part is in the inguinal canal and the other part projects from the deep inguinal ring into subperitoneal tissue.

Sportsman's Hernia

It is a groin pain in the absence of an obvious groin hernia. It usually occurs in athletes and sportsmen.
    Groin exploration may be helpful as sometimes occult hernia is found.
    In some persons, tenotomy of adductor tendon is helpful when strain over adductor muscles is the reason of groin pain.

Phantom Hernia (Fig. 18.17)

It is a muscle bulge due to paralysis of muscle which is due to the loss of its nerve supply. It is commonly seen in poliomyelitis.

Berger's Hernia

It is a hernia in the pouch of Douglas.
    Gilmore[13] attributed it to dilated superficial inguinal ring (Gilmore groin).

Gibbon's Hernia

It is a hernia associated with a hydrocele.

Beclard's Hernia

It is a type of femoral hernia. It occurs through saphenous opening.

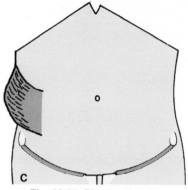

> **NOTE**
>
> *Experienced hernia surgeons must have clinical and operative knowledge of rare hernias also.*

Fig. 18.17. Phantom hernia.

> **KEY POINT**
>
> *Lumbar hernias are mostly secondary, primary lumbar hernia is extremely rare.*

REFERENCES

1. **Lower WE, Hicken NF.**, (1931). Interparietal hernias, *Ann. Surg.*, 94: 1070–1087.
2. **Altman B.**, (1989). Interparietal hernia. In: Nyhus LM, Condon RE, Editors. Hernia. Philadelphia, J.B., Lippincott, p. 380–387.
3. **Fuld JE.**, (1921), Interparietal inguinal hernia. *Int. J. Surg.*, 43: 132.
4. **Killeen KL,** *et al.*, (2000). Using CT to diagnose traumatic lumbar hernia. *AJR Am. J. Roentgenol* 174: 1413.
5. **Thor K.**, (1985). Lumbar hernia. *Acta Chir. Scand.* 151: 389.
6. **Habib E.**, (2003). Retroperitoneoscopic tension-free repair of lumbar hernia. Hernia. 7: 150.
7. **Skandalakis JE, Skandalakis LJ, Colborn GL, Androvlakins J,** *et al.*, (2007). Mastery of surgery, 5th edition, Lippincott Williams & Wilkins, p. 1871.
8. **Tucker JG, Wilson RA, Ramshaw BJ,** *et al.*, (1995). Laparoscopic herniorraphy: Technical concerns in prevention of complications and early recurrence. *Am. Surg.*, 61: 36.
9. **Hannington-Kiff JG.**, (1980). Absent thigh reflex in obturator hernia, Lancet; 1 (8161): p. 180.
10. **Naude G,** *et al.,* (1997). Obturator hernia is an unsuspected diagnosis, *Am. J. Surg.*, 174: 72.
11. **So JB,** *et al.,* (1997). Post operative perineal hernia. *Dis colon Rectum*, 40: 954.
12. **Warvi WN, Orr TG.**, (1940). Internal Supravasical hernias; *Surgery*, 312–325.
13. **Gilmor OJA.**, (1991). Gilmore groin. Ten years experience of groin disruption–A previously unsolved problem in sportsmen. Sports medicine and soft tissue trauma, 1: 3: 12–14.
14. **Salameh JR.**, (2008). Primary and unusual abdominal wall hernias. *Surg. Clin. N. Am.*, 88, 57.
15. **Bergstein JM, Condon RE.** (1996). Obturator hernia: current diagnosis and treatment. *Surgery*; 119(2):133–6.

Section 4
OPERATIVE SURGERY

"Courage is what it takes to standup & speak,
Courage is also what it takes to sitdown & listen"
-Winston Churchill

19

Operative Surgery

"The incision must be as long as necessary and as short as possible"

— **Theodor Kocher, Swiss Surgeon**

(Said more than 100 years back).
"You can judge the worth of a surgeon by the way he does a hernia"

— **Thomas Fair Bank (1876-1961)**

"One must remember that, whether one calls it "minimal access" or
what have you, incision heals from side to side, not end to end,
and in doing an operation it is necessary to make the incision
sufficiently long so one can do what one sets out to do easily."

— **Editor's Comment**
Mastery of Surgery, 5th Edition 2007

Surgery is the only curative treatment of a hernia (Figs. 19.1-19.4).

"When physiology is disrupted attempts at restoring anatomy are futile.
The preparation of the patient for surgery may be as crucial as the operation itself."
- **James C. Rucinski**

The goals of surgery in hernia are to relieve pain and cure the hernia to prevent complications.

PREOPERATIVE PREPARATIONS

• Aspirin and clopidogrel should be stopped at least seven days before the surgery and should not be started two weeks after operation.

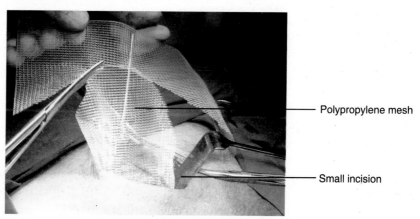

— Polypropylene mesh

— Small incision

Fig. 19.1. Open groin hernia repair.

- Obese patients must be asked to reduce weight if there is no emergency. Obese patients infact should be refused for operation until they reduce their weight substantially to reach their ideal weight. It is done so as to avoid recurrence.
- Chronic cough must be investigated. Bronchitis and bronchial asthma etc. must be controlled and treated as repeated coughing in post-operative period may contribute to recurrence. Hernia operation should be delayed in patients with acute or chronic cough until treated successfully, to avoid recurrence.

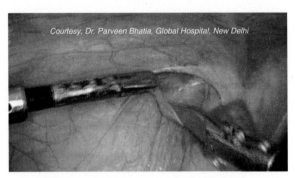

Fig. 19.2. Laparoscopic repair of groin hernia.

- Chronic smokers should be advised and motivated to stop smoking. Smoking must be stopped atleast six weeks before the surgery of hernia. Frequent intermittent positive-pressure breathing and chest physiotherapy are advised several days before the surgery.

- Skin infection should be treated and cleared before surgery. Intertrigo must be treated and controlled before the surgery.
- Prostatic enlargement should be tackled in elderly patients first then post them for hernia surgery.
- A mild laxative should be given two days before surgery and should be continued for a few days after surgery to avoid straining while defaecating. If the patient is suffering from chronic constipation, then advise high fibre diet.
- Urethral stricture in an young patient must also be treated before the patient is posted for surgery.
- Assess pulmonary function and respiratory reserve.

- Informed consent is to be taken.
- Consent for conversion from laparoscopic hernia repair to open repair must be taken from every patient.

SNIDER'S TEST

It is blowing of matchstick by patient keeping the matchstick one foot away from the patient. If the distance is less than 1 foot then respiratory reserve is very low.

It is a simple test of respiratory reserve.

- A child of less than five years of age should be psychologically prepared for hospital atmosphere for the surgery. Child should be gradually told with the help of booklets about hospitalization and operation so that no emotional trauma develops after the surgery.
- All patients going for surgery should be trained to get out of bed with minimum discomfort.

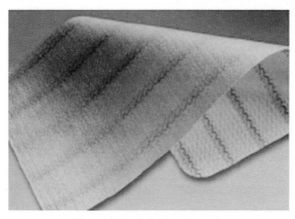

Fig. 19.3. Mesh for hernia repair.

• All elderly patients must undergo thorough medical evaluation including the history of medicines they are taking.

INTRAOPERATIVE PREPARATIONS (Fig. 19.4)

• Skin is shaved with electric hair shaver from umbilicus to upper thigh. Electric shaver avoids skin cuts which are caused if razor and blade are used. Skin of penis and scrotum should be shaved if the hernia is inguino-scrotal or if the hydrocele is also present.
• Patient is given preoperative antibiotics according to individual case. **Author uses single dose of preoperative antibiotic.**
• A nasogastric tube is passed for gastric decompression in strangulated hernias.
• A Foley catheter is introduced in laparoscopic hernia surgery.
• A sterile plastic transparent drape i.e. opsite, may be used to cover the operative area to avoid wound contamination from skin.
• Iodine should be avoided in case of inguino-scrotal hernia as it may cause severe excoriation of skin.

• Verify the side of hernia to be operated.

POSITION OF THE PATIENT

• Patient is placed in comfortable supine position.
• Legs are flexed at knees with a pillow. This keeps inguinal and abdominal muscles relaxed.
• Table is tilted with head down 10-15° to aid in reducing the contents of hernia. It also helps in retracting the thick abdominal wall by gravity in obese persons.
• An additional pillow should be kept under the neck and head of elderly patients.
• Legs of the patients should be slightly separated.
• A surgeon stands on the side of operation.

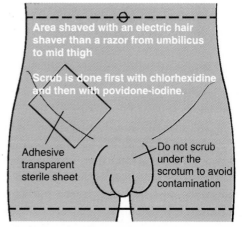

Area shaved with an electric hair shaver than a razor from umbilicus to mid thigh

Scrub is done first with chlorhexidine and then with povidone-iodine.

Adhesive transparent sterile sheet

Do not scrub under the scrotum to avoid contamination

Fig. 19.4. Intraoperative preparations for groin hernia repair.

ANAESTHESIA FOR ABDOMINAL WALL HERNIAS

"Dr Snow gave that blessed chloroform and the effect was soothing, quietening and delightful beyond measure."

— Queen Victoria
1853 at Queens 8th Child & Youngest Son,
Prince Leopold's birth.
Anaesthetist, Dr. John Snow of Edinburgh
World's First Anaesthesiologist

"Just as surgeons disagree about which is the best type of hernia repair, anaesthesiologists disagree on which is the best anaesthetic"

— William J Amado[116]

Hernia can be operated under local anaesthsia or regional anaesthesia or general anaesthesia.
- Most surgeons prefer operating under local anaesthesia due to its advantages.
- Spinal anaesthesia is preferred in large hernias because it provides excellent relaxation.
- General anaesthesia is also used in large hernias if not contraindicated.
- General anaesthesia is the anaesthesia of choice in children and apprehensive adults.
- In case of strangulated and obstructed hernias, general anaesthesia with endotracheal tube and cuff is recommended to avoid the tracheal aspiration.
- The amount of local anaesthetic agent is reduced in elderly persons.
- Abdominal wall hernias are one of the most common surgical problems. Hernia surgery can be a simple open primary tissue repair or open tension free mesh repair or a laparoscopic procedure. Hernia surgery may be elective or can be for an emergency presentation of hernia with strangulation which may require bowel resection. Nowadays, large percentage of hernia repairs are performed as a day case surgery and local anaethesia is required.

> The type of anaethesia required for particular type of hernia depends upon patient's general condition, patient's psychological status (highly anxious and uncooperative), type and size of hernia. Strangulated hernia requires general anaesthesia.

According to Rutkow, in 2003 in USA 7,70,000 inguinal hernia cases were operated most of them were out patients.[1]

General Anaesthesia

Before 1990, general anaesthesia was most widely used anaesthesia for abdominal wall hernia repair but due to shift of hernia surgery from inpatients to day case surgery the choice of anaesthesia technique also shifted to local and regional anaesthesia from general anaesthesia. Nowadays, general anaesthesia technique has become safer and less discomforting with latest drugs. Laryngeal mask airway (LMA) and Cuffed oropharyngeal airway (COPA) reduce the stimulation of vocal cords and trachea so reducing the incidence of bronchospasm and laryngospasm. Drugs like ondansetron can reduce the post-operative nausea and vomiting (PONV)[2,3], so nowadays general anaesthesia has become much smoother.

Regional Anaesthesia

Epidural and spinal anaesthesia used with low doses of sedation are smoother and speedy in recovery. Regional anaesthesia causes less PONV than general anaesthesia and are cheaper than general anaesthesia.

Post Dural Puncture Headache (PDPH)

It was first recognised by Bier in 1898 and Hildebrandt, his surgical resident, who performed spinal anaesthesia on each other.[4] It causes bifrontal and occipital headache whose intensity increases in upright posture and on coughing. The incidence is reducing with pencil point needle of No. 27. PDPH is treated with caffeine and sumatripta.

Transient Neruological Syndorme (TNS)

It is a feeling of aching and pain in buttocks and lower limbs after spinal anaesthesia. It occurs when surgery is done in lithotomy position. It is a self limiting condition.

Urinary retention

It develops in patients who have undergone hernia repair under spinal or epidural anaesthesia. In some hernia centres people required to void before discharge.[5]

LOCAL ANAESTHESIA (Figs. 19.5 & 19.6)

> • Nowadays local anaesthesia is the most commonly used technique in the repair of abdominal wall hernias in 'day case' surgery.
> • It has shortest post-operative interval to discharge.

In spite of so many advantages, some doctors are avoiding local anaesthesia for hernia surgery due to the following reasons:
• They do not want to give anaesthesia themselves.
• Patient has to be operated very gently and they cannot use retractors and other instruments freely.
• Electrocautry cannot be used freely.
• Local swelling appears due to infiltration of anaesthesia agent causing difficulty in identification of structures and their dissection.
• It takes longer time to operate under local anaesthesia.
• Difficult to teach trainees.

Advantages of Local Anaesthesia

A randomized trial of local, regional, and general anaesthesia in 611 adult patients undergoing open inguinal hernia repair in 10 hospitals found that local anaesthesia, was superior in the early post-operative period.[116]
• Lowest risk among all other methods of anaesthesia.
• Post-operative analgesics are required less in amount and frequency than in other anaesthesias.
• Almost no risk of post-operative urinary retention.
• Patients with cardiopulmonary diseases and other systemic diseases can be operated under local anaesthesia.

- Patient is conscious during the operation and repair can be checked by asking patient to cough.
- Early mobilization is easy.
- Shorter stay in hospital.
- Less post-operative vomiting than after general anaesthesia.
- It makes the surgeon gentle in his dissection.
- Less tension in suturing. It allows the approximation of the tissues at a more normal tension.
- Patient can walk in operation theatre and walk out after operation as a day care case. Local anaesthesia makes "come and go" hernia repair safe and effective. It is now a routine practice.
- Catheterization is eliminated.
- Deep sedation with an anxiolytic, narcotic and hypnotic along with local anaesthesia is commonly used nowaday. Drugs like midazolam, fentanyl and propofol are routinely used.

NOTE

It is better if adrenalin is not used during the opening of inguinal canal as it may obscure the bleeders which should be cauterized or ligated causing less hematoma and ecchymosis. During the closure of the wound, reinfiltrate with adrenalin. Adrenalin is not added in cardiac patients.

Local Anaesthetic Agents

- Use a mixture of short acting and long acting local anaesthetic agents. **Author prefers Inj. Lidocaine 1% with Adrenaline-1 in 200000 with Inj. Bupivacaine (0.25 to 0.5%).**
- The amount of local anaesthetic depends upon the size of hernia.
- Maximum dose of plain Lidocaine is 300 mg.
- Maximum dose of Lidocaine with adrenaline is 500 mg.
- Maximum dose of plain Bupivacaine is 175 mg.
- Maximum dose of Bupivacain with adrenaline is 225 mg.
- Local anaesthetic mixture is supplemented with I.V. propofol or midazolam or other sedative.

Before closing the wound infiltrate and splash some of local anaesthetic agent on wound which will have analgesic effect post-operatively. It gives benefit of:
- 4-6 hours local analgesia in post-operative period.
- Patient can be discharged on the same day.

	Local Anaesthesia		**General Anaesthesia**
1.	Cost effective method	1.	Costlier method
2.	Can be done by experienced surgeon	2.	Can be carried out by trainee surgeon
3.	Long "On-table time"	3.	Short "On-table time"
4.	No post-operative nausea, vomiting and retention of urine	4.	Post-operative nausea, vomiting and retention of urine happens
5.	No immediate post-operative pain	5.	Immediate post-operative pain is present
6.	Day care surgery possible	6.	Planned night stay surgery
7.	Not for strangulated hernia	7.	Good for strangulated hernia
8.	Not good for obese patient	8.	Good for obese patient
9.	Not good for very anxious patients and children	9.	Good for very anxious patients and children
10.	No effect on functions of other organs	10.	May affect functions of other organs

Contraindications of Local Anaesthesia

- Refusal by patient.
- Sensitivity to the drug.
- Irreducible and strangulated hernia, may require resection of bowel.
- Laparoscopic repair.
- Psychiatric factor or highly anxious and uncooperative patient.

Side Effects of Local Anaesthetic Agents

Toxicity with local anaesthetic agents is not common. The following side effects are observed:

Allergic reactions

Allergic reactions are uncommon. The following reactions happen rarely:

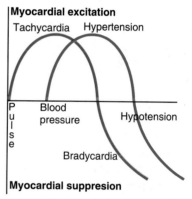

Fig. 19.5. CVS toxicity.

- Urticaria
- Bronchospasm
- Angioneurotic oedema

Treatment
- Oxygen inhalation
- Injection of epinephrine
- Injection of hydrocortisone

Neurological toxicity

Neurological toxicity of anaesthetic drugs affect CNS:
- Metallic taste
- Numbness on lips and around
- Dizziness
- Slurred speech
- Confusion
- Convulsions
- Respiratory arrest

Treatment
- Oxygen inhalation
- Injection of propofol

Convulsions and respiratory arrest usually occur after incidental I.V. administration, so keep the needle in vein only, change the syringe and give an injection of propofol. It will save the patient.

CVS Toxicity (Fig. 19.5)

It starts with excitation of myocardium leading to tachycardia and hypertension. It is followed by myocardial suppression leading to bradycardia and hypotension which may proceed to arrhythmias.

Treatment
- Oxygen inhalation
- Intubation
- Injection epinephrine

Technique of Local Anaesthesia (Figs. 19.6 & 19.7)

- **Anaesthetic agent**
  - 25 ml of 1% Lidocaine (Xylocaine).
  - 25 ml of 0.5% Bupivacaine (Marcaine) with 1/200,000 epinephrine.
  - 50 ml of this solution is injected locally in one inguinal region for unilateral inguinal hernia.
  - A mixture of lidocaine and bupivacaine gives post-operative relief of pain for 4-6 hours.
  - The infiltration is given in the following way with a 10 ml syringe with 26 G needle.
  - Three weals are raised.
  - First weal: 1.5 cm medial to ASIS.
  - Second weal: Over pubic tubercle.
  - Third weal: 1.5 cm above middle point of inguinal ligament.

- **First weal**
  The needle is introduced vertically down till it is felt to pierce external oblique aponeurosis.
- 15 ml of solution is deposited. It blocks ilioinguinal and iliohypogastric nerves.
- **Second weal**
  10 ml of solution is deposited in intradermal and subcutaneous layers in the direction of umbilicus. It blocks nerve twigs from opposite side.
- **Third weal**
  The needle is inserted perpendicular until it pierces external oblique aponeurosis. 15 ml of solution is deposited there. It blocks genital branch of genitofemoral nerve.
- 5 ml of solution is infiltrated intradermally and subcutaneously along the line of incision.
- 5 ml of solution is splashed in inguinal canal and subcutaneous layer before closure as it prolongs the local anaesthesia effect.
- In femoral hernia, the first weal is not near ASIS but 1.5 cm below midinguinal point and inguinal ligament.

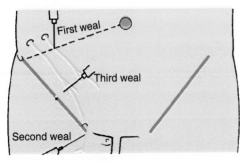

Fig. 19.6. Technique of local anaesthesia for inguinal hernia.

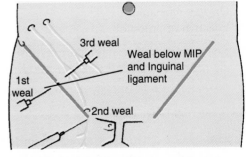

Fig. 19.7. Technique of local anaesthesia for femoral hernia.

Anaesthesia for Laparoscopic Repair

General anaesthesia is the anaesthesia of choice.
Pneumoperitoneum is created with carbon dioxide at 1-6 L/mt rate of pressure 10-18 mm of Hg.

Advantages of Carbon Dioxide

- It is highly soluble in blood.
- It does not support combustion.
- It is easily and quickly eliminated from blood.
- It is easily available.
- It is not very expensive.

Pathophysiological Changes During Laparoscopic Hernia Repair

Respiratory changes

- Reduction in tidal volume and functional residual capacity occurs due to lifting up of diaphragm.
- Decreased compliance with increased airway resistance happens.
- There is a distrubed ventilation – perfusion process.

Cardiovascular changes

- Low venous return occurs so low cardiac output results.
- Increased systemic vascular resistance develops.
- Tachycardia results.
- Arrhythmias may occur.

Renal changes

- Intra-abdominal pressure more than 20 mm of Hg may cause reduction in renal blood flow and in urine output.

NOTE

"All hernia surgeon, specialists or otherwise, should really be able to perform groin herniorrhaphy under local anaesthesia.

-Brian M Stephenson
General and colorectal surgeon

KEY POINT

"If there was one best technique for anaesthesia for hernia surgery it would be local."
-Ira M. Rutkow

OPERATIONS FOR INGUINAL HERNIA

"A single technique is not appropriate for all patients."

– Nyhus LM

"This is unfortunate because with the use of such things as plugs or tension-free anastomoses or combinations, a generation of residents and surgeons will grow up having no idea of what is the normal anatomy of the inguinal canal."

– Josef E. Fischer

Bassini did modernization of hernia surgery about 120 years back and since then only 20 years back we started modernization again.[6]

Basic techniques of inguinal hernia repair are the following (Fig. 19.8):

* Herniotomy
* Herniorrhaphy (Primary tissue repair)
* Hernioplasty with prosthetic mesh (open or laparoscopic procedure)

Anterior Approach for Posterior Wall of Inguinal Canal (Fig. 19.9)

* Primary tissue repairs
* Prosthetic repairs

Primary tissue repairs

* Bassini's repair
* Modified Bassini's repair
* Halsted's modification
* Ferguson's repair
* Willy-Andrew's modification
* Shouldice's repair
* Berliner modification of Shouldice's operation
* McVay's repair
* Nyhus procedure
* Condon procedure
* Kuntz procedure
* Hamilton-Bailey operation
* Bracey's modification
* Farquharson's modification
* Marcy repair
* Abrahamson's nylon darn repair
* Moloney darn repair

Prosthetic repairs

* Lichtenstein repair
* Sutureless mesh plug technique of Gilbert

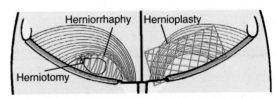

Fig. 19.8. Basic techniques of inguinal hernia repair.

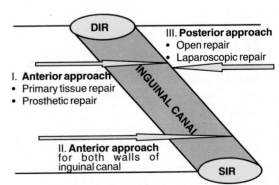

Fig. 19.9. Various approaches of repair of posterior wall of inguinal canal.

- Plug and patch technique of Rutkow and Robbins
- Trabucco tension-free sutureless pre-shaped mesh repair
- NRCH (Nigams' Reverse Curtain Hernioplasty)

Anterior Approach for Both Anterior and Posterior Repair of Posterior Wall of Inguinal Canal (Fig. 19.9)

- Prolene hernia system (PHS)

Posterior Approach for Repair of Posterior Wall of Inguinal Canal (Fig. 19.9)

- Open method
- Laparosocpic repair

Open methods

- Stoppa technique
- Nyhus technique
- Kugel repair
- Ugahari repair
- Wantz's technique
- Reed-Rives technique

Laparoscopic repairs

- TAPP (Transabdominal Preperitoneal) approach
- TEP (Total Extraperitoneal) approach
- IPOM (Intraperitoneal only mesh) repair

Advantages of Primary Tissue Repair

- No use of any foreign body.
- Easy and simple method, even a beginner can do it with little training.

Disadvantages of Primary Tissue Repair

- Recurrence rate of hernia is high, the recurrence is 5-10% in primary hernia and is 20-30% in recurrent hernia.
- Slow recovery in post-operative period. Slow return to normal activity and so higher man hour loss.

Fate of mesh

Fibroblasts and capillaries grow over the mesh. The mesh is converted into a thick fibrous sheet. The fibrous sheet may be hard (scarplate) or soft (scarmesh) depending upon the type of mesh used. Selection of mesh for hernia repair is important. Every surgeon doing hernia repair must enhance his knowledge about various meshes.[121]

HERNIOTOMY

"Every operation is an experiment in physiology."

                                                    - Tid Kommer

Herniotomy is the excision of the hernia sac. It is the part of both herniorrhaphy and hernioplasty.

Principle

The contents of the sac are reduced in peritoneal cavity and then neck of sac is transfixed, ligated and excised. Inguinal canal is not repaired.

Indications of Herniotomy

- In infants and children.
- In young adults with good musculature below 16 years age.
- It is the part of herniorrhaphy and hernioplasty.

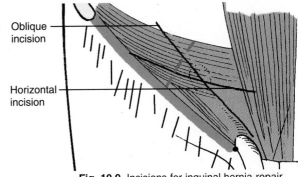

Fig. 19.9. Incisions for inguinal hernia repair.

Steps of Herniotomy:

- Incision (Fig. 19.9).
- Exposure of external oblique aponeurosis.
- Opening of inguinal canal.
- Identification of sac.
- Isolation of sac.
- Opening of sac.
- Reduction of contents of sac.
- Transfixation of neck of sac.
- Excision of sac.
- Closure of inguinal canal.
- Closure of wound.

Incision (Fig. 19.10)

- 5 to 6 cm long, 1.5-2 cm above and parallel to medial side of inguinal ligament.
  - A more horizontal incision in Langer's line gives better scar.
  - In bilateral cases, symmetrical incisions give better looking scar.

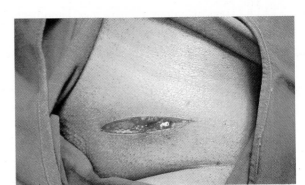

Fig. 19.10. Oblique incision for inguinal hernia repair.

NOTE

When you drape the patient with sterile towels, the positions of the following landmarks are kept in mind while putting the towel clips and exposing the area for operation:
(i) ASIS (ii) Pubic tubercle (iii) Inguinal ligament
This exercise will avoid making a too high or too low incision.

Exposure of external oblique aponeurosis (Figs. 19.11 A & B)

- Subcutaneous tissue is cut in the line of incision.
- Fascia of Camper is cut in the same line.

<table>
<tr><td>

The following three vessels are observed under fascia of Camper:

- Superficial epigastric vessels
- Superficial external pudendal vessles
- Superficial circumflex iliac vessles

</td></tr>
</table>

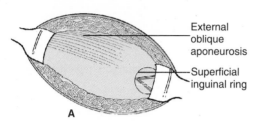

External
oblique
aponeurosis

Superficial
inguinal ring

A

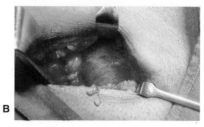

B

Fig. 19.11A. Exposure of external oblique fascia and aponeurosis, diagrammatic representation, **B.** On operation.

- These vessels are divided and ligated. In smaller incision, the superficial external iliac vessels are not met as they are more laterally placed.
  - Scarpa's fascia is cut in the same line and underlying external oblique aponeurosis is exposed.
  - The external oblique aponeurosis is cleansed of areolar tissue by blunt dissection with gauze wrapped on finger. It is recognized by its shiny fibres.

Opening of inguinal canal (Figs. 19.12 A & B)

- External oblique aponeurosis is cut. The incision is made from middle of apex of superficial inguinal ring to 2-3 cm lateral to deep inguinal ring. The superficial inguinal ring is divided in two parts to expose underlying structures adequately for further dissection.
- Two flaps of external oblique are mobilized and held with two artery forceps. Lower flap is raised to see femoral hernia.
- Ilioinguinal or iliohypogastric nerves come in picture, ilioinguinal nerve is commonly injured at superficial inguinal ring.
- Ilioinguinal nerve must be dissected free from tissues and kept on any one side of incision, away from the dissection by haemostates applied at edges of the wound.

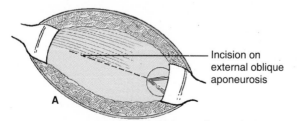

Incision on
external oblique
aponeurosis

A

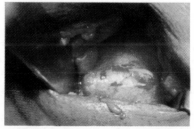

B

Fig. 19.12A. External oblique aponeurosis incised and inguinal canal opened, diagrammatic representation,
B. On operation.

- One bleeder is usually encountered along ilioinguinal nerve over the internal oblique muscle. It is caught and ligated to avoid hematoma formation. It should not be cauterized as it may cause thermal burn or injury to the ilioinguinal nerve.

- Iliohypogastric nerve is taken care of under upper flap of external oblique aponeurosis during dissection (Figs. 19.12 C & D).

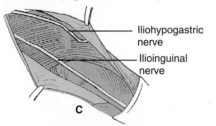
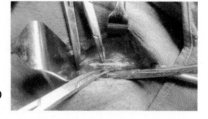

Fig. 19.12C. Iliohypogastric and Ilioinguinal nerves exposed and protected, diagrammatic representation, **D.** On operation.

Identification of sac

- The spermatic cord is isolated and care is taken to avoid injury to ilioinguinal nerve.
- An incision is made on cremasteric fascia and internal spermatic fascia. The incision is made longitudinally on medial side of midline to make lateral flap of cremaster muscle larger as it contains cremasteric vessels and genital branch of genitofemoral nerve. There are two ways to deal with cremasteric muscle and fascia covering the spermatic cord.
  - Make a longitudinal incision and dissect it away from vessels of spermatic cord.
  - Excise cremasteric fascia from the deep inguinal ring to the superficial inguinal ring.
- The margins of incision are separated and the sac is now seen. It looks pearly white and glistening.
- Sac is incorporated in spermatic cord in indirect inguinal hernia and lies separately in direct inguinal hernia.
- Spermatic cord is held and spread between fingers. Now the sac is clearly identified and seen.
- If you cannot identify the sac then ask the patient to cough if he is under spinal or local anaesthesia. If still cannot identify the sac then open the spermatic cord and search for the sac.

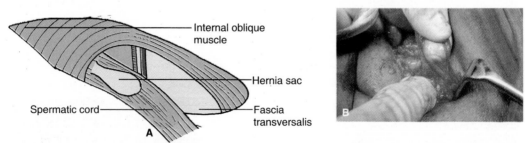

Fig. 19.13 A & B. Identification of the hernia sac.

Isolation of sac (Figs. 19.14, 19.15 A & B)

- Separation of the sac from cord structures is done up to the neck of the sac.
- The wall of the sac is held with two artery forceps. The sac is separated from spermatic cord structures by blunt and sharp dissection.

- The blunt dissection is done gradually with a pledget (a piece of gauze rolled and held by an artery forceps). This is done to minimize the injury to spermatic cord structures. The dissection is started at fundus of sac and is gradually taken towards deep inguinal ring and upto the neck of the hernia sac. The sac is completely separated from cord structures.

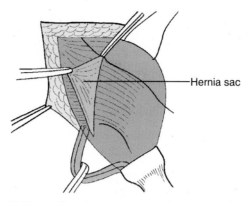

Fig. 19.14. Isolation of sac, diagrammatic representation.

Opening of the sac (Figs. 19.15 A - F)

- The sac is held with two artery forceps and lifted up.
- The sac is opened upto 3 cm of neck with scissors between two artery forceps.
- Search for pantaloon and direct hernia is made.
- Examine for:
  - Nature of the contents
  - Adhesions

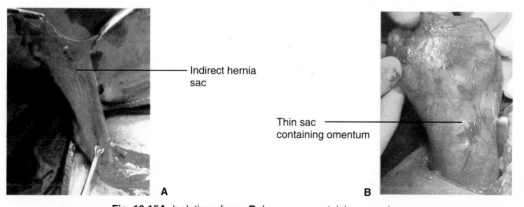

Fig. 19.15A. Isolation of sac, **B.** Large sac containing omentum.

NOTE

Do not separate contents from wall of the sac in sliding hernia.

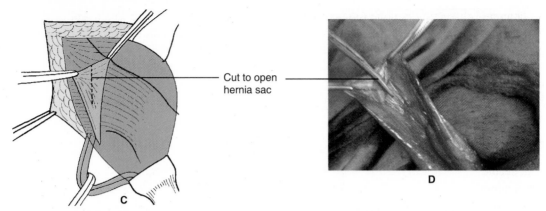

Fig. 19.15C. Opening of hernia sac, diagrammatic representation, **D.** Opening the sac with scissors.

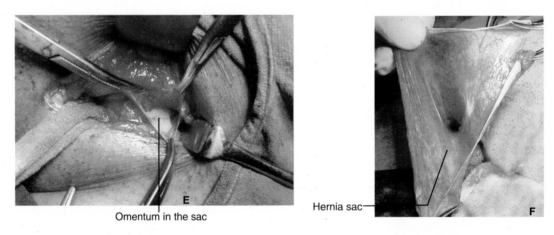

Fig. 19.15E. Hernia sac opened containing ometum, **F.** Empty hernia sac.

Reduction of contents of sac (Figs. 19.16 A & B)

• A finger is introduced inside the sac to make sure that no content is adherent to the sac at neck. The dissection is kept close to the sac wall, get in avascular plane. Sharp dissection separates vas

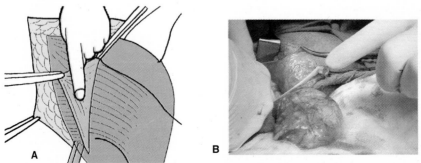

Fig. 19.16A. Reduction of the contents of hernia sac, diagrammatic representation, **B.** On operation.

deferens and vessels from sac wall. It reduces bleeding. Sweeping with gauze causes more bleeding and damage.

• Contents of the sac are reduced back to the peritoneal cavity.

Transfixation of the neck of the sac (Figs. 19.17A & B)

The sac if found empty can be transfixed directly but if it contains some contents then it is always better to twist it a few turns clockwise till the first turn reaches the neck; it empties the sac. Now the neck is transfixed.

The neck of the sac is transfixed with 1-0 non-absorbable suture i.e. black silk or polypropylene. The needle is passed through the neck of the sac and tied first on one side and then on other side so the ligature does not slip. Transfixation should be done under vision to avoid injury to intestine and omentum. It is better to do transfixation twice, second transfixation should be done 1 cm distal to first suture.

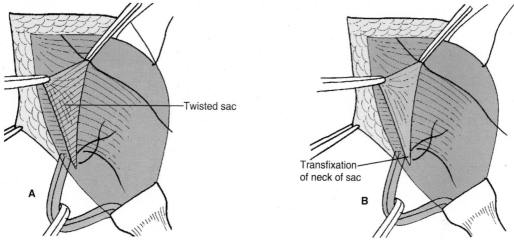

Fig. 19.17A. Twisting, **B.** Transfixation of neck of sac, diagrammatic representation.

Excision of the sac (Figs. 19.18 A & B)

• The sac is excised 1 cm distal to the ligature. Look for any bleeding from cut edge of the sac and

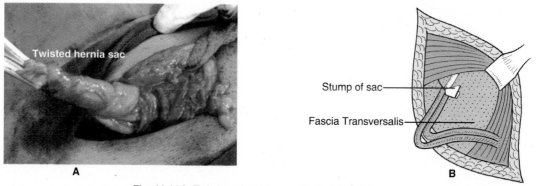

Fig. 19.18A. Twisting of hernia sac, **B.** Excision of the sac.

then cut the ligature. The neck of the sac will disappear under arched fibres of internal oblique and transversus abdominis muscles.

• Alternatively an electrocautery is used to cut the sac which minimizes bleeding and ecchymosis after operation.

> ### *High ligation of sac (Fig. 19.19)*
>
> • Some surgeons believe that it is useless to do high ligation of the sac. The sac is pulled and ligated proximal to the narrow thickened white ring of the sac.

• **Identification of neck of sac (Figs. 19.20 A & B)**

It is identified by the following features:

    – Constriction at the neck of sac.

    – Extraperitoneal pad of fat at and proximal to the neck as it becomes parietal peritoneum.

    – Inferior epigastric vessels are seen just medial to deep inguinal ring.

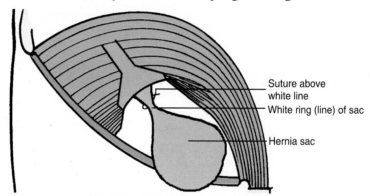

Fig. **19.19.** High ligation of sac.

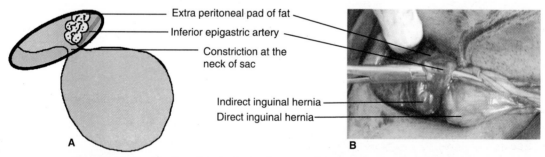

Fig. **19.20A.** Identification of neck of sac, diagrammatic representation, **B.** On operation.

Closure of inguinal canal (Fig. 19.21)

Before going further, look for other hernias in the following manner:

• Palpate the posterior wall of inguinal canal for direct hernia.

• Look for indirect hernia in case of direct hernia operation.

• Look for funicular direct hernia or Ogilvie hernia.

• Look for pantaloon hernia.

• Look for femoral hernia.

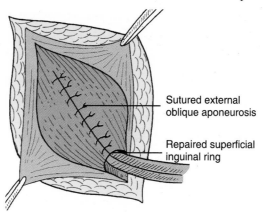

Fig. 19.21. Closure of inguinal canal.

- Search for lipoma of spermatic cord.
- The incised cremasteric muscle and fascia are approximated with 2-0 polyglactin suture.
- The spermatic cord is returned back to its normal position.
- The incised external oblique aponeurosis is sutured in front of spermatic cord with interrupted or continuous 2-0 polyglactin suture.
- The medial portion of external oblique aponeurosis is left open so as to form a new superficial inguinal ring allowing spermatic cord to pass. The newly made superficial inguinal ring should not be very tight. One can check it by passing the tip of the little finger through it. Only tip of the little finger can pass.

- The external ring now made must be kept loose enough to prevent strangulation of cord structures, but not so loose as an inexperienced surgeon may confuse a dilated ring with recurrence. This sometimes is referred to as "industrial hernia" as it causes problem at pre-employment checkup.

- It is better to avoid sutures in subcutaneous tissue except in obese persons as this layer does not give any strength to the wound.
- The wound is closed with staples or polypropylene sutures.

Other methods of dealing with sac

- Purse string sutures can be done instead of transfixation.
- Sac is cut at deep inguinal ring by electrocautery, explore with index finger and then close with 2-0 polypropylene. The rest of the sac is left as such, if it is the inguinoscrotal sac (Fig. 19.22) as the dissection may cause:
  - Seroma
  - Venous thrombosis
  - Testicular ischaemia
  - Hydrocele
  - Testicular atrophy

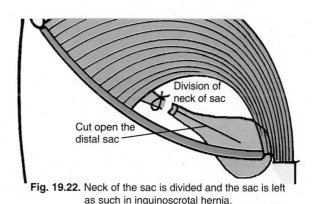

Fig. 19.22. Neck of the sac is divided and the sac is left as such in inguinoscrotal hernia.

When you leave the whole distal sac unremoved then the anterior wall is incised to avoid post-operative collection of fluid or hydrocele formation.[118]

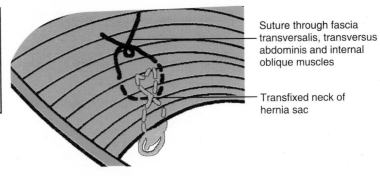

Suture through fascia transversalis, transversus abdominis and internal oblique muscles

Transfixed neck of hernia sac

Fig. 19.23. Misdirection of sac.

- The sac is opened and explored with index finger, then the opening is closed with 2-0 polypropylene or other non-absorbable suture. Now the neck of the sac is transfixed. Then the whole sac is pushed in preperitoneal space behind abdominal musculature.

- **Misdirection of the sac (Fig. 19.23)**
  - The sac is transfixed at the neck and the distal portion is excised then sutures are brought out through fascia transversalis, transversus abdominis and internal oblique muscles and tied over internal oblique muscle superolaterally. Inferior epigastric vessels are saved from injury.

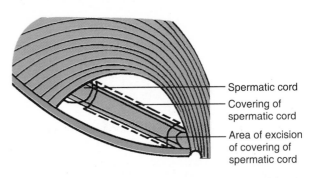

Spermatic cord

Covering of spermatic cord

Area of excision of covering of spermatic cord

Fig. 19.24. Parietalization of spermatic cord.

NOTE

- *Parietalization (Fig. 19.24)*
  - *This term was brought in use by Stoppa.*
  The term parietalization refers to "the dissection of spermatic cord to give sufficient length so that it can be mobilized more laterally without getting stretched".
- *Always the testis is pulled back in scrotum after hernia surgery.*

KEY POINT

Below 14-16 years of age herniotomy alone is sufficient. No repair is required.

PRIMARY TISSUE REPAIR (HERNIORRHAPHY)

"It is the reconstruction or strengthening of posterior wall of inguinal canal."

Bassini's Repair

"It reconstructs the inguinal canal as it is physiological".

- Edoardo Bassini

"In an Atlas of Hernia Surgery, all roads lead to Bassini".

- R. Bendavid (2005)

Edoardo Bassini was an Italian surgeon. His classical work on hernia was introduced in 1887 at the Italian Society of Surgery in Genoa. He is now known as "father of modern herniorrhaphy."

Approximation of conjoint tendon with inguinal ligament with non-absorbable sutures is done.

Indications for Bassini's herniorrhaphy

- Indirect inguinal hernia with good muscle tone.
- Direct inguinal hernia with good muscle tone.

  Bassini operated 206 cases of inguinal hernia by this method.
- He did a follow-up of 5 years in all patients, 1885-1890.[85]
- His results were as follows:
  - No mortality.
  - Wound infection in 11 cases.
  - Recurrence in 8 cases.
- He reported the recurrence rate of 2.7% at one year.[128]

Aim of Bassini's repair

To strengthen the posterior wall of inguinal canal by suturing arching fibres of internal oblique muscle and conjoint tendon with inguinal ligament behind the spermatic cord.

Principle of Bassini's repair

Repair of posterior wall of inguinal canal is done by suturing the conjoint tendon and internal oblique to inguinal ligament by interrupted or non-absorbable sutures behind the spermatic cord.

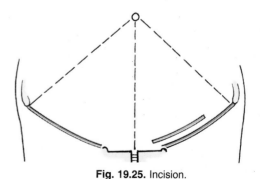

Fig. 19.25. Incision.

Criticism of Bassini's repair

- Silk or catgut is used for repair which causes infection.
- Suturing is continuous so as if it cuts through, the suture line becomes lax.
- Suturing of muscle to ligament causes weak scar.
- There is tension in the suture line.
- It is not a physiological method. It disturbs the shutter-like action of internal oblique muscle.

Steps of Bassini's Repair

Incision (Fig.19.25)

A 5-6 cm long incision is made approximately 2 cm long, parallel and above the medial part of inguinal ligament.

A cosmetic incision is made in one of the inguinal creases or Langer's line.

The incision is deepend down to external oblique aponeurosis.

Herniotomy

• It is done as earlier described.

Further steps (Figs. 19.26, 19.27 A & B)

• The suture of conjoint tendon with inguinal ligament is done with No. 1 polypropylene in 4 to 5 interrupted sutures.

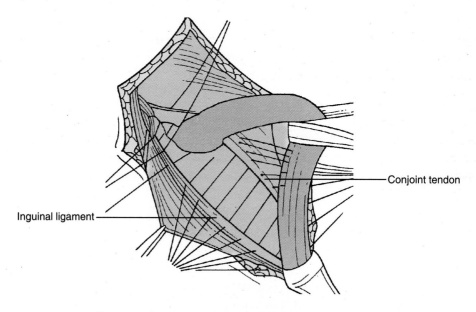

Fig. 19.26. Suturing of conjoint tendon and inguinal ligament.

• First the most medial suture is applied. It is called Bassini's stitch (Fig. 19.27A). The bite is taken from periosteum and not from inguinal ligament to give strength to this suture as most of recurrences occur here.
• Second suture is taken from inguinal ligament and through the transverse arch.
• While applying further sutures one must be careful for external iliac and femoral vessels as they can be injured in careless suturing.
• The best way to avoid injuries to vessels is that the bite is taken from inguinal ligament under vision and by passing the needle just under fibres of inguinal ligament.

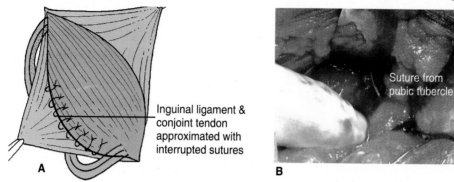

Fig. 19.27A. Bassini's repair, **B.** Bassini's stitch.

- The bite from inguinal ligament should be taken from different levels so to avoid avulsion of fibres of inguinal ligament.
- When the most lateral suture is applied one must take care that the spermatic cord does not get constricted and strangulated.
- Sutures should not be tied too tightly to cause undue tension which leads to poor healing and recurrence of hernia.
- Polypropylene suture material is slipping material so about seven knots are tied to avoid slipping of knots.
- If you see that the gap between transverse muscular arch and inguinal ligament is causing the tension on approximation which is unavoidable then you can go for "Tanner's muscle slide".
- Transverse fascia, transverse abdominis muscle and internal oblique muscle are called "Triple layer" by Bassini. He used to suture triple layer medially to the inguinal ligament and laterally to ileopubic tract. This step is suggested in drawings, but not clarified in original texts authored by Bassini[7] (Fig. 19.28).

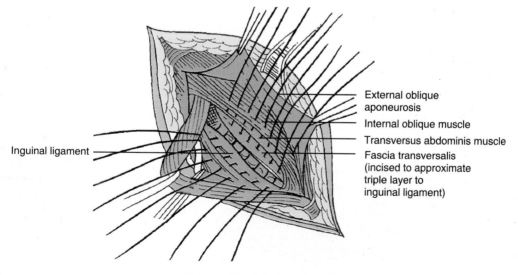

Fig. 19.28. Tripple layer of Bassini.

Repair of inguinal hernia in adult females

- The round ligament is cut and ligated. Bleeding may occur as it contains a small artery. The round ligament is fixed by including it in approximation of inguinal ligament and conjoint tendon. It is done for giving support to uterus.
- To avoid recurrence, the inguinal canal must be obliterated.

Post-operative care

- The patient is kept comfortably in supine position on the bed.
- Thighs are flexed slightly with a pillow underneath knees to avoid tension on operative site.
- Scrotum is supported by a suspensory bandage.
- Coughing is controlled by sedation.
- Mild laxatives are given to avoid straining at the time of defaecation.
- Patient must be ambulated as soon as possible.

Tanner's Slide Operation

Norman Cecil Tanner (1906-1982), Surgeon, Charring Cross Hospital, London, England introduced it.
- It is also called "Tanner's muscle slide" though it was first described by Wolfler in 1892. The incision is made just lateral to the attachment of external oblique aponeurosis to anterior lamina of rectus sheath.
- The incision starts at pubic crest and extends above approximately 6-8 cm.
- Take care to avoid linea alba and ileo-hypogastric nerve.
- Multiple small incisions can also be used instead of one large incision (Pie-crusting).[129]

Steps (Figs. 19.29 A-C)

- Lift and retract upper flap of the external oblique aponeurosis.
- The external oblique aponeurosis is separated from underlying internal oblique muscle by blunt dissection with a pledget on artery forceps or with index finger.
- Observe underlying fibres of internal oblique muscle. It fuses with the aponeurosis of transversus abdominis and forms anterior rectus sheath.
- A curved vertical incision is made in internal oblique and transversus aponeurosis. The lateral flap of the internal oblique retracts and becomes less tensed and relaxed.
- Repair of posterior wall of inguinal canal is done.

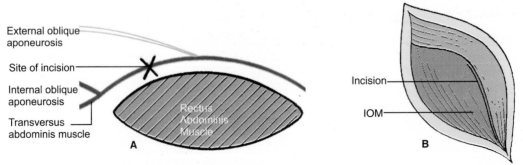

Fig. 19.29 A & B. Site of incision in "Tanner's slide" operation.

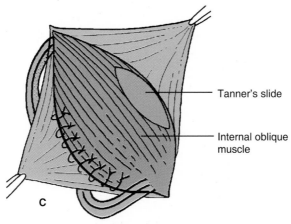

Fig. 19.29C. Tanner's slide.

- Spermatic cord is placed back to its normal position.
- External oblique aponeurosis is sutured back.

Lytle's Method

William James Lytle (1896-1986), Surgeon, Royal Infirmary, Sheffield, England (Fig. 19.30) introduced it.
- This procedure of narrowing of deep inguinal ring is named after James Lytle who started it. This procedure was published originally by Marcy in 1878.
- The spermatic cord is displaced laterally by suturing the two crura of deep inguinal ring medial to spermatic cord. It narrows the deep inguinal ring. Take care of inferior epigastric vessels while narrowing the inguinal ring.
- Narrowing of deep inguinal ring is done if it is dilated. (If it is wider than the base of little finger or proximal interphalangeal joint then it is called dilated deep inguinal ring.)

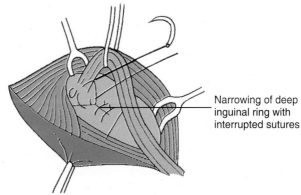

Narrowing of deep inguinal ring with interrupted sutures

Fig. 19.30. Lytle's method.

Modified Bassini's Repair (Fig. 19.31)

Indications of modified Bassini's repair

- Weak and patulous deep inguinal ring.
- Weak and lax posterior wall of inguinal canal.

Incision

As in Bassini repair.

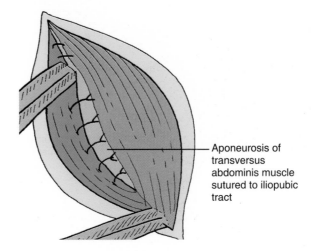

Aponeurosis of transversus abdominis muscle sutured to iliopubic tract

Fig. 19.31. Modified Bassini's repair.

Steps

- The conjoint tendon is retracted upwards so as to take good bite from aponeurosis of transversus abdominis muscle.
- Approximation of iliopubic tract and aponeurosis of transversus abdominis muscle is done with interrupted sutures. It removes the laxity of posterior wall of inguinal canal.
- Few sutures are also made between iliopubic tract and aponeurosis of transversus abdominis muscle lateral to the spermatic cord, to remove laxity of the deep inguinal ring.
- Second layer of interrupted sutures approximating conjoint tendon and inguinal ligament is started at pubic tubercle and extends upto deep inguinal ring.
- Care should be taken to avoid undue constriction of the spermatic cord.
- The external oblique aponeurosis is closed over the spermatic cord by a continuous suture.

Halsted's Modification

William Stewart Halsted, Professor of Surgery, Johns Hopkins Medical School, Baltimore, M.D., USA, (1852-1922) modified Bassini repair. Halsted pioneered the "Residency" teaching programme in USA. He was a tough teacher. He also gave Halsted's technique of mastectomy for breast cancer.
- Halsted operation is now of historical significance. Halsted operation is of two types:
    - **Halsted I operation:** It is the transplantation of spermatic cord in subcutaneous tissue.
In 1890, Halsted started placing spermatic cord in subcutaneous tissue. It was called Halsted one operation.[86]
    - **Halsted II operation:** Spermatic cord was transplanted under external oblique fascia.
In 1903, Halsted stopped doing Halsted I operation and started Halsted II operation.[87]

Transposition of spermatic cord (Figs. 19.32 A & B)

- In this method, the spermatic cord is brought in the subcutaneous tissue and the external oblique

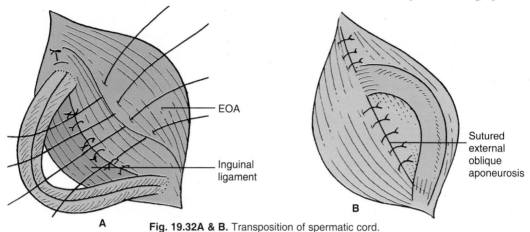

Fig. 19.32A & B. Transposition of spermatic cord.

aponeurosis is sutured behind the spermatic cord. This increases the strength of anterior wall of inguinal canal.

The classic Halsted operation

*   This method includes:
    *   Lateral mobilization of spermatic cord by sutures on medial side of deep inguinal ring.
    *   Spermatic cord is placed subcutaneously in front of sutured external oblique aponeurosis.
*   The two flaps of external oblique aponeurosis are overlapped (double breasted) to increase the strength of the anterior wall of inguinal canal.
*   The edge of the upper leaf of external oblique aponeurosis is sutured to the inner side of lower leaf as low as possible.
*   The margin of the lower leaf is sutured over the upper leaf in a double breasting manner.
*   Care is taken not to constrict the spermatic cord.

Ferguson Repair (Non-transplantation of Spermatic Cord) (Figs. 19.33 A-C)

It is named after Sir William Ferguson (1808-1877), British surgeon. He also gave "Ferguson's

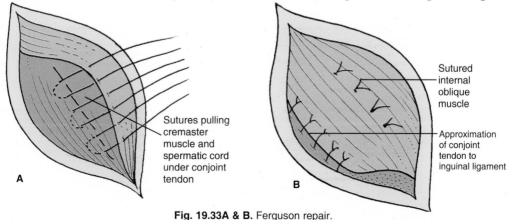

Fig. 19.33A & B. Ferguson repair.

Speculum", silvered glass vaginal speculum and "Ferguson's Incision", for removal of maxilla.
- Incised cremasteric fibres are approximated by 3-0 non-absorbable sutures.
- Cremaster muscle with spermatic cord is pulled under the upper flap of conjoint tendon and internal oblique muscle with multiple interrupted sutures. It gives strength.
- Now inguinal ligament is approximated with internal oblique muscle and conjoint tendon with 2-0 non-absorbable sutures.
- Care is taken to avoid injury to ilioinguinal nerve. It must not be included in the sutures.
- External oblique aponeurosis is sutured.

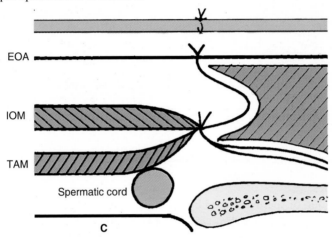

Fig. 19.33C. Ferguson repair, schematic representation.

Willys-Andrew's Modification (Fig. 19.34)

The operation has not been accepted because the obliquety of inguinal canal is lost as the spermatic cord directly comes from deep inguinal ring to newly formed superficial inguinal ring. In this procedure, the spermatic cord is sandwiched between two layers of external oblique aponeurosis.

It is a method of strengthening the anterior wall of inguinal canal by double breasting of external oblique aponeurosis.

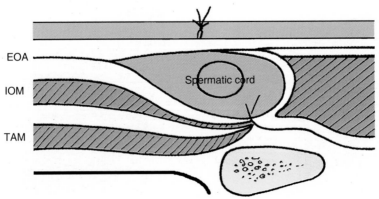

Fig. 19.34. Willys-Andrew's modification, schematic representation.

Steps of operation

- The spermatic cord is placed between the two layers of external oblique aponeurosis.
  - First the Bassini's repair is done.
  - Then upper layer of external oblique aponeurosis is sutured with inguinal ligament behind spermatic cord.
  - The lower layer of external oblique aponeurosis is brought in front of spermatic cord. So the spermatic cord is sandwiched between two layers of external oblique aponeurosis.

Shouldice Repair (Figs. 19.35 A-E)

This procedure was started by a Canadian surgeon, Edward Earl Shouldice (1890-1965).

Dr E. E. Shouldice was interested in inguinal hernia treatment since 1930s but introduced his technique of pure tissue repair for hernias in 1944, and reported his study for the first time at Ontario Medical Association meeting in 1944.[8] He published his study in 1953.[125]

Since 1945, 2,80,000 hernias have been repaired at Shouldice Hospital. Currently more than 150 abdominal wall hernias are repaired every week at Shouldice Hospital. E. E. Shouldice pioneered his approach to hernia repair and early ambulation, in the 1930s.[9]

It is a tension less double breasting of transversalis fascia, inguinal ligament and conjoint tendon with non-absorbable sutures in four layers. In Shouldice clinic, recurrence rate is less than 1% but recurrence rate is higher in non-specialized hernia centres. The low rate of recurrence is due to multiple factors such as principle of technique, pre-operative preparations, anaesthesia, comprehensive inguinal dissection and post-operative principles.[10]

Shouldice clinic principles of inguinal herniorrhaphy

- Weight reduction.
- Open technique with complete anatomic dissection.
- Use of local anaesthetic.
- Autologous tissue repairs.
- Early return to usual activity.

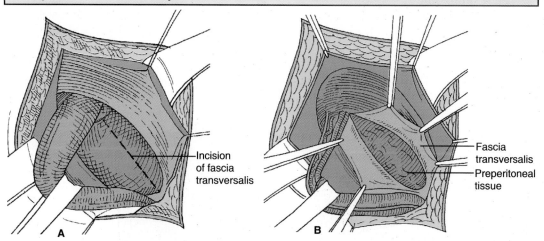

Fig. 19.35 A & B. Shouldice repair, opening of fascia transversalis.

The incidence of deep vein thrombosis, pulmonary embolism, and pulmonary atelectasis is well below 1%. The Shouldice series mortality is < 0.01%.[88] It is not the technique alone that makes Shouldice great, it is the strict adherence to the procedures, they like to call themselves a 'focussed factory'.[126]

Shouldice repair is not very widely used as extensive dissection is involved in it. It consists of:
- Double breasting of fascia transversalis in two layers.
- Narrowing of deep inguinal ring.
- Double breasting of conjoint tendon with inguinal ligament in two layers.

Incision

- 10 cm long incision is made 2 cm above and parallel to the medial part of inguinal ligament.

Herniotomy

- It is done as described earlier.

In this technique, the fascia transversalis is divided from inferior epigastric vessels to pubis. Then the divided fascia transversalis is sutured in double breasting manner in two layers. Now the arched fibres of transversus abdominis muscle and internal oblique muscle are sutured with inguinal ligament as in Bassini's repair. This technique has reduced the recurrence rate.

- Incise the posterior wall of inguinal canal from internal ring to pubic tubercle.
- Elevate the upper flap with blunt dissection.
- Do not elevate the lower flap.
- Now repair the posterior wall of inguinal canal with 3/0 polypropylene continuous suture in four layers.
- Use two sutures, one suture for first and second suture lines and another two sutures for third and fourth suture lines.

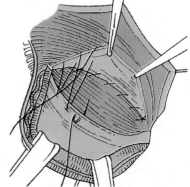

Fig. 19.35C. First and second suture lines.

  - **First suture line**
    Start from pubic tubercle side, put continuous suture, take deeper part of under surface of upper flap and edge of lower flap, go upto deep inguinal ring and put the knot but do not cut the suture.
  - **Second suture line**
    Now start from deep inguinal ring taking free edge of upper flap and folding edge of inguinal ligament upto pubic tubercle, tie a knot and cut the suture.

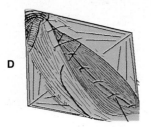
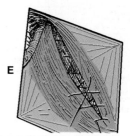

Fig. 19.35D & E. Shouldice repair, third and fourth suture lines.

- **Third suture line**

  Start a new suture from deep inguinal ring. Take conjoint tendon and approximate with inguinal ligament from deep ring to pubic tubercle then tie a knot but do not cut the suture.
- **Fourth suture line**

  Start same suture from pubic tubercle to the deep inguinal ring taking conjoined tendon and inguinal ligament. At deep inguinal ring tie a knot and cut the suture.
- Close the external oblique aponeurosis over spermatic cord.
- If tension is too much then external oblique aponeurosis can be closed behind spermatic cord.
- Close the wound in layers.

Berliner Modification of Shouldice's Operation

It is the repair of posterior wall of inguinal canal in six layers instead of four layers.

Indication

- Recurrent hernia with poor abdominal muscle tone in old age.

Procedure

- Spermatic cord is divided at deep inguinal ring and is removed along testis.
- It consists of three procedures:
  - Orchidectomy
  - Herniotomy
  - Herniorrhaphy: Repair of posterior wall of inguinal canal is done in six layers by apposing conjoint tendon and inguinal ligament by non-absorbable material i.e. polypropylene or silk.

McVay Repair or Cooper's Ligament Repair (Fig. 19.36)

The study by Anson and co-workers in 1940s proved that the transversalis fascia inserts on iliopectineal ligament of Cooper and not on inguinal ligament.[83] Chester McVay and Anson attributed the failure of Bassini's repair to absence of repair of transversalis facia.[84] McVay realised the importance of the iliopectineal ligament in fruitful repair of inguinal and femoral hernias.

Guisseppe Ruggi used Cooper's ligament for repair of femoral hernia a century back in 1892. McVay started performing this procedure 50 years after Guisseppe in 1942.

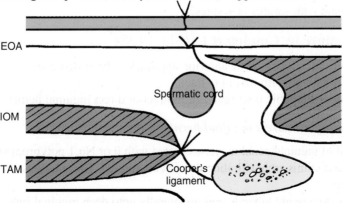

Fig. 19.36. McVay repair.

Transversalis fascia is sutured to Cooper's ligament medial to femoral vein and to inguinal ligament at the level of and lateral to femoral vein.

- It closes femoral space effectively and prevents femoral hernia also.
- The transversus fascia and aponeurotic area of transversus abdomen muscle are sutured with Cooper's ligament with 3-5 sutures.
- Thromboembolism may occur due to femoral vein narrowing.

Disadvantages of McVay or Cooper Ligament Repair

- The dissection is extensive.
- Recovery time is prolonged.

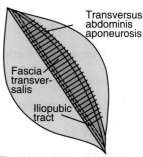

Fig. 19.37. Nyhus procedure.

Nyhus Procedure by L.M. Nyhus (Fig. 19.37)

- It is a preperitoneal approach where the iliopubic tract is sutured with fascia transversalis and transversus abdominis aponeurosis.

Steps

- A transverse incision is made 3-4 cm above the pubic symphysis.
- Skin and subcutaneous tissue are cut in the same line.
- Anterior rectus sheath is exposed.
- Deep inguinal ring is located by putting index finger into external inguinal ring. It is done to locate internal inguinal ring and then an incision is made in anterior rectus sheath just above the level of internal inguinal ring.
- A transverse incision is made over the mid rectus level on the side of hernia.
- Fascia and all the three abdominal muscles are cut in the same line.
- Now transversalis fascia is exposed.
- Now cut the transversalis fascia in the same line and preperitoneal space is approached.
- Sac is identified and isolated.
- Contents are pushed and the sac is ligated and excised.
- Now close the fused edges of transversus abdominis aponeurosis and fascia transversalis with iliopubic tract with 2-0 polypropylene.
- Close the wound with sutures or staples.

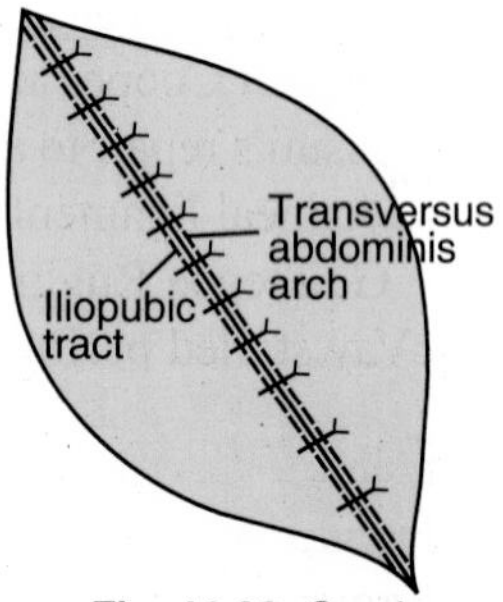

Fig. 19.38. Condon procedure.

Condon Procedure by Condon R.L. (Fig. 19.38)

It is an iliopubic tract repair with anterior approach. The transversus abdominis arch is sutured with iliopubic tract.

It is the anterior iliopubic tract repair of indirect or direct inguinal hernia.

Condon procedure for indirect inguinal hernia

- Posterior wall of inguinal canal is reconstructed with 0 or No.1 polypropylene.
- Transversus abdominis arch with iliopubic tract is sutured. The suture used is non-absorbable i.e. polypropylene.
- Start suturing from pubic tubercle and go laterally upto deep inguinal ring.
- One or two sutures are applied lateral to cord in deep inguinal ring to reconstruct it.

Condon procedure for direct inguinal hernia

- Make an incision in posterior wall of inguinal canal or bulge.
- Excise the loose and redundant tissue.
- Suture transverse abdominis arch with Cooper's ligament and iliopubic tract.
- If required a relaxing incision or Tanner's slide is made.
- First the Tanner's slide is made then sutures of reconstruction of posterior wall of inguinal canal are tied.

Kuntz Procedure (Fig. 19.39)

In this procedure testis is removed (orchidectomy) with spermatic cord from the level of deep inguinal ring.

Indications of Kuntz's procedure

It is done to avoid recurrence in old persons with weak musculature like:
- With very weak muscle tone.
- With very big hernia.
- With recurrence.

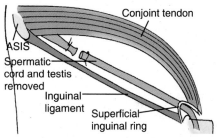

Fig. 19.39. Kuntz's procedure.

Aim

To prevent recurrence of hernia and preserve the strength of inguinal region.

Orchidectomy is done and spermatic cord is removed as pressure of spermatic cord causes weakness in inguinal area.

Procedures

- Orchidectomy
- Bassini's repair

Hamilton-Bailey Operation (Fig. 19.40)

It includes the following procedures:
- Herniotomy.
- Excision of spermatic cord after ligation at deep and superficial inguinal rings. Testis is not removed.
- Inguinal canal is closed.

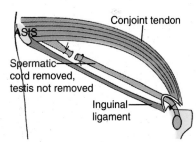

Fig. 19.40. Hamilton-Bailey operation.

Bracey's Modification (Fig. 19.41)

A Bassini's repair is done and then a releasing incision is made on fascia lata in the thigh below the inguinal ligament to relieve tension on suture line.

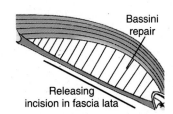

Fig. 19.41. Bracey's modification.

Farquharson's Modification (Fig. 19.42)

The overlapping of two flaps of external oblique aponeurosis is done and spermatic cord is placed between these two layers.

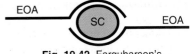

Fig. 19.42. Farquharson's modification.

Marcy's Technique (Fig. 19.43)

Henry Orlando Marcy (1837-1924) used to operate hernia by this technique. He was first who realised the protecting action of transversalis fascia in the beginning of the 19th century. He being a student of Joseph Lister, used carbolized catgut.[89,90]

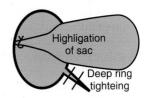

Fig. 19.43. Marcy technique.

It consists of two steps:
• High ligation of hernia sac.
• Tightening of deep inguinal ring by 1-2 sutures in the fascia transversalis.

It is smaller and more anatomically focussed than the Bassini repair.

Abrahamson's Nylon Darn Repair (Fig. 19.44)

The gap between musculoaponeurotic arch (conjoint tendon) and inguinal ligament and iliopubic tract is filled with multiple layers of polypropylene suture.

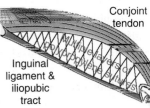

Fig. 19.44. Abrahamson's Nylon darn repair.

Moloney Darn Repair (1948) (Fig. 19.45)

Moloney was not satisfied with poor results of Bassini's repair of inguinal hernia, so he developed his "tension-free lattice" technique to fill the gap between transversus arch and inguinal ligament. The recurrence rate after his technique was lower than Bassini's repair.

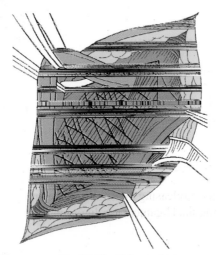

Fig. 19.45. Moloney darn.

In this method, continuous suturing is done with nylon suture which apposes fascia transversalis, transversus abdominis, rectus abdominis, internal oblique muscles to the inguinal ligament. Sutures are made either in parallel or in crisscross manner.

The rationale of the darn procedure is to form a mesh work of non-absorbable suture that is well-tolerated by the tissues. The interstices filled with fibrous connective tissue produces a buttress across the weakened area of the inguinal canal.[11]

Suture material in herniorrhaphy

- Absorbable sutures are not used in hernia repair due to the following reasons:
  - Catgut loses 50% of tensile strength within one week.
  - It gets absorbed in 90-100 days.
  - 80% wound tensile strength is achieved in 6 months and healing process takes 1 year.
- Braided silk is not used for hernia repair due to the following reasons:
  - Loses 40% of tensile strength in 6 weeks.
  - Polyfilament braided suture causes more tissue reaction.
  - It promotes infection as it harbours bacteria in the spaces between filaments.
- Monofilament non-absorbable synthetic suture like polypropylene is an ideal suture.

NOTE

Primary tissue repair procedures are losing their place in hernia surgery due to higher percentage of recurrence as compared to prosthetic repairs.

KEY POINT

Tension-free mesh repair is the operation of choice in open surgery for uncomplicated, unilateral, reducible inguinal hernias.

HERNIOPLASTY

"I know more than hundred surgeons whom I would cheerfully allow to remove my gall bladder but only one whom I should like to expose my inguinal canal."

- Sir William Henaege Ogilvie

"Tension-free repairs have become the "gold sandard" in hernia surgery"

- J. Stephenson Scott *et al.*,
Mastery of Surgery, 2007

"It is the reconstruction or strengthening of the posterior wall of the inguinal canal by filling the defect or weak area with autogenous or heterogenous material."

The commonest material used now is polypropylene mesh.

The various procedures of hernioplasty are as follows:

- **Lichtenstein's method or Gold standard method**
  - In it a tension-free implant of polypropylene mesh is done.
- **Stoppa's method**
  - Giant polypropylene mesh is used in preperitoneal space.
- **Gallie's method**
  - A strip of fascia lata is used to repair the weak area of posterior wall of inguinal canal.
- **Mair's method**
  - Skin strip is used to repair posterior wall of inguinal canal.
- **Blood good's method**
  - Anterior rectus sheath flap is used for repair.
- **Mac Arthur's method**
  - Flap is used from external oblique aponeurosis for repair.
- **NRCH (Nigam's Reverse Curtain Hernioplasty)**
  - Mesh is only sutured with three sutures to inguinal ligament and rest of the mesh is free like a "reverse curtain". The femoral canal is also closed to avoid femoral hernia.
- **"Plug and Patch" technique of Rutkow and Robbins**
  - A prosthetic mesh plug and mesh sheets are used.
- **Darning**
  - Usually a Gallie's needle is used with a big eye. The darning is done with the non-absorbable material between conjoint tendon and inguinal ligament.
- **Kugel's procedure**
  - A prosthetic patch in preperitoneal space.
- **Rives's repair**
  - The gap between the conjoint tendon and the inguinal ligament is filled with a mesh in preperitoneal space behind fascia transversalis.
- **Gosset's repair**
  - Silk ribbon is used.
- **Wantz posterior approach of open preperitoneal prosthetic repair**
  - A transverse incision is chosen, 2-3 cm below the level of ASIS, but above internal ring.[12]
- **Laparoscopic hernioplasty**
  - It is performed either by trans-abdominal approach or by total extraperitoneal approach.

Indications of Hernioplasty

- All direct inguinal hernia.
- Indirect inguinal hernia with poor muscle tone.
- Recurrent inguinal hernia.

Inguinal hernia repair is now questioned in asymptomatic hernias.[133,134]

Various Materials Used in Hernioplasty

- **Autogenous material or natural material** (patient's own tissues)
  The materials used are mentioned below:
  - Strip of fascia lata: It is taken by a fasciotome from lateral side of thigh.
  - Strip of external oblique aponeurosis.
  - Strip of anterior rectus sheath.
  - Skin is used in two ways:
    a) As skin ribbon and b) As skin flap (dermoplasty).
- **Heterogenous material**
  - **Metals**
    a) Stainless steel wire
    b) Stainless steel mesh
    c) Silver mesh
  - **Synthetic mesh**
    a) Polypropylene mesh
    b) Mersiline mesh
    c) Polyglactin mesh
    d) Composite mesh, polypropylene-polyglactin and polypropylene-polyglecaprone mesh.

> **KEY POINT**
>
> *The large inguinal scrotal sac should not be dissected beyond pubic tubercle to avoid chances of orchitis and post-operative atrophy of testis.*

Lichtenstein's Tension-free Hernioplasty (Figs. 19.46 A-E)

Irving L. Lichtenstein, pioneered "Tension-free hernioplasty", in 1984.[13]

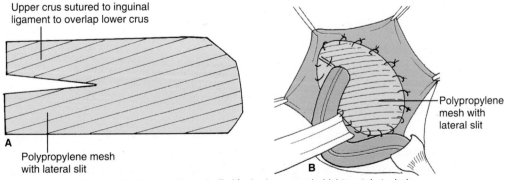

Upper crus sutured to inguinal
ligament to overlap lower crus

A
Polypropylene mesh
with lateral slit

Polypropylene
mesh with
lateral slit

B

Fig. 19.46A. Prosthetic mesh, **B.** Mesh placement in Lichtenstein technique.

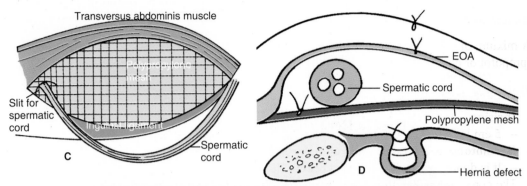

Fig. 19.46C & D. Mesh placement in Lichtenstein technique, schematic representation.

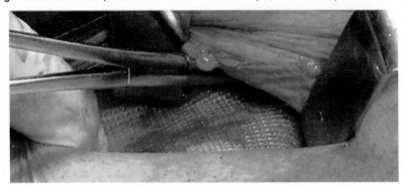

Fig. 19.46E. Mesh in Lichtenstein technique.

He realised that tension of suture line is the main cause of recurrence.

He wrote in 1964: **"We have found that if the mesh is used to bridge the defect instead of as a reinforcement for tissues approximated under stress, this factor of tension is eliminated and recurrence becomes less likely".**[14,15] He used tension-free mesh repair on 1000 patients with minimal complications and zero recurrence.

The same technique is used for both indirect and direct inguinal hernias and other groin hernias also. Lichtenstein was criticised badly by other surgeons for his tension-free mesh herniorrhaphy and now it has become a Gold Standard groin hernia repair.[15]

It is done under local anaesthesia.

Indications of Lichtenstein procedure

• All direct inguinal hernia.
• Indirect inguinal hernia with poor musculature.
• Recurrent inguinal hernia.

Principles of Lichtenstein hernioplasty

• A big polypropylene mesh is used to cover the Hesselbach's triangle, deep inguinal ring and an area 2-4 cm beyond this area on all sides without any tension.
• In this technique, a prosthetic implant is used without the repair of posterior wall of inguinal canal.

Anaesthesia

A mixture of 0.5% Lignocaine and 0.25% Bupivacaine is locally infiltrated. If required a sedative (propofol or midazolam) is given intravenously.

Technique

- **Incision**
  - 5 cm long incision 1.5 cm above the medial part of inguinal ligament.
- **Herniotomy**
  - It is done as described earlier.
- The conjoint tendon is not unphysiologically pulled down with tension to suture with inguinal ligament.
- A polypropylene mesh, 6×10 cm is placed on posterior wall of inguinal canal and is sutured with pubic tubercle, inguinal ligament and conjoint tendon with 2-0 polypropylene continuous sutures. Rectus sheath and conjoint tendon are sutured with continuous 3-0 polypropylene sutures.

> **NOTE**
>
> *The mesh should be relaxed and not kept tense. Nowadays a padded dome-shaped mesh is used which accommodates propulsive pressure on fascia transversalis during standing and straining. It avoids shrinkage and contraction of mesh.[16]*

- The inferiomedial corner of the mesh well overlaps the pubic tubercle upto 2-3 cm. Mesh must not be taut but kept relaxed.
- The lateral edge of the mesh is split to accommodate spermatic cord. The two crura are overlapped and sutured down to create new deep inguinal ring which fits snuggly around the spermatic cord.
- Care should be taken to avoid nerve injury.
- External oblique aponeurosis is sutured back in front of spermatic cord.
- If a direct inguinal hernia is found, usually the sac is not opened. The sac and preperitoneal fat are reduced and kept reduced with the help of forceps. A continuous non-absorbable 2-0 suture is used to repair the floor of the inguinal canal. The suture starts at the pubic tubercle and continues upto the deep inguinal ring by taking small bites in fascia transversalis. Now the sheet of mesh is placed and fixed.[17]

Advantages of Lichtenstein technique

- Recurrence rate is less than 1% (0.1%).
- Short learning curve.
- It does not require an experienced surgeon or expensive instruments.
- It is done under local anaesthesia.
- It is a physiological procedure.
- Lichtenstein advocates the routine use of tension-free mesh hernioplasty but other workers have advocated its selective use as there is not much work done about its long term biological compatibility.
- Lichtenstein hernia institute uses pre-shaped different meshes for right and left sides.
- Eggar *et al.* used skin staples for securing prosphetic mesh in Lichtenstein tension-free hernia repair. Stapling of mesh reduces the operation time than suturing the mesh.[18]

The Stoppa's Procedure (Figs. 19.47 A & B)

Invented by Dr Rene F. Stoppa.
• He uses the term GPRVS (Giant Prosthetic Reinforcement of Visceral Sac).
• The prosthesis replaces endopubic fascia.
• The hernia defect in anterior abdominal wall is reinforced with a big polypropylene mesh prosthesis in Bogro's space (preperitoneal space).
• Prosthesis is not fixed with sutures. The abdominal pressure keeps the prosthesis stable and then soon adhesions develop and prosthesis gets fixed.
• The term "parietalization of spermatic cord" was popularized by Stoppa, which needs thorough dissection of the spermatic cord to provide enough length, so that it can move laterally.

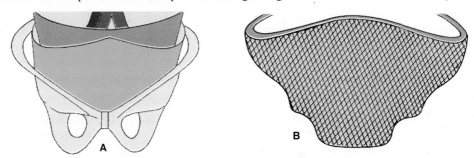

Fig. 19.47A. Stoppa's procedure, **B.** Prosthetic mesh used.

Indications of GPRVS

• Recurrent hernias
• Multiple groin hernias
• Groin hernia with lower abdominal incisional hernia
• Sliding hernia
• Huge inguinoscrotal hernia

Contraindications of GPRVS

• Skin infection
• Scarred lower abdomen due to multiple previous surgeries (relative contraindication)

Step

Position of patient
10-20° Trendelenberg position

Incision
• Subcutaneous tissue and fascia are cut in line of incision and two rectus muscles are retracted.
• Blunt dissection is done with gauze and finger and swab is mounted on sponge holder.
• Dissection proceeds to space of Retzius and space of Bogros, behind ileopubic tract, first on one side and then on the other side.
• Hernia sac is either excised or invaginated.
• Parietalization of spermatic cord is done.

- Measurements of mesh and pelvis are taken (distance between 2 ASIS minus 2 cm is equal to the transverse measurement of the mesh, vertical measurement is from umbilicus to pubis).
- Mesh is then placed with the help of long forceps.
- Mesh is fixed only by one absorbable suture to Richet's fascia in midline.
- Wound is closed with a drain or two.

Recurrence

- In 1989, 529 GPRVS repairs showed 0.56% recurrence in primary repair and 1.1% recurrence for recurrent hernia repair.[19,20,21]

Sutureless Mesh Plug Technique of Gilbert

It was invented by Dr Arthur I. Gilbert of Hernia Institute of Florida, USA. It was then modified by Rutkow and Robbins, Millikan and others.

Gilbert says that "The privilege of visiting and operating with Rene Stoppa in Amiens further convinced me that the ideal place to position mesh is in the properitoneal space, between the force of the hernia and the defect in the abdominal wall".[91]

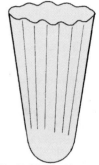

- Gilbert developed a technique of inverting the hernia sac and plugging the defect with the cone of a prosthetic mesh.[92] It looks like an upside-down umbrella[93] (Fig. 19.48).
- The polypropylene mesh is cut and folded in the shape of a cone to form plug according to the size of the defect.

Fig. 19.48. Mesh cone.

- The plug is introduced in the deep inguinal ring in indirect inguinal hernia.
- Dr Gilbert does not use any stitch to fix both the plug and the mesh sheet.

Plug and Patch Technique of Rutkow and Robbins

Invented by Dr Rutkow Ira M. and Dr Robbins Alan W of Rutkow Robbins Hernia Center, Freehold, New Jersey, USA (Figs. 19.41 & 19.42).

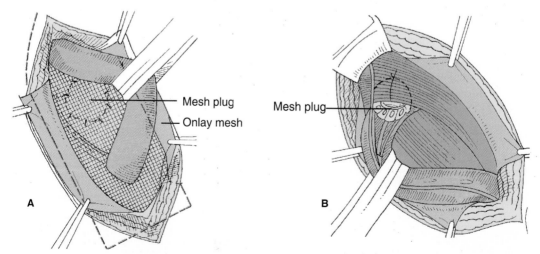

Fig. 19.49A. Cone plug and mesh in direct inguinal hernia repair, **B.** Cone plug and mesh in indirect inguinal hernia repair.

In this technique, a polypropylene mesh plug is used in hernia orifice, deep inguinal ring, and a patch of polypropylene mesh is used in posterior wall of inguinal canal.

- In 1995, Rutkow and Robbins wrote their first article about Per Fix plug.[94]
- Rutkow humorously calls it "Plugtenstein" technique as the result resembles Lichtenstein repair.
- Herniotomy is done as described earlier.
- Polypropylene mesh cone or plug is guided with surgeon's finger in the deep inguinal ring.[22]
- Plug is secured with 1-0 or 2-0 non-absorbable sutures to inguinal ligament.
- Onlay "patch" of mesh is placed on posterior wall of inguinal canal with lateral slit allowing spermatic cord to come out.
- Both tails are approximated with one 2-0 non-absorbable suture.
- Mesh patch is not sutured down.
- Indirect inguinal hernia sac is excised and the plug is placed in deep inguinal ring, sutures are applied at its periphery. Rest of the procedure is same.
- This method is used both in primary as well as in recurrent inguinal hernia.
- Rutkow and Robbins claim that the results and recurrence are comparable to Lichtenstein repair.[131]
- Rutkow does not suture the mesh patch but some surgeons suture it like Lichtenstein repair with inguinal ligament and internal oblique muscle.

Steps

Incision
- 5-6 cm incision 2 cm above and parallel to medial part of inguinal ligament.

Herniotomy

It is done as described earlier.
- Indirect inguinal hernia sac is invaginated and the lax transversalis fascia is reconstructed with 2-0, non-absorbable sutures from pubic tubercle to deep inguinal ring.
- A cone-shaped plug is made of polypropylene mesh. The deep inguinal ring is felt with the surgeon's finger to assess the size. The plug is introduced in the deep inguinal ring. The plug is secured to the conjoint tendon with 2-0 polyglactin suture. Plug should be placed behind the muscle and in such a way that preperitoneal fat and hernia sac cannot come out.
  Care of inferior epigastric vessels must be taken.
- Further steps of operation are same for both direct and indirect inguinal hernias.
  - A rectangular polypropylene mesh of 3×10 cm in size is used with a lateral slit for spermatic cord.
  - The mesh is placed on the floor of canal with its two crura encircling the spermatic cord.
  - A 2-0 polypropylene suture anchors the mesh with inguinal ligament from pubic tubercle to deep inguinal ring.
  - The upper margin is sutured with few interrupted sutures to underlying internal oblique muscle.
  - Two tails of the mesh are overlapped and sutured so a new deep inguinal ring of mesh is formed.

Rutkow and Robbins used an Umbrella plug (readymade) of polypropylene.[23] Gilbert used to prepare the plug for use at operation table. C. R. Bard Company marketed the preformed plug of Rutkow by the name "Per Fix Plug". This Per Fix Plug can be modified by the surgeon by removing few petals to suit the patient. The Per Fix Plug is inserted in the internal ring in indirect hernia, femoral ring in femoral hernia and hernia defect in direct inguinal hernia. One or two interrupted sutures are applied to fix the plug.

Kugel Hernia Repair (Preperitoneal Patch Repair)

Robert D. Kugel started using handmade polypropylene patches in 1994 by preperitoneal patch repair method. The forces available with the preperitoneal space secure the patch in place. These forces are:

* Intra-abdominal pressure
* Hydrostatic tissue forces

The Mesh Patch (Fig. 19.50)

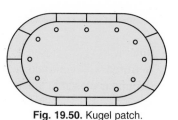

Fig. 19.50. Kugel patch.

Nowadays "Bard Kugel Patch", a two-layered monofilament of polypropylenes mesh patch is used. This oval-shaped patch has slits at periphery which allows it to unfold after placement and attain a suitable configuration.

* The patch also has multiple 'V'-shaped cuts which pop out when mesh is placed in hernia site and act as anchors for the prosthesis.
* The "Bard Kugel Patch" comes in the following two sizes:
    – 8 × 12 cm
    – 11 × 14 cm
* The open preperitoneal prosthetic repairs were developed to compete with laparoscopic repairs by using a small skin incision above the internal ring.[24, 25]

Technique

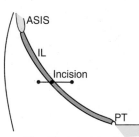

Fig. 19.51. Incision for Kugel hernia repair.

* A prosthetic patch is introduced in preperitoneal space.
* A 3 cm long incision (Fig. 19.51) is made with its centre at middle part of inguinal ligament or just above it after marking both ASIS and pubic tubercle.
* Underlying muscles are approached by dissecting in the same line and then muscle fibres are splitted, not cut.
* A similar vertical incision of about 3 cm length is made on fascia transversalis.
* A space is created in preperitoneal space by separating transversalis fascia and peritoneum by blunt dissection.
* The preperitoneal pocket so made is bounded as described below:
    – Medially: Pubic symphysis.
    – Laterally: 3 cm lateral to incision.
    – Posteriorly: Over iliac vessels.
    – Inferiorly: Inguinal ligament.
    – Superiorly: 3 cm above the incision.

Indirect inguinal hernia

Sac and peritoneum are dissected to separate from spermatic cord at approximately 3 cm posterior to deep inguinal ring.

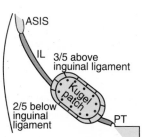

Fig. 19.52. Kugel patch in position.

Direct inguinal hernia

Dissection is done medially also. The patch is introduced by index finger. The patch is pushed in the pocket and is kept parallel to the inguinal ligament (Fig. 19.52).

- It is three-fifths above the inguinal ligament and two-fifths below it.
- Before the closure of the wound the patch is felt with index finger. It is opened properly and should be without any folds or wrinkles.
- Transversalis fascia wound is closed with single 2-0 polypropylene suture taking a bit of patch to fix it.
- Internal oblique muscle is not sutured to avoid nerve entrapment. External oblique aponeurosis is sutured with continuous absorbable suture.
- Wound is closed in layers as usual with 2-0 polyglactin sutures.

Post-operative recurrence

Between January 1, 1994 to September 9, 2004, a total of 1662 groin hernias were operated by Robert D Kugel for primary and recurrent groin hernia. 134 repairs were performed for recurrent hernia. Only 7 recurrences happened in primary hernia and no recurrence happened in group of recurrent hernia (0%).[96,97,98]

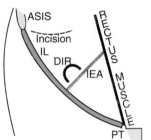

Fig. 19.53A. Incision, above and lateral to deep inguinal ring.

Ugahary Repair (Grid Iron Hernioplasty) (Figs. 19.53 A & B)

Franz Ugahary, Department of surgery, Rivierenland Ziekenhuis Tiel, the Netherlands.

The preperitoneal space is approached through a 3 cm incision similar to Kugel's operation. The space is held open by retractors. A 10 × 15 cm piece of polypropylene mesh is rolled on to a long forceps and introduced into the preperitoneal space, the mesh is then unrolled.[26]

Grid Iron hernioplasty is a minimally invasive, simple and rapid operation for the treatment of nearly all types of groin hernia.[27]

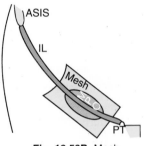

Fig. 19.53B. Mesh completely overlaping MPO.

NRCH (Nigam's Reverse Curtain Hernioplasty), Nigam V.K., Nigam, S., Surgeon, The Apollo Clinic, Gurgaon, India[28]

Principle

- It is a tension-free polypropylene mesh hernioplasty.
- Least number of sutures are used, as mesh is anchored to inguinal ligament with only three sutures and rest of the mesh remains free like an inverted curtain between the external oblique aponeurosis and internal oblique muscle.
- Middle suture on inguinal ligament also closes femoral canal so prevents future development of femoral hernia.
- NRCH does not distort the normal anatomy and physiology of inguinal area.

Advantages of NRCH

- It repairs IIH and DIH with least recurrence.
- It closes femoral ring and thus prevents future development of the femoral hernia.

Steps (Figs. 19.54 A-C)

Incision

A 5 cm long incision is made 2 cm above and parallel to medial part of inguinal ligament.

Herniotomy

It is done as described earlier.

- A 15 cm × 15 cm polypropylene mesh is used, which is fixed to inguinal ligament at base with only three 2/0 polypropylene sutures and the rest of the mesh remains free like an inverted curtain. It covers the groin hernia prone area well. Mesh is tailored after fixing it to the inguinal ligament.
- First suture is applied at pubic tubercle, not including the periosteum.
- Second suture, Nigam's suture, applied on inguinal ligament, medial to femoral vein anchors the mesh as well as narrows or closes the femoral ring thereby prevents the future development of femoral hernia. It is taken deep including Cooper's ligament.
- Third suture is from inguinal ligament lateral to deep inguinal ring.
- The mesh is cut from medial margin to make slit for spermatic cord. Deep inguinal ring narrowing and anchoring of two crura of mesh is done with the fourth suture. So one suture serves double purpose, reduces the dissection as well as number of sutures. Deep inguinal ring narrowing is done on lateral side to avoid injury to inferior epigastric vessels.

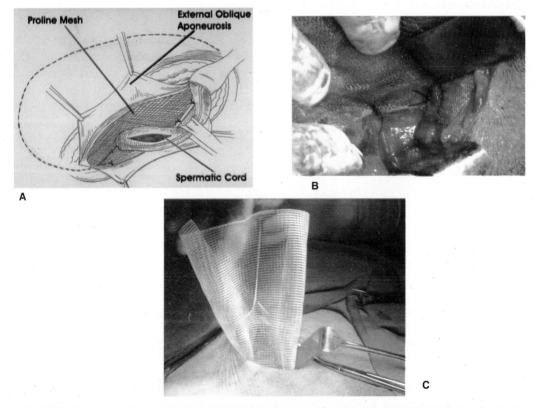

Fig. 19.54. Reverse curtain hernioplasty, NRCH, **A.** Schematic representation of NRCH, **B.** First and second sutures (second suture closes femoral canal), **C.** Mesh placement.

- A space is made with the index finger between the external oblique aponeurosis and the internal oblique muscles as anatomic cleavage between these two layers is avascular and dissection is done rapidly and non-traumatically.[130]
- Closure of the external oblique aponeurosis is done in semi-double breasting manner which serves the following dual purpose:
  - Keep the mesh in place by applying soft pressure, reduces haematoma.
  - Narros the superficial inguinal ring.

Prolene Hernia System, Ethicon, Somerville, New Jersey, USA (Figs. 19.55 A-C)

It is also known as "The Bilayer Mesh Hernioplasty". This system was developed by Dr Arthur I. Gilbert of Miami Clinic for Hernia, USA, in 1997 when he was a consultant to Ethicon Company (Somerville NJ). In its first generation, it was available in three sizes.[98]

It is a prosthetic system made by joining two meshes with a connector. One mesh remains outside the hernia prone area of anterior abdominal wall as onlay mesh and other mesh are inside the anterior abdominal wall and the connector is in the defect. Gilbert is of opinion that by introducing mesh on both sides of MPO, the area is permanently protected from hernia development.[29] It may be superior to open repair of inguinal hernia.[132]

- **Onlay patch** – It is of polypropylene. It covers MPO and lies under external oblique aponeurosis.
- **Underlay patch** – It has absorbable monocryl, lies in preperitoneal space and gives support.
- **Connector** – It is placed in deep inguinal ring.

Blunt dissection in preperitoneal space at the level of internal ring is done with the help of a finger to create space for internal layer of the mesh. The hernia sac is either invaginated or ligated and excised. The onlay patch is sutured with tissues medial to pubic tubercle, inguinal ligament and transversus arch. 6835 groin hernia repairs were done by PHS from April 1998 to June 2005 at the Hernia Institute of Florida, USA, by 4 surgeons and 5 cases of recurrence were reported.[99,100]

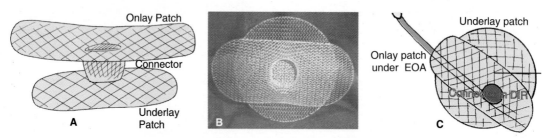

Fig. 19.55A. PHS, diagrammatic view, **B.** Photograph, **C.** In place.

Trabucco Tension-Free Suture Less Pre-shaped Mesh Repair (Figs. 19.56 A-C)

It is a tension free sutureless hernioplasty performed with a rigid pre-shaped polypropylene mesh.[30] Trabucco used a rigid preformed polypropylene mesh in inguinal box, a closed anatomical space so the mesh cannot migrate. Mesh is placed between external oblique muscle forming roof and internal oblique muscle with fascia transversalis forming floor of the inguinal box, mesh occupying as the middle layer. It has a low rate of complications and a low incidence of recurrence. Postoperative pain is minimal and the patient can quickly resume working and recreational activities.[31]

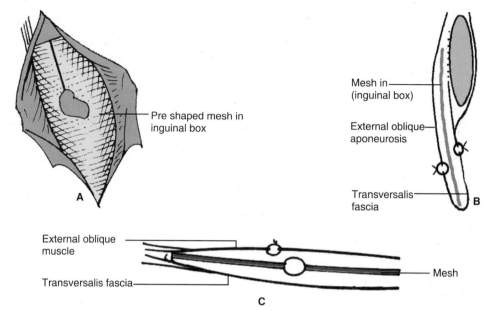

Fig. 19.56A. Sutureless pre-shaped mesh technique of Trabucco, anterior view,
B. Sagittal view, **C.** Horizontal-transverse view.

Reed-Rives Approach (Fig. 19.57)

It is like Bassini's repair except that fascia transversalis is opened and a
12 × 16 cm piece of mesh is pushed and spread on preperitoneal space.
The mesh is fixed with three sutures to pubic tubercle, inguinal ligament
and psoas major muscle.[32, 82]

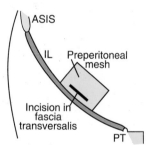

Fig. 19.57. Reed-Rives
approach.

Wantz's Approach (Fig. 19.58)

It is an unilateral preperitoneal approach. It is similar to Stoppa's
procedure using a giant prosthetic mesh in preperitoneal space covering
hernia prone area.[33, 81] The prosthesis is fixed with anterior abdominal
wall above the hernia defect. The lower border and corners of mesh
are unrolled with long clamps over MPO in preperitoneal space.

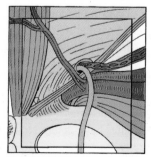

Fig. 19.58. Wantz's approach.

COMPLICATIONS OF OPEN INGUINAL HERNIA REPAIR

"If there is a possibility of several things going wrong, the one
that will cause the most damage will be the one to go wrong."

- Murphy's Law

"I do not seek kingdom; I do not seek heaven; I do not seek moksha; I pray that the
suffering humanity be relieved from pain."

- Mahatma Gandhi

The success of any method of herniorrhaphy is operator dependent and in the competent hands. Any standard technique gives good results and low recurrence rates.[34]

Intraoperative Complications

- Injury to ilioinguinal, iliohypogastric, genital branch of genitofemoral, lateral cutaneous nerves of the thigh and femoral nerve.
- Injury to inferior epigastric and femoral vessels, testicular artery and pampiniform plexus of veins.
- Injury to vas deferens.
- Injury to contents of hernia sac.
- Injury to external iliac vein or femoral vein. It usually occurs while taking bite from inguinal ligament. If there is only a prick to vein it usually subsides with application of hot and moist pack.
- Injury to urinary bladder.
  - Urinary bladder is sometimes injured in operation of direct inguinal hernia. Repair the bladder in two layers with absorbable sutures, put a drain in prevesical space and pass a Foley's catheter.

Post-operative Complications

Early

Haemorrhage
Haemorrhage occurs due to injury to the following structures:
- Femoral vein
- Long saphenous vein
- Abnormal obturator artery, during division of lacunar ligament in femoral hernia repair.
- Haemorrhage can cause bruising or haematoma.

Scrotal oedema

Retention of urine
Some surgeons prefer preoperative and intraoperative bladder catheterization as a routine procedure. Studies have demonstrated a higher rate of urinary tract complications with routine catheterization.

Haematoma of cord and scrotum
Haematoma can develop in retroperitoneum, scrotum, spermatic cord and wound.

Wound infection
It occurs specially in strangulated hernia operation. The incidence is 1-2%.

Robert Bendavid reported wound infection rate 0.27% to 1% with 7000 Shouldice inguinal herniorrhaphy performed every year.[101]

Even if the infection encroaches into the mesh itself, a conservative attempt is justifiable, provided the mesh is porous. Late infections appearing after months or even years are more challenging. They are often combined with complex fistulas including bowel. In these cases, preservation of the mesh is likely to fail and sooner or later most of the mesh has to be removed.[35]

> Studies have shown that the use of single dose antibiotic one-half hour before the surgery reduces the incidence of infection from 4% to 2%. Fischer applies his routine use of Hibiclens for three days, clipping rather shaving, use of Ioban after Iodine tincture, and prophylactic antibiotic as single dose and if the operation goes beyond three hours, a repeat dose is given.[102]

DVT (Deep Vein Thrombosis)

It occurs specially in the following conditions:
- If the patient is immobilized for long.
- If the femoral vein is compressed or injured.

Seroma (Fig. 19.59)

It is a self-limiting problem but sometimes requires several aspirations, but has a danger of introducing infection. So it must be done with aseptic precautions. Incidence of seroma is 1.2-10%. It is due to trauma to lymphatics due to dissection.

It is felt that abdominal binder reduces the chance of seroma or does not allow it to grow big.

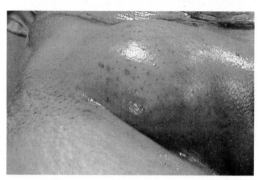

Fig. 19.59. Seroma, after inguinal hernia operation.

Daniel B Jones[103] states that "During the years, I have recommended an abdominal binder to potentially decrease the post-operative seroma" (Fig. 19.59).

Late

Neurologic pain (Iguinodynia) (Fig. 19.47)

It is common and is due to injury to any of these nerves:
- Ilioinguinal nerve.
- Iliohypogastric nerve.
- Genital branch of genitofemoral nerve.
- Lateral cutaneous nerve of the thigh (L2-L3)—It is the most common nerve involved in laparoscopic hernia surgery.

Cutaneous anaesthesia

Cutaneous anaethesia may persist for a few months and then it returns to normal.

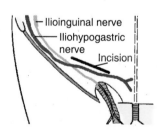

Fig. 19.60. Groin nerves injury by lateral extension or lateral placement of incision.

Recurrence

"A surgeon can do more for the community by operating on hernia cases, and seeing that his recurrence rate is lower, than he can by operating on cases of malignant diseases."

- Wakely

- 50% recurrence occurs after 5 years of operation.
- 20% recurrence is noticed after 15-25 years.
- So a long term follow-up of ten years is required.

Nowadays with tension-free hernia repair recurrence occurs in 1-2% cases. Recurrence rate is lower with tension-free repair and higher with anatomic repair.

- Early recurrence within few years is due to
  - Faulty technique
  - Missed hernia
  - Post-operative infection
- Late recurrence after few years is due to
  - Tissue weakness

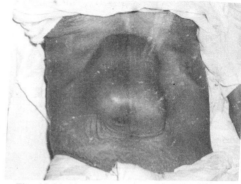

Fig. 19.61. Huge recurrence of incisional hernia.

- Recurrence is a challenge for a surgeon. The recurrence rate is kept below 2% which is the accepted rate of recurrence in hernia surgery (Fig. 19.61).

Kirk R.M. gave importance to following two factors in reducing recurrence rate:

- Enthusiasm for perfection from surgeon.
- Panistaking skill of surgeon.

NOTE

We now know that a percentage of recurrence in adults after hernia repair is due to collagen disorder. Considering the recurrence a problem of biology and collagens, one should not neglect technical failures directly leading to a poor outcome.[36]

Potential mechanisms for recurrence[37]

- Incomplete dissection
  - Missed hernias
  - Inadequate identification of landmarks
  - Prosthesis rolls up rather than lying flat
- Mesh too small
  - Incomplete coverage of all defects
- Migration of the mesh
- Mesh slit placed around cord
  - Slit may be the site of recurrence
- Folding or invagination of mesh into defect
- Displacement of mesh by hematoma

How to reduce recurrence

- Repair the hernia before it becomes big.
- High ligation of the neck of the sac.
- Narrowing of dilated deep inguinal ring.
- Exclude co-existing other hernias
- Treat diseases increasing intra-abdominal pressure in post-operative period.

> ### *Re-recurrence of inguinal hernia*
>
> Re-recurrence of inguinal hernia is a specialised problem and should be treated by experienced surgeon at a specialised hernia centre. Recurrence is more common after repair of recurrent hernias and it is directly related to the number of previous repair attempts.
>
> Large population based studies report overall re-recurrence rate of 4% to 5%. Tension-free and mesh based repairs have the lowest rate of reoperation after recurrence and provide a reduction in recurrence of approximately 60% as compared to the more traditional repairs.

Ischaemic orchitis

Ischaemic orchitis is defined as post-operative inflammation of the testicle occurring within one to five days after surgery. It occurs in about 1% primary hernioplasties, but is much more common with operations performed for recurrent hernias.[38] It is because of venous congestion rather than arterial damage.

Atrophy of testis

It occurs due to the damage to the spermatic cord. It occurs in 1-3% cases. Post-herniorrhaphy testicular orchitis may lead to testicular atrophy specially in recurrent hernia repair. Testicular atrophy rates with repairs of primary inguinal hernia was found 0.1% and after repair of recurrent inguinal hernia 0.9% by Robert Bendavid.[35] It is generally accepted that testicular complications can be decreased by division of large inguinio-scrotal sac rather than excision, leaving the distal sac open in situ.[34]

- It is seen that if the testis is brought to the wound testicular atrophy incidence increases.

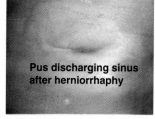

Pus discharging sinus after herniorrhaphy

Sinuses and Fistulae (Fig. 19.62)

Inter-position of omentum between mesh and intestine minimizes the chances of occurrence of enterocutaneous fistula.[117]

Fig. 19.62. Post-herniorrhaphy sinus (mesh was removed and sinus healed).

Painful scar

Epidermoid cyst

Hydrocele

It is due to extensive dissection in inguino-scrotal hernia. It is due to damage of lymphatics. Obney reported an incident of 0.7% after 14442 inguinal hernia repairs.[104]

Infertility and hernia

Groin hernia surgery can result in vas deferens obstruction in 1% of cases due to prosthetic mesh.
- Mesh used in hernia surgery may cause perivasal inflammation which increases the likelihood of vassal obstruction[39].

KEY POINT

Herniotomy, herniorrhaphy and hernioplasty are the three main operations for inguinal hernia.

OPERATION FOR GIANT INGUINAL HERNIA

Giant inguinal hernia should not be operated by a beginner but by experienced surgeon at special hernia centre.

General, spinal or epidural anaesthesia are preferred to local anaesthesia.

It is best operated in the following manner:

- Orcheidectomy with removal of spermatic cord
- Closure of deep inguinal ring
- Closure of inguinal canal
- Reinforcement of posterior wall of inguinal canal with a big prosthetic mesh (as usually the posterior wall of inguinal canal is lax and weak in such hernias).

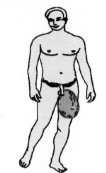

Fig. 19.63. Left giant indirect inguinal hernia.

LAPAROSCOPIC INGUINAL HERNIA SURGERY

"If you are too fond of new remedies, first you will not cure your patients;
secondly, you will have no patients to cure." ("Laparoscopic repair has proved it wrong")

- Astley Paston Cooper, 1768-1841

"What is now proved was once only imagined."

– Blake

Laparoscopic hernia surgery was first described by Ger in 1982 then by Schultz, Corbitt and Filipi in early 1990s[40,41,42,43]. In laparoscopic hernia repair, the experience of the surgeon is more important than the selection of the operative procedure.

The most extensive systematic review and meta-analysis of randomized controlled trials so far are those produced by the EU Hernia Trialists Collaborations. This group is a consortium of 70 investigators from 20 countries whose purpose is to analyse data from randomized controlled trials and report in meta-analysis form.[44] These studies indicate that laparoscopic inguinal hernia repair causes less post-operative pain and gives faster recovery than open mesh repair of inguinal hernia.

The cost, patient's satisfaction and quality of life (QOL) in relation to the laparoscopic inguinal surgery are well studied. Patient satisfaction and QOL are compensation for higher costs.

Principle of Laparoscopic Hernia Repair

The TAPP and TEP have the same basic principle of placing a piece of mesh in the preperitoneal space as described by Stoppa. The difference is that the former requires an incision in the peritoneum to access the preperitoneal space, whereas in the latter, dissection initiated and performed in the preperitoneal space.[124]

Equipment Required for Laparoscopic Hernia Repair

(1) Video monitor (Fig. 19.64)

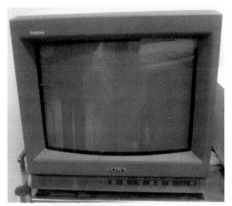

Fig. 19.64. Video monitor.

The resolution of video monitor and camera should be appropriate for a clear image. The size of monitor varies with the distance of monitor from the surgeon. A 17" monitor with resolution of 400 lines is sufficient.

(2) Telescope (Fig. 19.65)

A rod lens system is used in the telescope. Usually a 5 mm or 10 mm telescope is used with a view angle of 0° or 30°. The laparoscope can be sterilized by glutaraldehyde solution or steam autoclave.

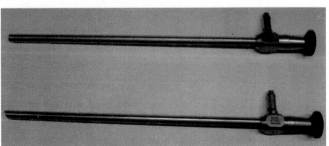

Fig.19.65. Telescopes, 0° and 30°.

(3) Camera (Fig. 19.66)

A single chip camera is commonly used. Triple chip camera is costlier but gives far better resolution. The camera should be compatible with the video monitor.

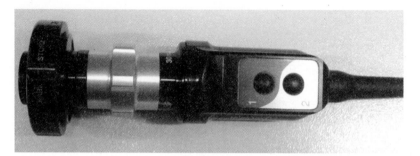

Fig.19.66. Camera.

(4) Light source – Xenon or halogen (Fig. 19.67)

Xenon or halogen light sources are used. Xenon light source of 300W or 175W is costlier but gives better and soothing light. Halogen light sources are commonly used as they are economical. These light sources are cold light sources.

    Nowadays light cables are fibre optic cables which are better than others.

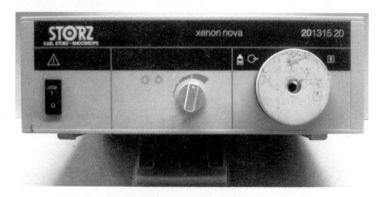

Fig.19.67. Light source – Xenon.

(5) Carbon dioxide insufflator (Fig. 19.68)

An insufflator is used to create pneumoperitoneum and to maintain pressure in the peritoneal cavity. Carbon dioxide gas is used as it is not combustible, is economical and easily available.

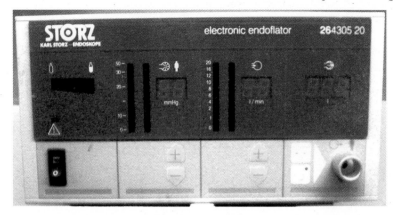

Fig.19.68. Carbon dioxide insufflator.

(6) Light cable

Fibre optic light cables are used.

(7) Suction and irrigation system

A simple suction machine of operation theatre is used for irrigation and suction purposes.

(8) Monopolar cautery

Both monopolar and bipolar cauteries are used. Bipolar cautery produces less heat to the surrounding area. One should be careful with the use of cautery as it can cause thermal injuries to the abdominal organs.

(9) Trocars and cannulas (Figs. 19.69 & 19.70)

Trocars and cannulas are both reusable and disposable. Following two sizes are commonly used:
• 10 mm Hasson Trocar – one

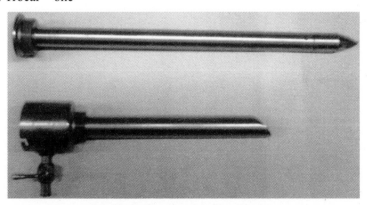

Fig.19.69. 10 mm trocar and cannula.

- 5 mm Trocar – two

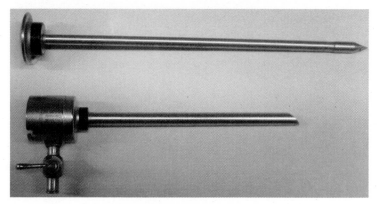

Fig.19.70. 5 mm trocar and cannula.

(10) Hand instruments

- Veress needle (Figs. 19.71 A & B) is used to create pneumoperitoneum. It is both disposable and reusable.

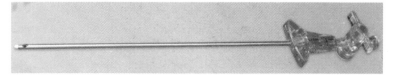

Fig.19.71A. Veress needle.

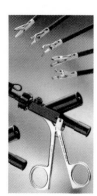

Fig.19.71B. Tips and handles of laparoscopic instruments

- Maryland dissector – 5 mm (Fig. 19.72)
- Grasper-traumatic – 5 mm. (Fig. 19.73)
- Grasper-atraumatic – 5 mm
- Scissors-curved – 5 mm (Fig. 19.72)

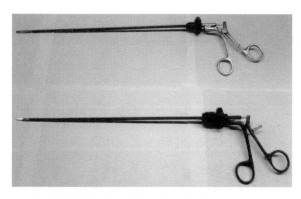

Fig.19.72. Maryland dissector and scissors.

- Suction tube and cannula 5 mm
- Endoloop and endoloop reducer
- Clip applicator (Fig. 19.73)
- Tacker with 5 mm helical tacks – Fixation device (Fig. 19.74)

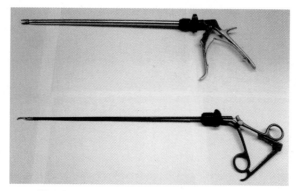

Fig.19.73. Clip applicator and grasper.

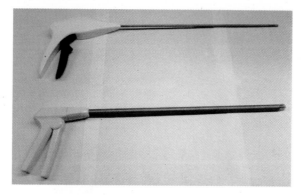

Fig.19.74. Tacker, 5 and 10 mm.

- Polypropylene mesh (Fig. 19.75)

- Clips and tacks (Fig. 19.75)

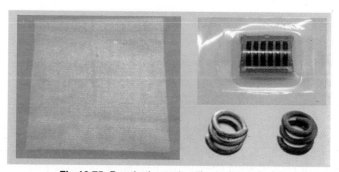

Fig.19.75. Prosthetic mesh, clips and tacks.

• Bipolar cautery (Fig. 19.76)

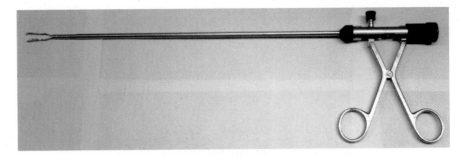

Fig.19.76. Bipolar cautery.

• Needle holder (Fig. 19.77)

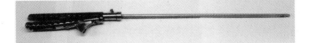

Fig.19.77. Needle holder.

• Balloons (Fig. 19.78)

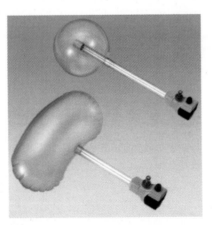

Fig.19.78. Balloons to create preperitoneal working space.

Indications (Fig. 19.79)

Several studies recently have shown benefits of laparoscopic over open hernia repair.[45]
Laparoscopic hernia surgery can be performed with unilateral and bilateral inguinal hernias. The clear indications of laparoscopic hernia repair is shown in Fig. 19.79.

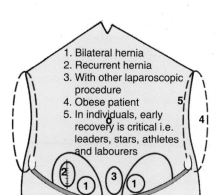

Fig.19.79. Indications of laparoscopic hernia repair.

- **Recurrent inguinal hernia**
  – In recurrent hernia, the normal anatomy is distorted due to scar tissue. Open repair of recurrent inguinal hernia has high failure rate upto 30% as it is done through scar tissue. On the other hand, the laparoscopic repair is done through healthy tissue so failure rate is considerably reduced.
- **Bilateral hernia**
  – Both sides hernia can be repaired by same ports and at same time.
- An inguinal hernia patient undergoing some other laparoscopic procedure can also be operated for hernia in same sitting.
- Obese patient.
- Patients in whom the early recovery is critical such as athletes and labourers.

   Large, randomized, prospective trials will be needed to definitively settle the questions of whether the added risks and costs are worth the benefit[46,136] and recurrence.[137]

Contraindications

- Strangulated and obstructed hernia.
- Intra-abdominal infection e.g peritonitis.
- Acute abdomen with strangulated or infarcted bowel.
- Coagulopathy.
- Inability to establish pneumoperitoneum safely.
- Pelvic radiation.
- Relative contraindications include:
  – Intra-abdominal adhesions from previous surgery.
  – Ascites.
  – Previous surgery in the space of Retzius, due to risk of bladder injury.
  – Severe medical illness as it adds risk to general anaesthesia.

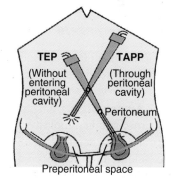

Fig. 19.80. TEP and TAPP techniques, diagrammatic representation.

Techniques to Perform Laparoscopic Hernia Surgery (Fig. 19.80)

- TAPP (Transabdominal Preperitoneal) hernia repair.

- TEP (Total Extraperitoneal) hernia repair.
- IPOM (Intraperitoneal Onlay Mesh) hernia repair.

Advantages of laparoscopic hernia repair over open hernia repair:

- Less post-operative complications, such as orchitis, epididymitis, neuralgia and wound infection.
- Faster return to normal activity.
- Good for bilateral and recurrent inguinal hernia.
- Contralateral hernia can be diagnosed and operated at the same time.

Disadvantages of laparoscopic hernia repair over open hernia repair:

- Risk of serious visceral or vascular injuries.
- Expensive.
- It has longer learning curve as it is difficult to learn.
- It requires general anaesthesia.
- In TAPP repair, peritoneal cavity is entered.
- Chances of port site hernia are there.

TAPP (Transabdominal Preperitoneal) Repair

"A beginner should not operate on obese patient, obstructed, reducible or complete hernia, patient unfit for general anaesthesia and patient with history of lower abdominal surgery".

– **Chowbey P.**

Principle

TAPP is the laparoscopic method of inguinal hernia repair through the abdominal cavity. Mesh is placed in preperitoneal space to cover MPO of Fruchaud to deal with direct, indirect and femoral hernia. The mesh is fixed with staples or tacks or sutures.

Indications of TAPP

- Reducible direct and indirect inguinal hernia
- Obstructed inguinal hernia
- Irreducible inguinal hernia
- Incarcerated inguinal hernia

Among all hernia repair techniques that utilize a preperitoneal placement of mesh, the laparoscopic hernioplasty (TAPP) is the most advantageous as it can be used to treat any type of groin hernia safely. Precondition for excellent results is the strict application of a standardized technique. In experienced hands, all types of hernias, including large scrotal hernias and recurrent hernias after previous preperitoneal repair, can be operated with low morbidity and recurrence rate.[47]

Evidence-based data show that laparoscopic hernia repair is significantly better than the conventional operation, specially with respect to the pain associated parameters.[48]

Contraindications of TAPP

- Patient unfit for general anesthesia.
- Pregnancy.
- Coagulopathy.

Operative technique

Anaesthesia

- General anaesthesia

Position of patient

- Supine in trendelenberg position.
- Ask the patient to pass urine or catheterise the patient before surgery.

Position of surgeon (Fig. 19.81)

Surgeon stands opposite to the side of hernia.

Assistant with camera stands opposite to surgeon's side.

TV monitor is kept near footend of the operation table.

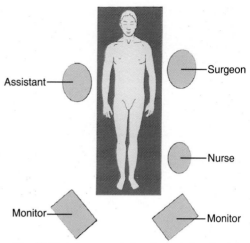

Fig. 19.81. Laparoscopic hernia operation theatre setup in TAPP.

Pneumoperitoneum establishment

Pneumoperitoneum is established with Veress's needle, (J. Veress, German Surgeon, 20th century).

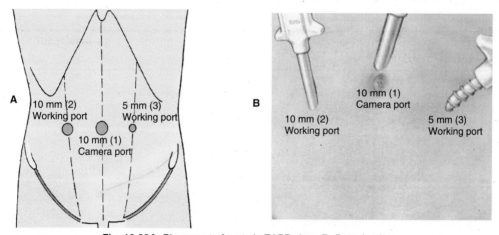

Fig. 19.82A. Placement of ports in TAPP sites, **B.** Ports in place.

Placement of ports (Figs. 19.82 A & B)

- First port is placed in the midline below the umbilicus. It is 5 mm or 10 mm port for laparoscope.
- Two 5 mm ports are placed lateral to rectus sheath on either side at a level just below the umbilicus.

Exploration

- Inspect both inguinal areas.
- Make orientation of abdominal fossae and folds and MPO of Fruchaud.
- Inspect both the indirect and direct inguinal hernia sites as well as femoral hernia site.
- Reduce the hernia after clearing adhesions if they are present.
- Peritoneum is incised 3-4 cm above the hernia defect (Figs. 19.83 A-D).

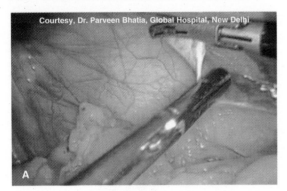
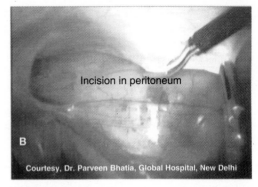

Fig. 19.83 A & B. Incision in peritoneum.

- The incision is extended from median umbilical fold to ASIS.
- Flaps are raised with blunt and sharp dissection.
- Preperitoneal space is prepared and the landmarks are to be identified. The first landmark is pubic bone, second is Cooper's ligament, third is inferior epigastric vessels and so on other landmarks are to be identified.
- As a rough guide the extent of dissection is 3-4 cm from the margin of defect on all sides. Do not cross medial umbilical fold and do not dissect in "Trapezoid of Doom."

Learning surgeons should only operate non-obese thin patients with small unilateral uncomplicated hernia.[122]

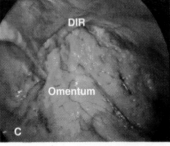

Courtesy, Dr. Pradeep Chowbey, SGRH, New Delhi

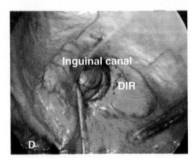

Fig. 19.83C. Indirect inguinal hernia, **D.** After reduction.

KEY POINT

Incision over lateral umbilical fold should be given delicately as injury to inferior epigastric vessels can be caused.

- Identify the following structures:
  - Pubic bone
  - Psoas muscle
  - Lateral cutaneous nerve of thigh
  - External iliac vessels
  - Testicular or genital vessels
  - Cooper's ligament
  - Genitofemoral nerve
  - Inferior epigastric vessels
  - Vas deferens

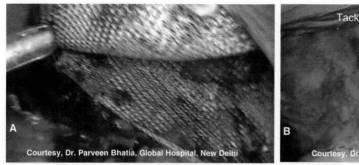
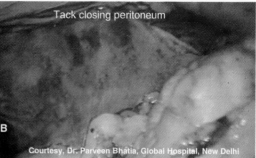

Fig. 19.84A & B. Placing of mesh and closure of peritoneum.

> **NOTE**
>
> • *If indirect hernia sac is big then it is dissected at deep inguinal ring and ligated. The distal part of the sac is left like that. Attempt should not be made to dissect and remove distal part of the sac. It causes haematoma.*
> • *If the direct hernia sac is not big then it may not be visible through laparoscope. Then palpate and apply pressure from hand on Hesselbach's triangle from outside then a direct hernia will be easily recognised.*

KEY POINT

Use of cautery is to be minimized to avoid thermal injury to bowel and nerves.

• A 15 cm × 15 cm polypropylene mesh is placed over MPO to cover sites of all hernias (Figs. 19.84 A & B).
• The mesh is first fixed at (Fig. 19.85).
  – Pubic symphysis or pubic bone.
  – Cooper's ligament (dissection and placing tacks over Cooper's ligament can cause trauma to puedendal vein, so be careful).

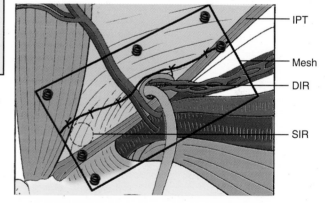

Fig. 19.85. TAPP, a diagrammatic representation.

  – On lateral side, the mesh is fixed to anterior abdominal wall, above the iliopubic tract, by applying pressure and feel it from outside to avoid injury to vessels and nerves in "Trapezoid of Disaster".
• The peritoneal flaps are now sutured back or fixed with fixation device over the mesh. Since the mesh is now fixed in "Preperitoneal space of Bogros" ports are removed.
• Local anaesthetic is injected in all port sites for reduction of post-operative pain.
• For bilateral hernia two meshes are placed, one on either side.
• Bilateral hernias can be dealt with either of the two methods:
  – One peritoneal incision and one big mesh.
  – Two peritoneal incisions and two meshes.

- Bittner *et al.*[127] gave TAPP- Stuttgart technique having the following special features:
  - Use of non-disposable instruments, blunt trocars, clips, glue and closer of peritoneum by running suture.
  - Meticulous dissection of entire pelvic floor after complete reduction of sac, wide parietalization of peritoneal sac and use of large mesh of 15×10 cm size.

NOTE

TAPPWR

- *TAPP without reperitonealization (TAPPWR) with new mesh having one side rough and another side smooth surface, peritoneal closer over mesh is not required. The reperitonealization process begins within few hours and the neoperitoneum should completely cover the mesh within 7 to 10 days.*[105]

KEY POINTS

- *Do not dissect medial to medial umbilical fold, as it may damage urinary bladder.*
- *Do not use tacks lateral to lateral umbilical fold to avoid injury to nerves.*

TOTAL EXTRAPERITONEAL (TEP) HERNIA REPAIR

"Everything in surgery, is complicated until one learns to do it well, then it is easy."
- Robert E. Condon

Principle

A mesh is placed in preperitoneal space to cover MPO of Fruchaud without going through the peritoneal cavity. Mesh gets sandwiched between the layers of tissues of anterior abdominal wall.

Advantages of TEP over TAPP

- Early return to normal activity.
- Reduced post-operative pain and complications.
- Bigger working space.
- A bigger mesh can be introduced so better coverage of MPO of Fruchaud.
- Dissection is easy.
- Avoids intraperitoneal adhesions as it stays out of peritoneal cavity.
- Avoids bowel and vascular injuries which are more with TAPP.[105]

Advantages of TAPP over TEP

- Easier technique than TEP.
- Has a shorter learning curve than TEP.
- In TAPP anatomical landmark identification is easier than in TEP.
- In TEP if peritoneum is opened then it leads to conversion to TAPP or open repair. In experienced hands, the conversion rate for laparoscopic to open repair is extremely low (<1%).[106]
- Extraperitoneal adhesions are minimum.
- Irreducible hernia can be reduced without any injury to the contents of the sac.
- Sliding hernia can be recognized easily.
- Better vizualization of inguinal area and simultaneous screening of intra-abdominal organs and recognition of occult intra-abdominal pathology.
- TAPP can be combined with other intra-peritoneal surgeries such as adhesiolysis and cholecystectomy.
- A recent metaanalysis could not find support for TEP as superior than TAPP.[135]

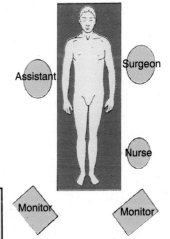

Fig. 19.86. Operation theatre setup for TEP.

- Experts report that an inadequate dissection of the peritoneum away from the posterior inguinal wall is the most common reason for recurrent hernias following TEP repairs.[107]

OPERATIVE TECHNIQUE (Figs. 19.86)

The prosthetic mesh is placed in preperitoneal space without opening the peritoneum.

Placement of Ports (Figs. 19.87A & B)

The following three ports are placed:
- 10 mm port of Hasson – Telescopic port or camera port.
- 5 mm port – Working port.
- 5 mm port – Working port.

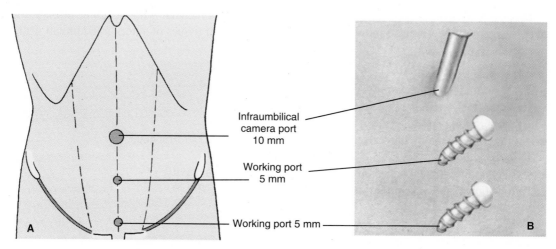

Fig. 19.87A. Placement of ports in TEP sites, **B.** Ports in place.

Access to Extraperitoneal Area

Incision

1.2 cm infraumbilical, transverse incision on one side of the midline.

Steps

- Rectus sheath is incised on the side of hernia.
- Two margins of incision of anterior rectus sheath are held with two stay sutures.
- Blunt dissection is done with index finger through anterior rectus sheath incision to create space between rectus muscle and posterior rectus sheath. It is pushed downwards so as to reach arcuate line and then below it to preperitoneal area.
- A trocar with balloon is introduced then and the balloon is inflated with 200 ml of normal saline.
- The balloon remains inflated for 5 minutes and then deflated.
- Now a 10 mm blunt tip Hasson's cannula is introduced in this space through subumbilical incision.
- Hasson's cannula is now secured and fixed with stay sutures.
- Now carbon dioxide insufflation is done with 12 mm pressure.
- A 10 mm 30 degree laparoscope with camera is now introduced through Hasson's cannula.
- A 5 mm working port is placed 2 cm above the pubic symphysis in midline.
- Second 5 mm working port is placed in the midline midway between first two ports.

KEY POINT

In TEP repair force at the time of introducing the trocars should be guarded to avoid peritoneal penetration.

Dissection (Figs. 19.88 A & B)

• Dissection is done with graspers and curved scissors.
• Cut and clear all loose areolar tissues in the midline.

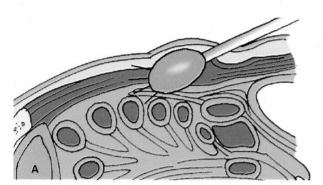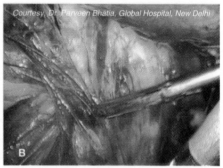

Fig. 19.88 A & B. Introduction of trocar with balloon and dissection in preperitoneal space.

NOTE

Blunt dissection with blunt instruments is encouraged and sharp dissection with sharp instruments and cautery is discouraged.

Now identify

• Pubic bone – White glistening surface, which is hard on touch with forceps.
• Cooper's ligament – Extending from pubic bone laterally and downwards.
  – Clear the area and cauterize the small vessels and identify inferior epigastric vessels.

Take care of

• Urinary bladder
• Prostatic plexus of veins

KEY POINTS

Dissection over Cooper's ligament and beyond is cautiously done to avoid injury to:
• *Pudendal veins*
• *Obturator vessels*
• *Obturator nerves*

• Now dissect gradually laterally towards the side of hernia. More and more anatomical landmarks will be gradually visible. Now identify:

- Pubic bone
- Iliopubic tract
- Cooper's ligament
- Inferior epigastric vessels
- Spermatic cord
- Direct hernia sac or indirect hernia sac or both (if present)
- Vas deferens
- Testicular vessels

> Pubic bone, iliopubic tract, Cooper's ligament make a transverse "Y"-shaped structure where femoral canal is situated between its two legs (iliopubic tract and Cooper's ligament).

- **Mesh application (Figs. 19.89 A & B, 19.90)**
  - A 15 cm × 15cm rolled mesh is introduced through subumbilical port.
  - The mesh is unfolded and spread over hernia prone areas.
  - It is fixed with 5 mm tacks with pubic bone and Cooper's ligament.
  - Mesh is not fixed laterally to avoid injury to lateral cutaneous nerve of the thigh.
  - Pneumoperitoneum is reversed.
  - All ports are removed.
  - The stay sutures of Hasson's cannula are cut.
  - All three wounds are closed with skin clips.
- **Post-operative advice**
  - Liquids are orally started after 2-3 hours.
  - Patient is discharged next morning.

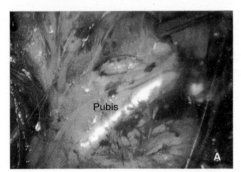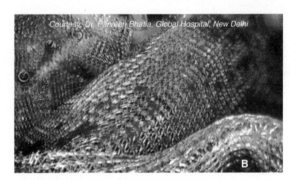

Fig. 19.89A & B. Preperitoneal dissection and placement of mesh.

> ## KEY POINT
>
> *TEP is recommended by NICE (National Institute of Clinical Excellence) for recurrent inguinal hernias and bilateral primary inguinal hernias.*

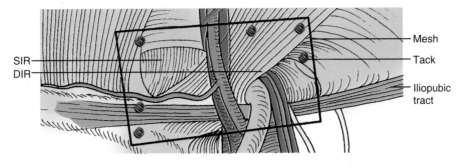

Fig. 19.90. TEP repair, diagrammatic representation.

TEP—Sir Ganga Ram Hospital (SGRH) Technique (Figs. 19.91 A-C)

It is a cost-effective simple technique with prevention of recurrence. It has the following features:
- Indigenous glove finger balloon
- Unrolling of mesh is simple
- Fruchaud's MPO is covered well

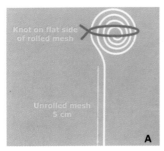 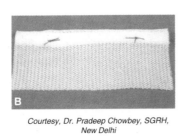 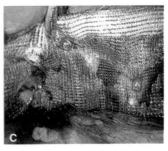

Courtesy, Dr. Pradeep Chowbey, SGRH, New Delhi

Fig. 19.91A. TEP, **B.** SGRH technique, **C.** diagrammatic representation.

With the modified SGRH technique we have found TEP to be safe, cost effective, reproducible and without significant complications.[123]

IPOM (Intraperitoneal Onlay Mesh) Repair

In this procedure, the prosthesis is placed directly on the peritoneum. Thus no peritoneal dissection is required and the hernia sac is undisturbed. This procedure was developed by Franklin, Rosenthal and Fitzgibbons in 1992.

The IPOM method had the highest incidence of neuralgia. The procedure was abandoned.[49]

POST-OPERATIVE COMPLICATIONS OF LAPAROSCOPIC HERNIA SURGERY

"Nothing so prevents the occurrence of complications as
one's awareness and fear of them."

- R.Bendavid[50]

"It is important for surgeons in the learning curve to be cautious and ideally supervised by experts so that potentially fatal complications do not put the procedure in disrepute."

Davide Lomento, *et al.*[51]

"Conversion to an open procedure is alway an option and should not be considerd a failure."

Bruce Ram Shaw

NOTE

Ninety percent complications occur in the first 50% cases of a surgeon. Felix et al.[52,55], found post-operative complication rate of 2.7% in 6 years. But it showed that first 3 years had 5.6% complications and the next 3 years had 0.5% which shows that experience reduces the rate of complications. The incidence of complication has decreased with time.[53]

Chronic Groin Pain (Inguinodynia) (Fig. 19.92)

"Pain management is a necessity in the work of each physician".

F. Sauerbruch, 1936

"Chronic post-herniorrhaphy groin pain is the pain occurring with greater frequency than was previously thought and lasting for more than three months."

Chronic groin pain is caused due to the following factors but the aetiology is unclear:
• Reaction to prosthetic material, studies show lack of evidence.[139]
• Involvement of nerve in staples and sutures.
• Scar tissue pain.

The incidence of chronic post-herniorrhaphy groin pain is less with the prosthetic repair.[54]

"Mesh inguinodynia" term was first used by Heise and Starling[55]. They descibed it as a new clinical syndrome.[107] It is less common in laparoscopic mesh repair than open mesh repair. There is evidence that ... upto 30% patients will have some degree of discomfort or pain, one year or more after inguinal hernia repair,[56] incidence of inguinodynia commonly is 4-5%.[140]

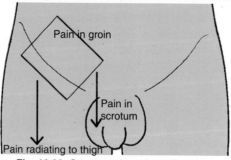

Fig. 19.92. Common sites of inguinodynia.

Chronic groin pain is a recognized complication after inguinal hernia repair. It can be mild, severe, even disabling and can adversely affect QOL.[57]

The surgical technique of closing external oblique fascia or aponeurosis and avoiding injury or entrapment of ilioinguinal or iliohypogastric nerve in open mesh repair and avoiding entrapment of lateral cutaneous nerve of thigh and genitofemoral nerve during stapling in laparoscopic method, are the important factors in preventing inguinodynia.

This pain is of two types:

- **Nociceptive pain:** It is caused by tissue damage. It can be:
  - Somatic pain: It is due to the damage to ligaments, tendons and muscles.
  - Visceral pain: It is due to the injury to some viscera.
- **Neuropathic pain:** It is due to direct nerve injury.

  Pain is described as stabbing, shooting, tearing, throbbing, dull or pulling, sometimes disabling.

To avoid post-operative neuralgia avoid introperative fiddling in the Triangle of Pain.

Types of Neuralgia (Fig. 19.93)

Chevrel[120] has described following four types of neuralgia:

- **Neuroma neuralgia:** Pain is like an electric shock. It is due to neuroma formation in nerve.
- **Differentiation neuralgia:** It is burning sensation, due to partial or complete division of nerve.
- **Projected neuralgia:** Touching at the nerve site at the site of entrapment causes pain.
- **Referred neuralgia:** Pain is felt at the other site. It is due to granuloma formation over suture.

Orchalgia

Pain felt in the scrotum lasting three months after hernia surgery may be due to by prosthetic mesh.

Ramus genitalis syndrome

It is a form of inguinodynia caused by entrapment of genital branch of genitofemoral nerve. It occurs after the groin hernia surgery. Pain occurs in the area of distribution of the nerve.

Ilioinguinalis syndrome

Pain is due to entrapment of ilioinguinal nerve during the groin hernia surgery, is in its distribution.

Treatment

- Reassurance, anti-inflammatory drugs, Local nerve blockers, neurolysis and neurectomy

How to avoid post hernia operation chronic groin pain

Amid PK described six maneuvers to reduce the risk of nerve injury. (i) avoiding indiscriminate division of subcutaneous tissue. (ii) avoiding removal of cremasteric muscle fibers. (iii) avoiding extensive dissection of the ilioinguinal nerve. (iv) dentifying and preserving all neural structure. (v) avoiding making the inguinal ring too tight. (vi) avoiding placement of sutures in the lower edge of the internal oblique muscle.[56]

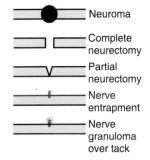

Fig. 19.93. Causes of neuralgia after laparoscopic hernia repair.

Triple Neurectomy

The patient who gets severe pain in post-operative period requires re-exploration. Neurectomy is performed. When treatment fails, wound should be explored and the division of three groin nerves to be undertaken,[57] If after one year patient continuous to suffer, operation is the only solution.[138]

Three large series of neurectomy showed success rate of 80% (Madura, 100 patient) and of 95% (Amid and Starling—Triple neurectomy).[57,109,110]

- Neuropathic pain can be caused by compression of one or more nerves by perineural fibrosis, suture material, staples and tacks or by nerve injury so if possible limit the use of sutures and fixation devices. Fibrin sealant glu can be used in place of fixation devices.[58]
- Manipulation and lifting the nerve from its bed will increase the risk of perineural fibrosis and chronic post-herniorrhaphy inguinodynia.[111]

Nerve Injury

The true incidence of post-herniorrhaphy neuropathic pain is not known, but published reports present incidence rates from 0% to more than 30%.[112]

The most commonly injured nerves in laparoscopic herinoplasty are:

- Lateral cutaneous nerve of thigh.
- Femoral branch of genitofemoral nerve.
- Intermediate branch of anterior branch of femoral nerve.
    Other nerves injured during laparoscopic hernioplasty are:
- Iliohypogastric nerve.
- Ilioinguinal nerve.
- Femoral nerve.
    These nerves are injured due to:
- Improper stapling.
- Non-meticulous dissection.
- Non-recognition of nerves.
- Nerve entrapment can be diagnosed by:
    - "Arch and Twist" maneuver[113] (Fig. 19.94), hyperextension and rotation of trunk causes pain.
    - Injection of local anaesthetic agent to nerve will relieve pain in the area of nerve distribution.

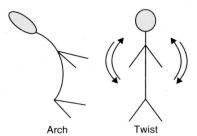

Arch   Twist

Fig. 19.94. Arch and Twist maneuver.

Treatment

- Re-exploration and removal of staple or tack causing injury.
- Anti-inflammatory drugs.

Vascular Injuries

- Intra-abdominal vascular injuries.
- Retroperitoneal vascular injuries.
- Abdominal wall vascular injuries.
- Gas embolism due to vascular injuries.

Inferior epigastric and spermatic vessels are the most common vessels injured during laparoscopic surgery.

Vascular injuries can be avoided by:
– Clear understanding of anatomy.
– Meticulous display of important landmarks.
– Avoiding unnecessary use of electrocautery.

Treatment of vascular injuries

• Immediate repair is required for external iliac vessels.
• Inferior epigastric and other vessels can be ligated.

KEY POINT

If you find any dangerous abnormality such as iliac artery aneurysm then stop and convert to open tension-free mesh repair.

Urinary Tract Injuries

Commonest injury is urinary bladder injury, specially in space of Retizus if there is history of some previous surgery such as open prostatectomy. Due to open prostatectomy, adhesions and fibrosis develop hence it becomes difficult to dissect the space of Retzius.

Treatment

• Catheterization
• Antibiotics
• Repair of the bladder injury

Bowel Injury

It occurs while separating adhesions of bowel loops.

Treatment

Convert to open procedure and close the bowel perforation.

KEY POINT

Do not place tacks below iliopubic tract.

Vas Deferens and Testicular Complications

• Transection of vas deferens
• Orchitis
• Testicular atrophy
• Testicular pain
• Epididymitis
• Hydrocele

- Dysejaculation
- Infertility

> The **dysejaculation syndrome** is explained as a burning and painful sensation occurring just before, during or after ejaculation. It may be caused by stenotic lesion of vas deferens. It is a self-limiting condition. The mechanism is not well understood. The prognosis is excellent. Symptoms begin in 2 to 3 week after surgery and clear in 1 to 5 years.[114]

"**Infertility**" after bilateral inguinal herniorrhaphy is rare but a devastating complication. Reanastamosis of vas deferens should be done if it is transected during herniorrhaphy.

Treatment

- Transection of vas deferens is repaired by vaso-vasal anastomosis.
- Bilateral testicular atrophy is treated by testosterone injection (intramuscular).
- Rest of the testicular problems are treated with analgesics, scrotal support and rest.

> **KEY POINT**
>
> *If you can palpate the tip of tacker or stapler while applying tacks or staples then you are above IPT so apply the tacks, if tacker is not palpable then do not apply tacks, as you are below the IPT.*

Mesh Complications

These are:
- Migration of mesh
- Contraction of mesh – Contracture of mesh must be kept in mind by the surgeon. Sufficient overlap anticipating a 20% contracture is accepted by most.
- Erosion of mesh
- Rejection
- Fracture
- Infection
  - Chronic mesh sepsis or chronic groin sepsis is usually not common, it occurs in 0.1% mesh hernioplasties[54] (Fig. 19.95).
  - Infection of mesh can be prevented by the following precautions:
    a) Strict asepsis.
    b) Proper sterilization of hand instruments and ports.
    c) Mesh and instruments must not come in contact with skin.
    d) Gloves must be changed before the mesh is taken out of its container and handled.
- Mass lesion
- Adhesions
- Seroma formation
- Haematoma
- "Meshoma" (The word used by Amid PK), is caused by folding and wadding of the mesh which can cause chronic pain and recurrence of the hernia[111] (Fig. 19.96).

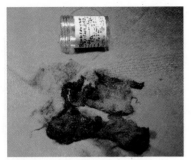

Fig. 19.95. Mesh removal after chronic infection.

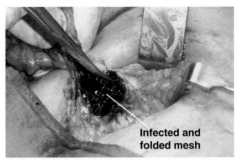

Fig. 19.96. Infected Meshoma.

Treatment

* Migration of mesh is avoided by proper fixation of mesh.
* Infection is prevented by preoperative and post-operative antibiotics.
* Mass lesion requires extraction of mesh.

KEY POINTS

As a rule excessive force must not be used while applying tacks especially in thin patients as it can cause ilioinguinal and iliohypogastric nerves entrapment and skin puckering

Recurrence of Hernia

"Although all surgeons must be prepared to admit that recurrence will occur, the only proper attitude to take is that any recurrence is the fault of the surgeon".   *– MM Ravitch*

A followup of atleast 10 years showed that 50% of recurrences do not appear before 5 years and 20% of recurrences appear after 15 years or so.

Usual causes of recurrence of hernia after laparoscopic hernioplasty are:
* Missed hernia – A hernia which was already there but was overlooked or not treated.
* Migration of mesh.
* Too small mesh – If the mesh size is inadequate to completely cover the MPO of Fruchaud, then recurrence develops.
* Rolling of mesh.
* Risk factors responsible for recurrence in laparoscopic inguinal hernia repair include collagen disease, smoking, obesity, malnutrition, diabetes type II, chronic lung diseases, coagulopathy, steroids, radiotherapy, chemotherapy, jaundice, male gender and anaemia.[59]

KEY POINT

Large series have reported a recurrence rate of less than 1% in laparoscopic hernioplasty, TAPP 0.8% and TEP 0%.

Treatment

Recurrence will require re-operation either by laparoscopic or open method.

Port Site Hernia (Fig. 19.97)

Umbilical trocar site hernias occur about 1% of the time after laparoscopic herniorrhaphy and the incidence is the same for secondary trocar sites, varying in relation to the size of the cannula. Factors responsible for port site hernias are:

- Port site hernia occurs in 10 mm ports or wider ports if fascial opening is not closed. It can be prevented by closing the port site opening.
- Obesity.

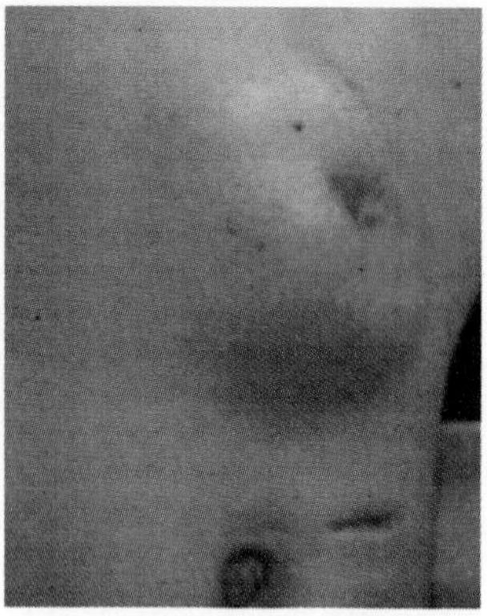

How to avoid port site hernia

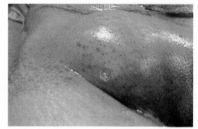

Fig. 19.97. Epigastric port site hernia.

- Use ports of smaller diameter, less then 10 mm.
- Fascial defects should be closed properly.
- Avoid unnecessary and forceful manipulation of ports, specially 10 mm ports, which may enlarge the fascial defect.
- Desufflation of the peritoneal cavity should be done slowly to avoid sucking of intestine loop or omentum in port sites.

Groin Seroma and Haematoma (Fig. 19.98)

They develop due to:
- Improper haemostasis.
- Extensive tissue dissection causing lymphatic damage.
  There is no proof that polypropylene mesh forms a seroma.

Treatment

Most surgeons believe that seroma should not be regarded as a post-operative complication unless it persists for more than 6-8 weeks.

Fig. 19.98. Groin seroma after hernia surgery.

Application of abdominal binder post operation in ventral hernia repair reduces it significantly.

Aspiration of seroma is helpful to resolve it. This should be done under antibiotic cover to avoid infection. Aspiration may be required several times.

Osteitis Pubis

It is caused due to placement of staples or sutures through the periosteum of the pubis. It is a painful inflammatory condition of the pubic symphysis. It is most often caused by repeated traumatic or exertional stresses on the fascia and joint.

Treatment

- Anti-inflammatory drugs.
- Local heat and ultrasound diathermy application.
- Corticosteroid injections.
- Sometimes surgical exploration is required to remove the causative staple or suture.

Miscellaneous Complications

- Nausea and vomiting
- Paralytic ileus
- Aspiration pneumonia
- Trocar site keloid
- Diaphragmatic dysfunction
- Pneumoscrotum
  - It is due to preperitoneal insufflation. It is a self-limiting condition.

Mortality in Laparoscopic Hernia Surgery

Mortality in laparoscopic hernia repair is due to direct injury to major blood vessels in "Triangle of Doom". But the mortality has considerably reduced due to proper training in laparoscopic surgery. Crowfield (1995) has reported 0.06% mortality in his series.

Conversion to Open from Laparoscopic Operation

It is difficult to reach to a correct rate of conversion to open due to under reporting but European Association of Endoscopic Surgeons (EAES) have reported 2.7% when they studied 3130 patients of laparoscopic hernia repair and found 85 patients were converted to open operation.[119] In experienced hand, the conversion is less than 1%.

Reasons of conversion

- Inability to gain access to the groin.
- Intraoperative difficulties and complications specially in TEP.
- Anaesthetic complications due to excessive absorption of carbon dioxide, especially in obstructive lung disease and heart patients and when time taken by operation was prolonged.

Re-exploration

Re-exploration is usually required in following conditions.
- Post-operative vascular complication i.e. bleeding and haematoma. It is required when conservative treatment fails to check bleeding and spread of haematoma.
- Neuralgia in immediate post-operative period.

KEY POINT

Laparoscopic repair for recurrent and bilateral inguinal hernia is better than open hernia repair.

OPERATIONS FOR FEMORAL HERNIA

"Surgery is like making love, must be done gently and with adequate exposure"

- Anonymous

> In 1804, Astley Cooper described the anatomy of the transversalis fascia and the superior pubic ligament, which later came to bear his name. Cooper's ligament was later on used in femoral hernia repair.[60]

There are three approaches of femoral hernias repair: (Figs. 19.99 & 19.100)
* Extraperitoneal approach
* Inguinal approach
* Femoral approach

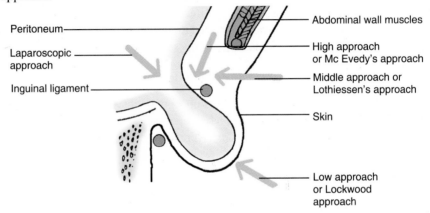

Fig. 19.99. Various operative approaches of femoral hernia.

High Approach or McEvedy Operation (Extraperitoneal approach)

It is named after Peter George McEvedy (1890-1951), Surgeon, Ancoats Hospital, Manchester, England.

Incision

A 7-8 cm long vertical incision over femoral canal extending above the inguinal ligament, 1-5 cm medial to linea semilunaris.

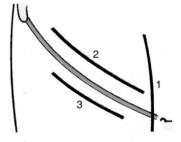

Fig. 19.100. Incisions for femoral hernia. (1) High, (2) middle, (3) low approaches.

Steps

* Upper part of incision is deepened.
* Anterior rectus sheath is incised.
* Rectus muscle is retracted medially.
* Fascia transversalis is divided.
* Sac entering the femoral ring is identified and pulled upward (Fig. 19.101).
* Neck of the sac is ligated and the sac is excised.
* Repair of femoral ring is done by suturing conjoint tendon down to Cooper's ligament with non-absorbable sutures.

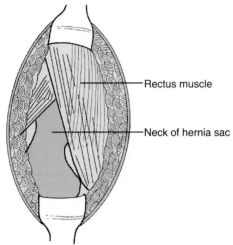

Fig. 19.101. McEvedy operation.

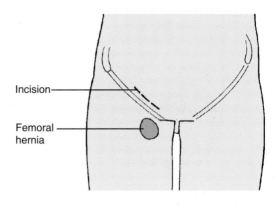

Fig. 19.102. Incision in Lotheissen's operation.

• Nyhus in 1960, started operating femoral hernia by preperitoneal approach and approximated iliopubic tract to Cooper's ligament. His recurrence rate is 1%.[61]

Middle Approach or Inguinal Approach or Lotheissen's Operation

It is named after George Lotheissen (1898-1941) surgeon, Kaiser Franz Joseph Hospital, Vienna, Austria. George Lotheissen was first to suture the conjoint tendon and the Cooper's ligament in a recurrent hernia case.[62] Infact Lotheissen learned this operation from Professor Narath of Amsterdam.

Incision (Fig. 19.102)

Transverse incision, as applied for inguinal hernia but nearer to inguinal ligament.

Steps

• External oblique aponeurosis is incised and inguinal canal is opened.
• Spermatic cord and conjoint tendon are retracted upwards.
• Fascia transversalis is also incised in the same line but care should be taken of inferior epigastric vessels at its lateral end.
• Here blunt dissection with gauze is done to push extraperitoneal tissue aside and identify the sac entering the femoral ring.
• The sac is pulled up (Fig. 19.103A).
• Ligate the neck of the sac and excise the sac (Fig. 19.103B).
• Repair of femoral ring is done by suturing conjoint tendon or inguinal ligament to the pectineal ligament.
• Repair is done with three interrupted non-absorbable sutures.
• The posterior wall of inguinal canal is strengthened by Bassini repair.
• Spermatic cord is placed back.
• External oblique aponeurosis is sutured back.
• Skin is closed with staples.

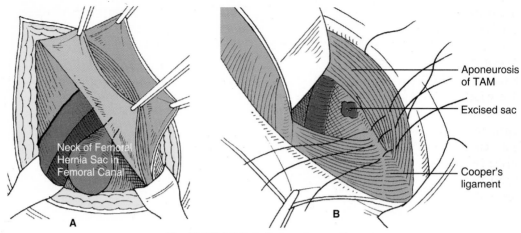

Fig. 19.103A & B. Lotheissen's operation.

Low Approach or Femoral Approach or Lockwood Operation (Figs. 19.104 A & B)

It is named after Charles Barrett Lockwood (1856-1914), Surgeon, St. Bartholomew's Hospital, London, England. The femoral approach was abandoned and replaced by the inguinal approach.[63]

Socin was the first surgeon who described a femoral approach to femoral hernia repair in 1879.[64]

Incision

An incision in groin crease is made 1.25 cm below and parallel to inguinal ligament.

Steps

• All layers are incised till the sac.

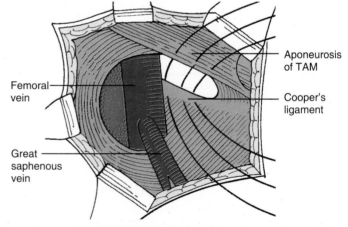

Fig. 19.104A. Lockwood operation, interrupted sutures.

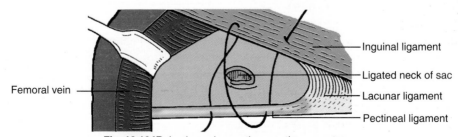

Fig. 19.104B. Lockwood operation, continuous sutures.

- Sac is freed by blunt dissection with gauze.
- Sac is opened at fundus.
- Contents of the sac are pushed back to peritoneal cavity.
- Transfix the neck as high as possible.
- Excise the sac below the ligature (Fig. 19.105).
- Three interrupted non-absorbable sutures are applied on the fascia forming the floor and lateral margin of saphenous opening.
- Take care of femoral vein. Protect it by a finger.
- In the 19th century, renowned surgeons as Bassini[65], Marcy[66], and Cushing[67] wrote papers about femoral approach to femoral hernia. It was later replaced by inguinal approach.

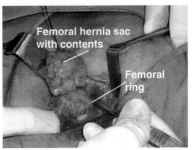

Fig. 19.105. Low approach operation.

Operation for Strangulated Femoral Hernia

- High approach operation or McEvedy's operation is operation of choice.
- First open the sac at the fundus and examine the contents.
- Expose the femoral ring above the inguinal ligament.
- If constriction is found at femoral ring then cut the lacunar ligament and avoid injury to abnormal
  - obturator artery. Abnormal obturator artery is present in 20% of cases either on medial side or lateral side of the neck of the sac.
  - Contents are now drawn above the inguinal ligament and dealt with according to the viability.
  - Repair is done with three interrupted non-absorbable sutures.

Mesh Repair of Femoral Hernia (Figs. 19.106 A & B)

In 1974, Lichtenstein introduced the idea of tension-free femoral hernioplasty. He rolled a piece of mesh and formed a plug and inserted in femoral canal from the femoral side.[68] It was called "Cigarette plug".

In late 1980's, Arther Gilbert used a cone-shaped plug and believed it worked better than Lichtenstein's, cylindrical plug.[69] At the same time Rutkow and Robbin designed "Per Fix Plug" used to operate both the inguinal and femoral hernias.[70]

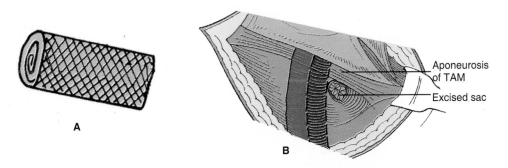

A

B

Fig. 19.106A. Prolene mesh plug, **B.** Its application in femoral ring.

Incision

Same as for inguinal hernia.

Steps

Incision is deepened.
- External oblique aponeurosis is incised along its fibres.
- Spermatic cord or round ligament is retracted superiorly.
- Inferior flap of external oblique aponeurosis is retracted up.
- Sac is grasped and dissected with blunt and sharp dissection from the fat of the thigh.
- A plug of 2 × 15 cm polypropylene mesh is made by rolling it.
- Hold the plug with Babcock's forceps and introduce it in hole of femoral ring.
- The mesh plug is fixed with three sutures.
  - One suture is tied to inguinal ligament, second is fixed to lacunar ligament and the third is fixed to pectineus muscle.
- The wound is now closed.

KEY POINT

Conservative treatment has no place in treatment of femoral hernia. The treatment of choice is early operation.

LAPAROSCOPIC VENTRAL HERNIA REPAIR (LVHR)

(Umbilical, Paraumbilical, Epigastric and Incisional Hernia)

"One should advise surgery only if there is a reasonable chance of success.
To operate without having a chance means to prostitute the beautiful art and science of surgery"
                                                                   - Theodor Billroth, 1829-1894

"Herniation of omentum, intestine and other abdominal organs through anterior abdominal wall except groin hernias is called ventral hernia. Ventral hernia is also called abdominal hernia and laparocele."

Ventral hernias represent defects in the parietal abdominal wall, fascia and muscles through which intra-abdominal or preperitoneal contents can protrude.

> Ventral hernias include incisional hernias and primary defects in the abdominal fascia, which can cause umbilical, epigastric or Spigelian hernia.[71]

Ventral hernia can be:
- Congenital
- Acquired
  Ventral hernia can also be classified as:
- Primary or true or non-incisional ventral hernia e.g.
  – Epigastric
  – Umbilical
  – Paraumbilical
  – Spigelian
- Secondary or incisional hernia

Indications of Laparoscopic Repair

- **Spontaneous hernia**
  – Umbilical hernia and paraumbilical hernia
  – Epigastric hernia
  – Spigelian hernia
- **Delayed hernia or incisional hernia**

Treatment plan of ventral hernia

- **Hernia less than 2 cm in diameter**
  – Primary tissue repair.
- **Hernia more than 2 cm in diameter**
  – Mesh hernia repair
  – 2-10% of all abdominal operations result in incisional hernia.
  – 30% of hernia, bigger than 2 cm size develop recurrence if repaired by primary tissue repair.

Advantages of Laparoscopic Repair of Ventral Hernia

The use of prosthetic mesh in ventral hernia repair has reduced the recurrence rate as compared to primary tissue repair but more extensive dissection is necessary which increases the risk of wound healing complications.[72,73]

- Less pain.
- Faster return to normal activity.
- Early return to work so less "manhour loss".
- Laparoscopy enables to detect multiple defects in incisional hernia which are commonly present in midline incisional hernia and may be missed in open repair (Swiss cheese hernia), (Figs. 19.107 & 19.108).

Disadvantages of Laparoscopic Repair of Ventral Hernia

- Expensive.
- Difficult in the following situations:
  - Extremely big hernia
  - Extensive adhesions
  - Hernia with loss of domain

The study by Park[74] compared the laparoscopic repair of incisional hernia with open incisional hernia repair. The operation time was long with laparoscopic group (95 min versus 78 min) whereas the hospital stay and perioperative complications were lower in laparoscopic group.

Contraindications of Laparoscopic repair of ventral hernia[75]

- Extensive scarring in abdomen
- Inability to produce pneumoperitoneum
- Acute abdomen with peritonitis and strangulation
- Big hernia involving large part of anterior abdominal wall leaving no place to introduce lateral trocars

---

Anaesthesia

General anaesthesia with an endotracheal tube.

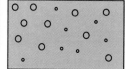

Fig. 19.107. Swiss cheese hernia, diagrammatic representation.

Position

- Patient is placed in supine position.
- A pillow is placed under knees to produce some flexion of hips and knees to relax abdominal wall muscles.

Operative preparations

- Perioperative antibiotics are given.
- Nasogastric tube is passed to decompress the stomach.
- A Foley's catheter is passed.
- Skin is prepared in routine manner.

Courtesy, Dr. Parveen Bhatia, Global Hospital, New Delhi

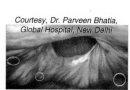

Fig. 19.108. Swiss cheese hernia, laparoscopic view.

Technique

The mesh can be placed in any of the following ways:
- **Onlay mesh placement or anterior mesh placement**
  - Mesh is placed on rectus sheath and defect.

- **Sublay mesh placement or posterior mesh placement**
  - Mesh is placed posterior to rectus muscle and fascia: It is better than onlay mesh placement.
- **Inlay mesh placement**
  - Nowadays dual-sided mesh are in use such as polypropylene-polyglactin composite mesh (Vypro). These meshes do not cause harm to internal viscera as the intraperitoneal surface is non-adherent to PTFE surface whereas the outer surface has polypropylene mesh, which causes adherence to peritoneum and posterior abdominal wall quickly.

Placement of ports

- **Camera port**–10 mm laparoscope is introduced above or below the hernia site.
- **Working ports**– Two 5 mm ports are placed for operative instrument on lateral sides of hernia.
- All ports are placed according to "Principle of Triangulations" that means to make a triangle with all three ports.
- Bruce Ramshaw advocates three relatively safe sites for peritoneal access in laparoscopic ventral hernia repair.[76]
- Subxiphoid midline.
- Right subcostal space at anterior axillary line.
- Left subcostal space at anterior axillary line (Palmar's point).

Steps (Figs. 19.109 A - E)

- Release adhesions between omentum, bowel and anterior abdominal wall carefully.
- At least 5 cm of area around the defect must be cleared of any adhesion.
- Use of electrocautery is not encouraged. It should be minimum as it can cause thermal injury to intestine.
- The dissection and release of adhesions can be assisted by external pressure on hernia sac and by inversion of sac.
- Assess the size of defect.
- Marks on skin – Reduce the pressure of CO_2 from 15 mm to 6-8 mm, so that proper assessment of the size of defect can be made (Fig. 19.113).
- Four small stab wounds of 2-3 mm size are made with a 11 no. blade at 4 corners of proposed site of mesh (Figs. 19.110-19.113).
- The mesh is unfolded and spread over omentum.

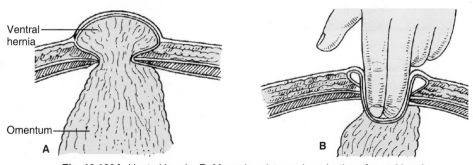

Fig. 19.109A. Ventral hernia, **B.** Manual assistance in reduction of vental hernia.

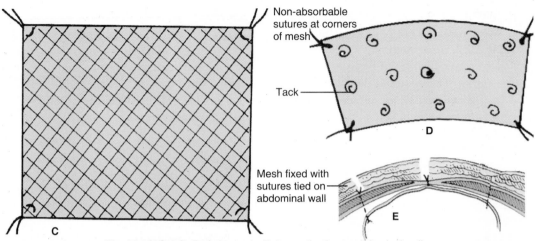

Fig. 19.109C & D. Prolene mesh, **E.** Its application to abdominal wall.

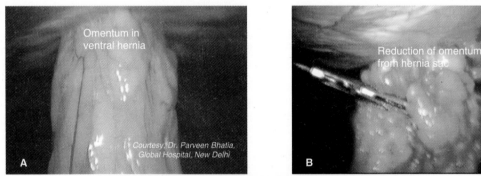

Fig. 19.110A. Ventral hernia containing omentum, **B.** Its reduction.

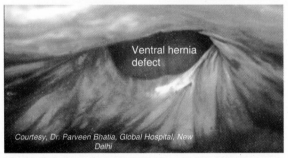

Fig. 19.111. Ventral hernia defect in anterior abdominal wall.

- Now with a Keith needle or a special suture needle (Shoeman's needle) four long sutures of 2-0 polypropylene are made out from four corners of mesh and tied outside (Figs. 19.113 B & C).
- The rest of the mesh is fixed by multiple tacks with a 5 mm tacker.
- The omentum must cover the intestinal loops at the end of the operation to avoid contact of mesh with intestines (Fig. 19.113D).
- "Double Crowning" of mesh: The mesh is fixed with fixation device at the periphery of the mesh and also at the periphery of the hernia defect.

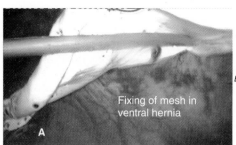

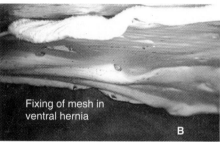

Courtesy, Dr. Parveen Bhatia, Global Hospital, New Delhi

Fixing of mesh in ventral hernia

Fixing of mesh in ventral hernia

Fig. 19.102A & B. Mesh placement in ventral hernia.

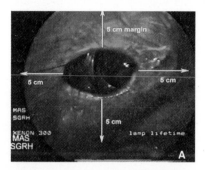

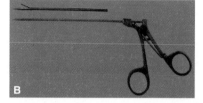

Courtesy, Dr. Pradeep Chowbey, SGRH, New Delhi

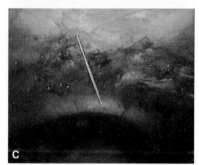

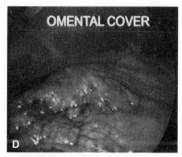

Courtesy, Dr. Pradeep Chowbey, SGRH, New Delhi

Fig. 19.113A. Measurement of hernia defect, **B.** Shoeman's needle, **C.** Shoeman's needle piercing abdominal wall and entering peritoneal cavity, **D.** Omentum is covering intestines.

KEY POINT

While performing LVHR, remain near anterior abdominal wall, to avoid bowel injury.

OPERATIONS FOR UMBILICAL HERNIA

"Modern doctors regrettably prefer to look at the results on a piece of computer paper than to listen to the credible, consistent and seasoned observations of their patients who after all live with their bodies."

- John Dwyer, 1993

Indications

Operation for umbilical hernia in an infant is rarely indicated as 80% of defects will close by the age of 2 years.
- In children, if the umbilical fascial ring is large enough to admit index finger, the hernia should be repaired before the child goes to school.
- Umbilical hernia in adult is repaired due to the risk of strangulation.

Anaesthesia

Spinal anaethesia is preferred in large hernias in adults as it gives good relaxation.
    General anaesthesia is the method of choice for children.

Position

Supine.

Incision

A curved incision is placed above or below the umbilicus.
    Umbilicus should be retained in skin flap.

Steps

- Incision is deepened.
- Sac is mobilised, umbilical skin is carefully dissected so as to avoid creating a button hole.
- Neck of hernia sac is dissected out.
- If omentum is adherent to the sac, remove it carefully.
- If the defect is less than 2 cm in diameter, then sac is excised and the peritoneum and fascial defect are closed with 2-0 non-absorbable sutures.
- If the defect is 2-4 cm, then Mayo's repair is done (Vest-over-trousers).
- If the defect is more than 4 cm, then it is repaired with polypropylene mesh.

Closure

Haemostasis is secured.
    Subcutaneous dead space is obliterated with absorbable sutures.
    If the hernia is quite large, then Radivac suction drain negative pressure is introduced.
    Skin is closed with staples.

Mayo's Operation (Vest-over Trousers)[76] (Figs. 19.114 A - D)

William James Mayo, 1861-1939, (The Mayo Clinic, Rochester, M.N., U.S.A.), described this

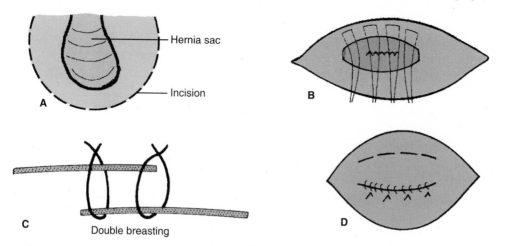

Hernia sac

Incision

A

B

C

Double breasting

D

Fig. 19.114 A - D. Mayo's vest-over-trousers operation.

operation in 1901, though the operation was performed since 1895. He performed 25 operations without any recurrence[115]. Mayo's technique is still one of the most commonly used surgical techniques performed routinely in hospitals all over the world.

There is a high rate of recurrence reported after Mayo's repair, 20%-28%,[77] but Mayo's repair is still in use due to lack of a Gold Standard technique.

Incision

Transverse elliptical incision is given encircling the umbilicus and hernia.

Steps

- Sac is opened at neck.
- Contents are returned back to peritoneal cavity.
- Sac with skin is removed.
- Neck of the sac is closed with interrupted sutures.
- Neck of the sac is usually found free from adhesions so the neck is dealt first before fundus of sac (neck first method).
- The linea alba is incised 2.5 cm laterally so that overlapping can be done.
- The lower flap is pulled up with mattress and non-absorbable sutures are tied under upper flap.
- Now the free margin of upper flap is sutured to the outer surface of lower flap with interrupted non-absorbable sutures.
- A suction drain is introduced to remove oozed blood.
- Skin is approximated.

Mesh Repair of Umbilical Hernia (Figs. 19.115 A & B)

Position

In comfortable supine position.

Incision

Curved incision around umbilicus either above or below.

In large umbilical hernia sometimes a vertical incision is also made.

Steps

Incision is deepened.
- Skin of umbilicus is preserved and not sacrificed.
- Sac is dissected out easily except at umbilical skin attachment.
- Neck is well-defined by blunt and sharp dissection.
- Sac is opened and adhesions are divided.
- Polypropylene (prolene) mesh is placed between peritoneum and posterior rectus sheath (in open mesh repair).
- Prolene mesh is placed in intraperitoneal position as in incisional hernia. The mesh used here should be dual-sided composite mesh. On inner side, it has PTFE (poly tetrafluoroethylene) and on outer side, it has polypropylene layer so not to develop adhesions with bowel and omentum and develop adhesions with fascia. Alternatively, a mesh plug is also used.

Arroyo and co-workers performed 200 operations, resulted in recurrence rate of 11% in primary repair and 1 % in tension-free mesh repair.[78]

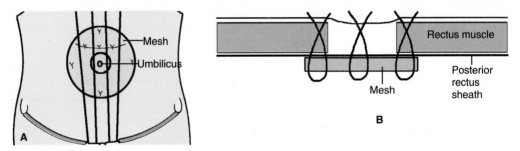

Fig. 19.115 A & B. Mesh repair of umbilical hernia.

KEY POINT

Adhesions in umbilical hernia are usually at fundus and the neck is free so "neck first" is the principle of umbilical hernia surgery.

OPERATIONS FOR PARAUMBILICAL HERNIA

All cases of paraumbilical hernia require operations due to following reasons:
- Hernia will increase in size and discomfort.
- Hernia may strangulate.
Two important points must be kept in mind while operating for paraumbilical hernia:
- Most of the patients of paraumbilical hernia are obese so lipectomy or abdominoplasty should be considered with hernia repair.

- Adhesions are very common in paraumbilical hernia. Adhesions are commonly found between fundus and body of the sac and the contents. Neck remains free. Neck should be tackled first during operation, "neck first method" is used (Fig. 19.116C).

    Following procedures are advised for paraumbilical hernia operation:

- **Primary apposition of edges:** This method has maximum recurrence rate, hence is not practised nowadays.
- **Mayo's repair:** It is a good method for hernias smaller than 4 cm.
- **Prosthetic mesh hernioplasty:** It is the method of choice. It is indicated in the following cases:
    - Paraumbilical hernia more than 4 cm in diameter.
    - Recurrent paraumbilical hernia.

Prosthetic mesh hernioplasty can be performed by two methods:
- Open method (Figs. 19.116 A - C)
- Laparoscopic method.

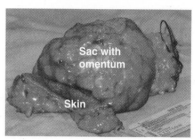

Fig. 19.116A. Open prosthetic mesh hernioplasty, excised omentum and skin

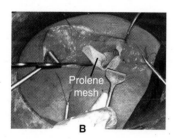

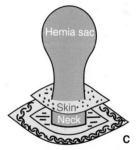

Fig. 19.116B. Open umbilical hernia prosthetic hernioplasty, mesh with four corner sutures is introduced, **C.** "Neck first method" of dealing paraumbilical hernia sac.

NOTE

Application of a negative pressure drain is a must in open prosthetic paraumbilical hernio plasty. Drain is applied for two purposes:
- *To remove oozing blood*
- *To remove liquid fat*

OPERATIONS FOR EPIGASTRIC HERNIA (FIG. 19.117)

"A minor complication is one that happens to somebody else."

— Anonymous

Position

Supine

Anaesthesia

General anaesthesia.

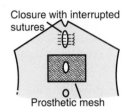

Fig. 19.117. Operative procedures of epigastric hernia.

Incision

Vertical or transverse incision is made over hernia swelling exposing linea alba.

Steps

Protruding or herniating extraperitoneal fat or lump or sac is cleared from all surroundings upto its neck by blunt dissection.

- **If there is no sac**
  - Pedicle is ligated and fat nodule is excised.
  - Opening in linea alba is closed with non-absorbable sutures.
- **If the hernia sac is present**
  - Hernia sac is opened.
  - Contents of the sac are reduced.
  - Neck of the sac is transfixed and the sac is excised.
  - The defect in the linea alba is closed with a few interrupted non-absorbable sutures.
- **If the hernia sac is more than 4 cm**
  - A tension-free mesh hernioplasty is done. The mesh is placed behind muscles.

NOTE

Recurrence rate of epigastric hernia repair is 10%-20% higher than other groin hernia repair. This high recurrence rate may be partly due to failure to recognize and repair multiple small defects.[79] There is advantage of tension-free prosthetic repair of epigastric hernia[80] over primary tissue repair.

KEY POINT

Operative repair of epigastric hernia is only needed if it is causing symptoms.

OPERATIONS FOR INCISIONAL HERNIA

Refer to Page no. 171-182

REFERENCE

1. **Rutkow Ira M.**, (2003). Demographic and socioeconomic aspects of hernia repair in the United States in 2003, *Surg. Clin. North Am.*, 1042.
2. **Kehlit H, White PF.**, (2001). Optimising anaesthesia for inguinal herniorrhaphy: General, regional or local anaesthesia; *Anaesth Analg.*, 93: 1367–1369.
3. **Song D, Grelich NB, White PE, Watcha MF, Tongier WK.**, (2000). Recovery profits and cost of anaesthesia for outpatient unilateral inguinal herniorrhaphy, *Anaesth Analog.* 91: 876–878.
4. **NJH Davies, and Carhman JN.**, (2006). Post-dural puncture headache, Lee's synopsis of anaesthesia, p. 517.
5. **Mulraj MF, Salinas FV, Larkin KL, Polissar NL.**, (2004). Ambulatory surgery patients may be discharged before voiding after short acting spinal and epidural anaesthesia. *Anaesthology*, 97: 315–319.
6. **Bassini E.**, (1887). Nuoro metodo Sulla cura radicale dell ernia enguinale, *Arch SOC Ital. Chir.*, 4: 380.
7. **Castrine G, Pappalardo G, Trentino P,** *et al.,* (1986). The original Bassini technique in the surgical treatment of inguinal hernia. *Int. Surg.*, 71: 141.
8. **Shouldice EE.**, (1944). Surgical treatment of hernia-presented at the Annual Meeting of the Ontario Medical Association, Districts No. 9 and 10.
9. **Shouldice EB.**, (2003). The shouldice repair for groin hernias, *Surg. Clin. North Am.*, 83: 1163–1187.
10. **Chin Keung Chang, Gubriel Chan.**, (2006). The shouldice technique for the treatment of inguinal hernia. *Journal of Minimus Access Surgery*, 124.
11. **Lifscutz H.**, (1986). The inguinal darn, *Arch. Surg.*, 121: 717.
12. **Wantz GE.**, (1989). Giant prosthetic reinforcement of the visceral sac, *Surg. Gynecol. Obstet.*, 169: 408–417.
13. **Lichtenstein IL.**, (1986). Hernia repair without disability, 200, editor St. Louis, Tokyo: Isheyaku, Euroamerica, Ine.
14. **Usher FC.**, (1960). A new technique for the repair of ingunal and incisional hernia. *Arch. Surg.*, 81: 847–855.
15. **Martin Kurzer.**, (2003). The Lichtenstein repair for groin hernias, *Surg. Clin. North Am.*, 83: pp. 1099–1117.
16. **Amid PK.**, (2004). Lichtenstein tension-free hernioplasty, New procedures in open hernia surgery, Springer, pp. 1–12.
17. **Arned RK.**, (2002). How to avoid recurrence in a Lichtenstein tension-free hernioplasty, *Am. J. Surg.*, 184: 259–260.
18. **Eggar B, Fawall D, Dowling BL.**, (1996). Use of skin staples for securing the mesh in Lichtenstein tension-free hernia repair of inguinal hernia, *Ann. R. Coll. Surg. Engl.*, 78(1): 63–64.

19. **Gilbert AI.**, (2002). Generation of the plug and patch repair: Its development and lesson for history. In: **Baker RJ, Ficher JE**, Editors; Master of surgery **2,** 4th edition, Philadelphia: Lippincott, Williams & Wilkins: pp. 1975–1982.

20. **Gilbert AI.**, (1992). Suture less repair of inguinal hernias. *AMJ Surg.,* 163: 331.

21. **Rutkow IM, Robbins AW.**, (1995). Mesh plug hernia repair: A followup report. *Surgery,* 117: 597–598.

22. **Rutkow IM, Robbins AW.**, (1995). Open mesh plug hernioplasty. *Prob. Gen. Surg.,* 12: 121–127.

23. **Rutkow IM, Robbins AW.**, (1996). Open tensionless mesh plug hernioplasty. In: Skandalakis L, Gadacz T, Mansberger A, Editors. Modern hernia repair. New York: Parthenon, pp. 204–210.

24. **Skandalakis JE, Skandalakis PN, Skandalakis LJ.**, Abdominal wall hernias. In: Surgical anatomy and technique, New York, Springer-Verlag: 200; pp. 133–135.

25. **Kugel RD.**, (1999). Minimally invasive, nonlaparoscopic, preperitoneal and sutureless inguinal herniorrhaphy. *Am. J. Surg.,* 178: 298–302.

26. **Ugahary F.**, (2001). The grid iron hernioplasty, in Bendavid R Abramson J, Arrigui M, Flament J.B., Philips hernias of the abdominal wall: principles and management. New York: Springer-Verlag, p. 219.

27. **Ugahary F, Simmer Macher PKJ.**, (1998). Groin hernia repair via a grid iron incision: An alternative technique for preperitoneal mesh insertion, 2: 123–5.

28. **Nigam VK.**, (2006). Nigam's Reverse Curtain Hernioplasty (NRCH). A new approach to inguinal hernia repair, Second Congress of Asia Pacific Hernia Society; 6-8, Asia Pacific Hernia Congress, New Delhi, India.

29. **Gilbert Al, Graham MF, Voigt WJ.**, (2001). Gilbert's repair of inguinal hernias. In abdominal wall hernias. Robert Bendavid, Springer NY 377–381.

30. **Trabucco EE, Trabucco AF.**, (1998). Flat plug and mesh hernioplasty in the "Inguinal Box": description of the surgical technique: Hernia 2: 133–138.

31. **Rollino RAM.**, (2004). Trabucco inguinal hernioplasty with tension-free sutureless pre-shaped mesh, new procedures in open hernia surgery, p. 23.

32. **Brunicardi FC,** *et al.,* (2005). Schwartz's principles of surgery, McGraw-Hill, 8th edition, p. 1374.

33. **Wantz GE.**, (1989). Giant prosthetic reinforcement of the visceral sac, *Surg. Gynecol. Obstet.,* 169: 408–417.

34. **Basoglu M, Yildirgam MI, Yilmaz I, Balik A, Celebi F, Atamanalp SS,** *et al.,* (2004). Late complications of incisional hernias following prosthetic mesh repair. *Acta Chir. Belg.,* 104: 425–428.

35. **Yerdil MA, Akin EB, Dolalan S,** *et al.,* (2001). Effects of single dose prophylactic ampicillin and sulbactum on wound infection after tension free inguinal hernia repair with polypropylene mesh. The randomised, double blind prospective trial. *Ann. Surg.,* 233: 26–33.

36. **Israilsson LA,** *et al.,* (2006). Incisional hernia repair in Sweden, 2002, Hernia 10: 258–61.

37. **Memon MA, Fitzgibbons RJ.**, (2006). Laparoscopic inguinal hernia repair: Transabdominal preperitoneal (TAPP) and Totally extraperitoneal (TEP), The SAGES Manual, 2nd edition, p. 480.

38. **Want GE.**, (1982). Testicular atrophy as risk of inguinoplasty. *Surg. Gynacol. Obstet.,* 154: 570.

39. **Turek PJ.**, (2004). Male infertility, Smith's general urology, 16th edition, p. 701.

40. **Ger R**., (1991). The laparoscopic management of groin hernias. *Contamp. Surg.*, 39(4): 15–19
41. **Schultz L, Garber J, Pietrafitta J**, *et al*., (1990). Laser laparoscopic herniorrhaphy: A clinical trial, preliminary results. *J. Laparoendose Surg.*, 1: 41–45.
42. **Corbett J**., (1991). Laparoscopic herniorrhaphy. *Surg. Laparose Endose*, 1(1): 23–25.
43. **Filipe C, Fitzgibbons RJ, Salerno GM**, *et al*., (1992). The laparoscopic herniorrhaphy, *Surg. Clin. North Am.*, 172: 1109–1124.
44. **Grant A**., (2000). EV hernia, Trialists collaboration laparoscopic compared with open methods of groin hernia repair: systematic review of randomised control trials. *Br. J. Surg.*, 87(7): 860–867.
45. **McCormack K, Scott NW**., 60 PMNYH, *et al*. on behalf of EU hernia trialists collaboration (2001). Laparoscopic techniques versus open techniques for inguinal hernia repair. (Cochrane Database of Systematic Reviews) AN. 00075320-100000000-0050. In update Software-Cochrane Library, Oxford.
46. **Douek M, Smith G, Oshowo A, Soker D, Wellwood J**., (2003). Prospective randomised controlled trial of laparoscopic versus open inguinal hernia mesh repair: Five-year followup BMJ, 326: 1012–1013.
47. **Bittner R**, *et al*., (2006) TAPP – Stuttgart technique and result of a large single center service, *Journal of Minimum Access Surgery*, **3**, p. 155.
48. **Schmedt CG**, *et al*., (2005). Comparison of endoscopic procedures versus Lichtenstein and other open mesh techniques for inguinal hernia repair: A meta-analysis of randomized controlled trials. *Surg. Endosc.*, 19: 188–189.
49. **Amid PK**., (2002). A-I Stage surgical treatment for post herniorrhaphy nuropathic pain. *Arch. Surg.*, 137: 100–104.
50. **Bendavid R**., (1998). Complications of groin hernia surgery. *Surg. Clin. North Am.*, 78: 1089.
51. **Davide Lomanto**, *et al*., (2006). Managing intra-operative complications during totally extraperitoneal repair of inguinal hernia, *Journal of Minimal Access Surgery*, **2**, 169.
52. **Carol EH, Scott-Conner**., (2007). The SAGES manual, I Indian reprint, p. 467.
53. **Davis C J, Arregui ME**., (2003). Laparoscopic repair for groin hernia, *Surg. Clin. North Am.*, 83: 1141–1161.
54. **Fitzgibbons RJ, Jr. Cornet DA**, *et al*., (1995). Laparoscopic inguinal herniorrhaphy: Results of a multicenter trial, *Ann. Surg.*, 221(1): 3–13.
55. **Felix**, *et al*., (1995). Laparoscopic hernioplasty, TAPPVs TEP, *Surgical Endoscopy*, 9(9), 984–989.
56. **Amid PK**., (2004). Causes, prevention and surgical treatment of post herniorrhaphy neuropathic inguinodynia: Triple neurectomy with proximal end implantation, Hernia, 8: 343–349.
57. **Amid PK**., (2004). Causes, prevention and surgical treatment of post herniorrhaphy neuropathic inguinodynia: Triple neurectomy with proximal end implantation, Hernia, 8: 343–349.
58. **Cannonico S**, *et al*.. (2005). Mesh fixation with human fibrin glu (Tissucol) in open tension-free inguinal hernia repair: A preliminary report. Hernias, 9: 330–333.
59. **Kukleta JF**., (2006). Causes of recurrence in laparoscopic inguinal hernia repair, *Journal of Minimal Access Surgery*, **2**, 190.
60. **Cooper A**., Anatomy and surgical treatment of inguinal and congenital hernia. London : JT Cox: 1804.
61. **Nyhus LM**., (1993). Iliopubic tract repair of inguinal and femoral hernia. The posterior (preperitoneal) approach. *Surg. Clin. North Am.*, 73: 487–499.
62. **Lotheissen G**., (1898). Zur Radikal Operation der Schenkelhernian, *Central be Chir.*, 25: 548.

63. **Hachisuka T.**, (2003). Femoral hernia repair, *Surg. Clin. North Am.*, 83: 1192–1203.
64. **Socin A.**, (1879). Ueber Redicaloperation der Herniea. *Arch. F. Klin. Chir.*, 24: 391.
65. **Bassini E.**, (1894). New operation: Method zur Radikal behandlung der Shenkelhernie. *Arch Klin Chir.*, 47: 1.
66. **Marcy HO.**, The anatomy and surgical treatment of hernia. New York; Appleton: 1982
67. **Cushing HW**: (1888). An improved method of radical cure of femoral hernia. *Boston Med. Surg. J.*, 119: 546.
68. **Lichtenstein IL, Shore JM.**, (1974). Simplified repair of femoral and recurrent inguinal hernias by a "plug" technique. *Am. J. Surg.*, 128: 439.
69. **Gilbert AI.**, (1992). Sutureless repair of inguinal hernia, *Am. J. Surg.*, 163: 331.
70. **Robbins AW, Rutkow IM.**, (1998). Repair of femoral hernias with "plug" technique. Hernia 2: 73.
71. **Larson GM.**, (2000). Ventral hernia repair by the laparoscopic approach, *Surg. Clin. North Am.*, 80, 4, 1329.
72. **Costanza MJ, Hemiford BT, Arca MJ,** *et al.*, (1998). Laparoscopic repair of recurrent ventral hernias. *Am. Surg.*, 64: 1121–1127.
73. **Larson GM, Harvower HW.**, (1978). Plastic mesh repair of incisional hernia. *Am. J. Surg.*, 135: 559–563.
74. **Park A, Berch DW, Lovrics, P,** *et al.*, (1998). Laparoscopic and open incisional hernia repair: A comparative study, *Surgery*, 124: 816–822.
75. **Holzman MD, Purut CM, Reintgen K,** *et al.*, (1997). Laparoscopic ventral and incisional hernioplasty: *Surg. Endosc.*, 11: 32–35.
76. **Mayo, WJ.**, (1901). An operation for the radical cure of umbilical hernia. *Am. Surg.*, 34: 276–280.
77. **Celdran A, Bazire P, Garcia-urena MA,** *et al.*, (1995). Hernioplasty; A tension free repair for umbilical hernia, *Br. J. Surg.*, 82: 371–372.
78. **Arroyo A, Gracia P, Perez F,** *et al.*, (2001). Randomized clinical trial comparing suture and mesh repair of umbilical hernia in adults B. *J. Surg.*, 88(10): 1321–1323.
79. **Muschaweck U.**, (2003). Umbilical and epigastric hernia repair, *Surg. Clin. North Am.*, 83: 1207–1221.
80. **Brancato G, Privitera A, Donate M,** *et al.*, (2003). Tension-free prosthetic repair in surgery treatment of epigastric hernia, 83, *Surg. Cl. North Am.*
81. **Wantz GE, Fischer E.**, (2002). Clinilateral giant prosthetic reinforcement of the visceral sac, in Fitzgibbon RJ Jr. Greenberg AG (Eds): Nyhus and Condon's hernia, 5th edition, Philadelphia, Lippincott, Williams and Wilkins, p. 219.
82. **Reed RC.**, (1994). Prosthesis in abdominal wall hernia surgery, in Bendavid R (Ed): Austin TX: RG Lands Co, p. 2.
83. **Anson BJ, Morgan EH, McVay CB.**, (1960). Surgical anatomy of the inguinal region based upon a study of 500 body halves. *Surg. Gynaecol. Obestet.*, 11: 707–725.
84. **Anson BJ, McVay CB.**, (1940). *Anat. Rec.*, 76: 213.
85. **Bassini E.**, (1887). *Atti. Cong. Assosci. Med. Hal.*, 2: 179.
86. **Halsted WS.**, (1890). *Bull. Johns Hopkins Hosp.*, 1: 12.
87. **Halsted WS.**, (1903). *Bull. Johns Hopkins Hosp.*, 14: 208.
88. **Franz GM.**, (2007). Complications in Surgery, Lippincott Williams & Wilkins, 532.

89. **Griffith CA.**, (1971). *Surg. Clin. North Am.*, 1: 1309.

90. **Read RC.**, (1989). *World J. Surg.*, 13: 532.

91. **Gilbert AI.**, (2007). Generation of the plug and patch repair: Its development and lessons from history, Mastery of surgery, 5th edition, Lippincott Williams & Wilkins, p. 1941.

92. **Stoppa RE.**, (2007). Giant prothesis for Reinforcement of the visceral sac in the repair of groin and incisional hernias; Mastery of surgery, 5th edition, p. 1923–1931.

93. **Stoppa R., Ralamiaramanana F. Henry X.** *et al.*; (1999). Evaluation of large ventral incisional repair. The French contribution to a difficult problem, hernia, 3: 1.

94. **Warlaumont CR.**, (1989). The preperitoneal approach and prosthetic repair of groin hernias. In: Nyhus LM, Condon RE, Eds. Hernia, 3rd edition. Philadelphia: JB Lippincott, 199.

95. **Kugel RD.**, (2007). Groin Hernia Repair. Kugel technique, Mastery of surgery, 5th edition, Lippincott Williams & Wilkins, pp. 1912–1923.

96. **Kugel RD.**, (2003). The Kugel repair for Groin Hernias. *Surg. Clin. North Am.*, 83: 1119.

97. **Kugel RD.**, (2002). Minimally invasive repair of groin and ventral hernias using a self-expanding mesh patch. *Surg. Technol. Int.*, 10: 81.

98. **Gilbert AI.**, (2007). Generation of the plug and patch repair: Its development and lesson from history, Mastery of surgery, 5th edition, Lippincott Williams & Wilkins, p. 1942.

99. **Gilbert AI.**, (1987). Overnight hernia repair, *South Med. J.*, 80: 191.

100. **Gilbert AI.**, (2004). Combined anterior and posterior inguinal hernia repair: Intermediate recurrent rates with three groups of surgeons. Hernia, 88(3): 203.

101. **Bendavid R.**, (2007). The shouldice method of inguinal herniorrhaphy, Mastery of surgery, 5th edition, Lippincott Williams & Wilkins, p. 1897.

102. **Fischer JE, Bland KI.**, (2007). Editor's comment, Mastery of surgery, 5th Edition., 1957.

103. **Jones DB.**, (2007). Editor's comment, Mastery of surgery, 5th edition, p. 1965.

104. **Obney N.**, (1956). Hydroceles of the testicle complicating inguinal hernias. *Can. Med. Ass. J.*, 75: 733.

105. **Scott JS, DeLatorre RA, Ramshaw B.**, (2007). Laparoscopic transabdominal preperitoneal inguinal hernia repair, Mastery of surgery, 5th edition, pp. 1899–1904.

106. **Rattner D, Noord MV.**, (2007). Totally extraperitoneal inguinal hernia repair, Mastery of surgery, 5th edition, Lippincott, Williams & Wilkins, pp. 1905–1911.

107. **Franz GM.**, (2007). Complications in surgery, Lippincott Williams & Wilkins, pp. 537.

108. **Heise CP, Sterling JR.**, (1998). Mesh inguinodynia: A new clinical syndrome after inguinal herniorrhaphy, *J. Am. Coll. Surg.*, 187: 514.

109. **Madura JA, Madura II JA, Copper CM,** *et al.*, (2005). Inguinal neurectomy for inguinal nerve entrapment; an experience with 100 patients. *Am. J. Surg.*, 189: 283.

110. **Starling JR, Harms BA.**, (1994). Ilioinguinal, iliohypogastric, and genitofemoral neuralgia. In: Bendavid R, Eds. prostheses and abdominal wall hernia, Austin, Tx: Landes; 351.

111. **Amid PK.**, (2007). Lichtenstein tension-free hernioplasty, Mastery of surgery, 5th Edn., 1936.

112. **Madura JA.**, (2007). Inguinal neurectomy for postinguinal nerve entraptment, Mastery of surgery, 5th edition, Lippincott Williams & Wilkins, p. 1969.

113. **Madura JA.**, (2007). Inguinal neurectomy for postinguinal nerve entraptment, Mastery of surgery, 5th edition, Lippincott Williams & Wilkins, p. 1971.

114. **Bendavid R.**, (1992). Dysejeaculation, an unsual complication of inguinal herniorrhaphy. *Postgrad. Gen. Surg.*, 4: 139.

115. **Ramshaw BJ.**, (2007). Laparoscopic ventral hernia repair, Mastery of surgery, 5th Edn, 1959.
116. **Nordin P, Zenerstrom H, Gunnarsson U,** *et al.*, (2003). Local, regional, or general anaesthesia in groin hernia repair: multicentre randomised trial. *Lancet.* 362: 853.
117. **Townsend CM.** *et al.*, (2004). Hernias, Sabiston textbook of surgery, **2**, Elvisier, p. 213.
118. **Brunicardi FC** *et al.*, (2005). Schwartz's principles of surgery, 8th edition, p. 1369.
119. **Laparoscopic hernia repair versus open repair of groin hernia; A randomised comparison; The MRC Laparoscopic Groin Hernia Trial Group.** (1999). The Lancet, **354,** 185–190.
120. **Chevrel JP.**, Post operative complications; hernia and surgery of the abdominal wall; 98–102.
121. **Lifscutz H.**, (1986). The inguinal darn, *Arch. Surg.*, 121: 353.
122. **Chowbey P.**, (2004). Endoscopic repair of abdominal wall hernias, 1st Edn., ByWord, p. 78
123. **Chowbey P,** *et al.*, (2006). Totally extraperitoneal repair of inguinal hernia, Sir Ganga Ram Hospital Technique, *Jour. MAS,* **2,** 162–164.
124. **Bhatia P.**, (2008). Current status of laparoscopic inguinal hernia surgery, *GIS.,* 1st ed. 923.
125. **Shouldice EE.**, (1953). *Ont. Med. Rev.*, 20: 670.
126. **Gawande A.**, (2002). Complications, Penguin Books, pp. 32–33.
127. **Bittner R,** *et al.,* (2006). TAPP–Stuttgart technique and result of a large single center service, *Journal of Minimum Acum. Surgery,* **3,** p. 155.
128. **Kuntz AR.**, (1963). Hernia, New York, Appleton-Century-Crofts.
129. **Fischer JE, Bland KI.**, (2007). Editor's comment, Mastery of surgery, 5th edition, 1891.
130. **Amid PK.**, (2007). Lichtenstein tension-free hernioplasty, Mastery of surgery, 5th Ed., 111.
131. **Frey D.M., Wildisen A., Hamel C.T.,** *et al.* (2007). Randomized clinical trial of Lichtenstein's operation versus mesh plug for inguinal hernia repair. *Br. J. Surg.* 94(1): 36–41.
132. **Awad S.S., Yallalampalli S., Srour A.M.,** *et al.* (2007). Improved outcomes with the Prolene Hernia System mesh compared with the time-honoured Lichtenstein onlay mesh repair for inguinal hernia repair. *Am. J. Surg.* 193(6): 697–701.
133. **Fitzgibbons R.J. Jr. Giobbie-Hurder A., Gibbs J.O.,** *et al.* (2006). Watchful waiting vs repair of inguinal hernia in minimally symptomatic: randomized clinical trial. *JAMA* 295(3): 285–92.
134. **Witt W.P., Gibbs J., Wang J.,** *et al.* (2006). Impact of inguinal hernia repair on family and other informall caregivers. *Arch. Surg.* 141(9): 925-30.
135. **Wake B.L., McCormack K., Fraser C.,** *et al.* (2005). Transabdominal pre-peritoneal (TAPP) vs totally extraperitoneal (TEP) laparoscopic techniques for inguinal hernia repair. *Cochrane Database Syst. Rev.* 1: CD004703.
136. **Hynes D.M.,** *et al.* (2006). Cost effectiveness of laparoscopic versus open mesh hernia operation: results of a Department of Veterans Affairs randomized clinical trial. *JACS*; 203(4): 447–57.
137. **Arvidsson D., Berndsen F.H., Larsson L.G.,** *et al.* (2005). Randomized clinical trial comparing 5-year recurrent rate after laparoscopic versus Shouldice repair of primary inguinal hernia. *Br. J. Surg.* 92(9): 1085–91.
138. **Ferzli GS.,** *et al.*, (2008). Postherniorrhaphy groin pain and how to avoid it. *Surg. Clin. N. Am.*, 88, 214.
139. **Poobalan AS, Bruce J, King MP,** *et al.*, (2001). Chronic pain and quality of life following open inguinal hernia repair. Br J. Surg.; (88): 1122–6.
140. **Weyhe D, Belyaev O, Muller C.,** *et al.*, (2007). Improving outcomes in hernia repair by the use of light meshes-a comparision of different implant constructions based on a critical appraisal of the literature. World J Surg.; 31(1):234–44.

Section 5

MISCELLANEOUS ASPECTS OF ABDOMINAL WALL HERNIAS

"The habit of persistence is the habit of victory"
-Herbert Kaufman

20 Abdominal Wall Hernia "Day Case Surgery"

Physician heals, Nature cures
— **Aristotle**

Day case hernia surgery is also known as ambulatory hernia surgery.

It is a planned investigation or procedure on patients who are admitted and discharged home on the same day of their surgery but who require some facilities and time for recovery.

Abdominal wall hernia day surgery is fast becoming popular globally for elective hernia surgery. It is increasing due to following factors:
• Advancement in pain control and anaesthesia
• Increasing minimal invasive surgery
• Changing attitude of patients and doctors
• Increasing cost of in-patient treatment
• Long waiting list of hernia surgery
• Better utilization of funds[1]

HISTORICAL BACKGROUND

The concept of "Day Hernia Surgery" was started in 1909 by James Nicholl. He started DSU "Day Surgery Unit",[2] to save resources and utilize the existing resources in a better way. He was surgeon at Western Infirmary, Glasgow, Scotland. In 1912, Ralph Waters, anaesthetist, Iowa, USA, opened "Down-town anaesthesia clinic".[3] It was a day surgery unit. In 1969, Walter Reed, surgeon, started "Phoenix Surgicenter", a DSU where hernia cases were also operated with same day discharge.[4]

Benefits of Day Surgery were realised after World War II. Hernia cases were discharged on the same day of operation and dangers of prolonged bed rest and economic benefits of day surgery were realised.[5]

Eric Farquharson described in 1955 consecutive 458 inguinal hernia repairs performed as day cases.[6]

A concept of "Basket" of 20 surgical procedures, including inguinal hernia repair was given by Audit Commission of UK.[7]

INDICATIONS OF DAY CASE HERNIA SURGERY

The day hernia surgery is becoming important day by day and more and more hospitals are adopting it.

Following are the indications of day hernia surgery:
• Inguinal hernia

- Femoral hernia
- Umbilical hernia
- Epigastric hernia
- Small incisional hernia

Day care hernia or "come and go" hernia surgery is a routine procedure nowadays. Open mesh repair of primary unilateral inguinal hernia under local anaesthesia is an ideal day case surgery.

BENEFITS OF DAY CASE HERNIA SURGERY

Day care rate in UK for hernia repair are improving but are still below the recommended guidelines. In UK only less than 6% of hernia are repaired under LA. Yet in NHS units where surgeons have expressed an interest, the number of cases carried out under LA will rise over 30% and in dedicated consultant-led units this figure can reach over 80%.[6]

Following are the benefits of day hernia surgery:

- Cost reduction and better utilization of resources. Day case surgery can cut the cost for hernia operation considerably.
- Day case surgery provides high quality, patient-centred treatment that is safe, efficient and effective and is accompanied by a lower incidence of hospital acquired infection and an earlier return to normal activity compared with in-patient treatment.
- Waiting lists of hernia surgery patient are reduced.
- Reduced incidence of DVT as prolonged bed rest is not needed.
- Hospital acquired infections are avoided.
- Early return to work reduces the manhour loss.

POST-OPERATIVE MORBIDITY AND MORTALITY AFTER DAY CASE SURGERY

Mayo Clinic reported in 1993 that the mortality and major morbidity around 0.0007% in day case surgery. Usually the post-operative morbidity in DSU are minor problems. The post-operative morbidity is related to the type of surgery and the type of anaesthesia. The selection of patients for surgery and the selection of anaesthesia for patients are two important factors in reducing the post-operative morbidity and mortality.

REQUIREMENTS OF DAY CASE SURGERY

- Try to select ideal patient and ideal standard surgical procedure.
- Preadmission surgical, medical and anaesthetic assessment.
- Clear post-operative instructions.
- Post-operative medications must be in oral form.
- Maximum duration of surgery should be 1-2 hours.
- Surgery should not have much blood loss.
- Patient should be conscious and ambulatory before discharged to go home.
- Attendent should go home with patient if general anaesthesia was given.
- No excessive pain or vomiting or bleeding at the time of discharge.
- It is better if the patient voids before discharge specially if general anaesthesia was given.

SELF CONTAINED DAY CASE HERNIA SURGERY UNIT

The day case surgery unit should be self-sufficient, dedicated and specially planned. Following is the plan for day case hernia surgery unit:

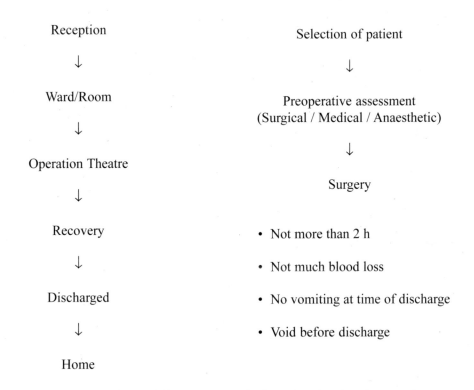

Reception   Selection of patient

↓   ↓

Ward/Room   Preoperative assessment
(Surgical / Medical / Anaesthetic)

↓   ↓

Operation Theatre   Surgery

↓

Recovery   • Not more than 2 h

↓   • Not much blood loss

Discharged   • No vomiting at time of discharge

↓   • Void before discharge

Home

A day hernia surgery unit should have an anaesthetic and analgesic unit, consultant room, small laboratory and standard equipment.

SELECTION OF PATIENTS FOR DAY CASE HERNIA SURGERY

The selection of patients and surgical procedure for hernia are two important factors for successful day hernia surgery programme. Age is no bar for day case hernia surgery. Following factors must be considered for patient selection:

Obesity

BMI is usually checked to determine the obesity as obesity can cause some complications in day case hernia surgery which may lead to extended stay. BMI upto 35 or even 40 is nowadays taken as upper limit for day hernia surgery[8].

Obesity related complications in day hernia surgery are given below:
- Pulmonary infection.
- Wound infection.
- Bleeding in subcutaneous plane leading to haematoma formation.

- Hernia repair in depth will require more amount of anaesthetic drugs—local or general.
- Difficult intubation in general anaesthesia.

Smoking

Smokers must stop smoking at least one week before surgery but if due to certain reasons surgery is to be done early then there must be a smoke free period of 12 hours before the surgery which helps to improve lung functions. Ideally smoking should be stopped six weeks before the surgery and breathing exercises should be started.

Medical Sicknesses

Diabetes mellitus, hypertension, ischaemic heart disease, bronchial asthma, bleeding diathesis and renal insufficiency should be detected at day case surgery medical assessment.

History of Drugs

History of drugs specially aspirin and clopidogrel must be asked to avoid operative and post-operative bleeding. These drugs must be stopped at least one week before the surgery.

History of allergy to drugs is mandatory.

Physical Fitness

Physical status of the patient can be assessed by using ASA (American Society of Anaesthesiologists) guidelines.[9]

ASA has divided the day surgery cases into following five classes from healthy patient to moribund patient:

Class I (ASA-I)   – Healthy patient
Class II (ASA-II)   – Mild to moderate systemic disease without functional limitation
Class III (ASA-III)   – Severe systemic disease with functional limitation
Class IV (ASA-IV)   – Severe systemic disease with a constant threat to life
Class V (ASA-V)   – Moribund patient
Day hernia surgery can be done for patients from Class I to Class III.

ANAESTHESIA FOR DAY CASE HERNIA SURGERY

Day case surgery for abdominal wall hernia can be performed by both open and laparoscopic techniques. So it can be done under general, regional and local anaesthesia. Local anaesthesia is the method of choice and most preferred one. Local anaesthesia with sedation gives good response from patient. The sedation removes the anxiety of the patient which is common even in day hernia surgery. There were fewer unplanned overnight admissions (3% versus 14% and 22% respectively)[10] with local anaesthesia than regional and general anaesthesia. Anaesthetic technique of Lichtenstein results in uniformly anaesthetized operation field independent of the operator.[13]

UNPLANNED OVERSTAY (OVERNIGHT STAY)

In hernia surgery, unplanned overstay is usually after general anaesthesia or regional block post-anaesthesia complications. Some overstays can be avoided if proper preassessment is done.

Following are the common causes of unplanned over-stay:

- Post-anaesthetic problems e.g.
  - PONV (Post Operative Nausea Vomiting)
  - Urinary retention
  - Dizziness
  - Dead leg after incidental femoral nerve block
- Pain
- Post-operative complication
  - Bleeding at hernia operation site. It is more in patients who take aspirin or clopidogrel and drugs were not stopped seven days before the surgery.
- Miscellaneous
  - Patient was admitted late.
  - Operation started late due to busy operation theatre.
  - Patient wanted to stay.

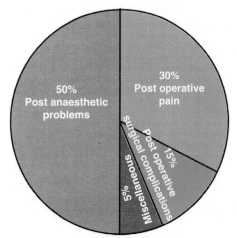

Fig. 20.1. Reasons for unplanned overstay.

KEY POINT

Local anaesthesia is the ideal anaesthesia for day case hernia surgery.

REFERENCES

1. **RCG Russell,** *et al.,* (2004). Bailey and Love's short practice of surgery, 24th edition, p. 228.
2. **Nicholl JH.,** (1909). The surgery of infancy. *Br. Med. J.,* II: 753–6.
3. **Waters RM.,** (1919). The down-town anaesthesia Clinic. *Am. J. Surg.,* 33(Supl.): 71–3.
4. **RCG Russell,** *et al.,* (2004). Bailey and Love's short practice of surgery, 24th edition, p. 228.
5. **Palumbo LT, Laul RE, Emery FB.,** (1952). Results of primary inguinal hernioplasty. *Arch. Surg.,* 64: 384–94.
6. **Farquharson EL.,** (1955). Early ambulation with special references to herniorrhaphy as an out-patient procedure. *Lancet.* II : 517–19.
7. **Audit Commission.,** (1990). A short cut to better services: Day surgery in England and Wales. London: HMSO.
8. **Davies KE, Houghton K, Montgomery J.,** (2001). Obesity and day case surgery. *Anaesthesia,* 56: 1090–115.
9. **American Society of Anaesthesiology.,** (1991). ASA classification of surgical patients. *Chicago.*
10. **Mackenzie JW.,** (1989). Day case anaesthesia and anxiety. *Anaesthesia,* 44: 437–40.
11. **NHS Management Executive.,** (1993). Day surgery, reports by the day surgery task force, BAPS, Health Publications Unit, Heywood, Lancashire.
12. **The Royal College of Surgeons of England.,** (1992). Guidelines for day case surgery, the Royal College of Surgeons of England.
13. **Woods B.,** *et al.,* (2008). Open repair of inquinal hernia: An evidence based review, *Surg. Clin N. Am.,* 88, 148.

21 Prosthesis for Hernia Repair

"If only the proper material could be created to artificially produce tissues of density and toughness of fascia and tendon, the secret of the radical cure for hernia would be discoverd,"
— **Billroth**[1]

"Since no single ideal operation exists for the cure of hernia, it is unlikely that a single ideal prosthesis to aurgument hernia repair will be developed that is universally adaptated"
— **James R. Debord and Lisa A Whitty**
Mastery of Surgery, 2007

CHARACTERISTICS OF PROSTHETIC MESH

Nowadays various biomaterials are used as prosthetic material to form mesh for hernia repair.

The ideal biomaterial for mesh must be compatible with the criteria of "Cumberland and Scale". This criteria was given in 1950.[2] The ideal prosthetic should be chosen based on following criteria:
- It should be chemically inert.
- It should not excite an inflammatory or foreign body reaction.
- It should not produce hypersensitivity reaction.
- It should not evoke a carcinogenic response.
- It should resist mechanical strains.
- It should not react with body tissue fluid.
- It should be easily sterilized.
- It should be able to be fabricated in the form required.
- It must be resistant to infection.
- It must provide barrier to adhesions with abdominal viscera.
- The mesh must develop some adhesion to tissue immediately soon after its application and not move or slip.

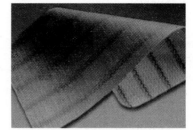

Fig. 21.1. Partially absorbable light weight soft flexible mesh.

The following biomaterials are currently in use which are found very near to the criteria of Cumberland and Scale:

(1) Polypropylene Mesh (PPM) (Fig. 21.1)

Polypropylene mesh is most widely used for the past twenty years because of its strength, stability, inertness and handling qualities.[3]
- It has high tensile strength (50,000-150,000 lb/sq in).

In order to rupture polypropylene mesh, an intra-abdominal pressure of more than 10 times the maximum pressure would be required.[4]
- It resists water, chemicals and high temperature (260° F).
- It is pliable and can be readily introduced into any defect without getting fragmented.

- It is tolerant to bending and flex stresses and can be used in groin without problem and it withstands infection.
- Polypropylene (Ethicon, Somerville, NJ, USA) and Marlex (CR Bard, Somerville, NJ, USA) are common brands in use (Figs. 21.2, 21.3 & 21.4). Atrium and Surgipro are other brands.
- Shrinkage of mesh occurs 40% and plug shrinks up to 70%.

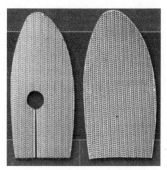

Fig. 21.2. Pre-shaped PPM mesh.

(2) Expanded Polytetra Fluoroethylene (e-PTFE)

It was discovered in 1938 by Plunkett of El du Pont de Nemonis and Company. The characteristics of e-PTFE are:

- It is almost chemically inert.
- It produces minimal inflammatory reaction, so low rate of adhesion formation.
- It is strong, soft and flexible.
- It withstands infection well.
- Tissue ingrowth is good.
- The common e-PTFE brands are:
  - Goretex STP (Soft Tissue Patch) and Gortex Micromesh

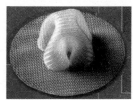

Fig. 21.3. Prosthetic mesh with plug.

(3) Polyethylene (Polyster, Dacron, Marsilene) Mesh

It was used by Stoppa in 1975 and Wantz in 1989. It has following features:
- Suppleness
- Early fibroelastic response for early fixation of mesh
    The common brand in use is Parietex (Sofradin Inc., Lyon, France)

(4) Composite Meshes

- They reduce the amount of non-absorbable polypropylene by 70%
- Polypropylene-polyglactin mesh (Vipro I/II)
- Polypropylene - Polyglecaprone (Ultrapro)
- Polypropylene-oxidized with regenerated cellulose
- Polypropylene - Omega-3 fatty acid (C-Qur, Atrium)
- Polypropylene - Titanium (Ti MESH)
- Polypropylene - Oat beta glucan (GLUCAMESH)
- It gives tough scar.
- Polyglactin usually gets absorbed within 120 to 180 days.
- Parietex Composite Mesh (PCM) has a collagen coating on one side which acts as antiadhesive layer, so can be in contact with abdominal viscera inside peritoneal cavity.
- Ventralax patch: It has two discs, larger disc is of PTFE towards viscera and smaller disc of PPM is against abdominal wall.

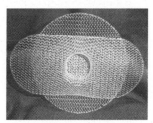

Fig. 21.4. PHS.

Surgeon should consider raw material, design, technique and clinical condition in selection of mesh.

RECENT DEVELOPMENTS IN MESH PROSTHESIS

Seprafilm or sepracoat

- It is a three-dimensional polyester mesh with coating of sodium hyaluronate. It enhances the rapid ingrowth of tissue and causes least visceral adhesions.

Light weight polypropylene mesh (Figs. 21.5 & 21.6)

- These meshes also have self-gripping quality. Heavy weight meshes cause inflammatory reactions leading to shrinking of mesh. To reduce these drawbacks, low weight meshes are advised.[5]

Biologic Meshes

Biologic meshes made up of acellular collagen matrix have inherited tensile strength but allow host angiogenesis and cellular ingrowth.[6,7]

- Human as well as animal tissues are used except cellular component to prevent allergic reaction.

The examples of biologic meshes are:

- Surgisis: It is made from porcine gut submucosa.
- Alloderm: It is made from cadaver dermis tissue.
- Permacol: It is made from porcine dermis.

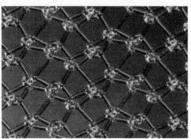

Fig. 21.5. Polypropylene monofilament mesh

Disadvantages of Biologic Mesh

- All these biologic meshes are expensive.
- No proper long term evaluation is done, so long term evaluation is required.
- Latest prosthetic meshes could not become popular due to cost.

Partially absorbable Hernia Mesh System is now available (Ultrapro, Ethicon).

- It is a stronger mesh.
- Excellent tissue ingrowth.
- Partially absorbable so 50% less foreign material remains in body of patient as compared to usual polypropylene mesh.
- It is a polypropylene mesh with an absorbable film of Monocryl (Poliglecaprone – 25), gets absorbed fully within 84 days.
- Excessive healing of peritoneum can cause adhesions with bowel loops if the prosthetic mesh is in contact with it.[8]

> **NOTE**
>
> *"Placement of polypropylene mesh in the abdominal cavity is not a problem for the surgeon placing the mesh, but it can be a disaster for the surgeon who has to do the next operation on the patient."*
>   **- Guy Voeller**

- Peritoneal healing differs from that of skin healing, which heals gradually by epithelialization, from the border. Defects in the parietal peritoneum, in contrast, heal by simultaneous epithelialization of the entire surface. Hence, complete mesothelialization, developing from multiple points throughout the defect, occurs just as rapidly for large and small defects.[9] It takes 14 days to complete mesotheliazation.

- Development of intraperitoneal adhesions is a dynamic process that actually begins at the time of incision when surgically traumatized tissues in apposition have their first opportunity to bind through fibrin bridges,[10] and causes chronic pain and discomfort.[20]

- "A pore size lower than 800–600 μm results in a fibrous tissue reaction response similar to "bridging reaction" between pores, thus rather leading to a scar plate than a scar net. We therefore recommended the use of large pored mesh materials[11]."

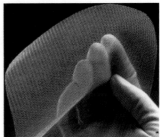

Fig. 21.6. Latest mesh are flexible smooth and strong.

- The new macroporous compound meshes present both the successful reduction of the overall foreign body amount and the preservation of mesh elasticity after the scar tissue ingrowth due to very limited shrinkage and reduced bridging effect. These meshes provide the possibility of forming a scar net instead of a stiff scar plate and therefore help to avoid former known mesh complications.[11]

- Timothy W Judge et al.[12] studied a comparison between Parietex composite mesh (PCM, a polyester mesh with an absorbable coating of polyethylene glycol and glycerol) and Sepramesh (SM, macroporous polypropylene mesh coated on one side with bioresorbable sodium hyaluronate and carboxy methyl cellulose on other side). PCM showed stronger SOI (strength of incorporation) and superior adhesion preservation but PCM showed more shrinkage than SM. Coda[13] et al. also found increased shrinkage with PCM.

- All meshes show a decrease in abdominal wall compliance, measured by patient's complaints and three-dimensional stereography, in ventral hernia repair. Marlex is the worst offender and vipro is the least.[14,15]

Mesh failure occurs, almost always at the mesh fascia interface rather than mesh material failure.[16]

Tissue Adhesives to Fix Prosthesis[18]

Hard fixation devices such as staples and tacks are blamed for inguinodynia and other post-operative problems, so tissue adhesives are developed to avoid these problems.

- **Surgical glue:** It is n-butyl -2-cyanoacrylate which is haemostatic and an effective adhesive. It is a polymer and its film binds tissues with mesh. It has following side effects:
  - May induce foreign body reaction.
  - Cannot be used in patients having hypersensitivity to it.
  - Sometimes it may produce hot sensations due to exothermic reaction.
- **Fibrin sealant:** It is combination of human derived fibrinogen and thrombin activated by calcium chloride leading to formation of polymerized fibrin chain. Fibrinogen gives:
  - Tensile strength.
  - Adhesive properties.
  Thrombin promotes fibroblast proliferation.
  "Our preliminary observational study has shown that the use of fibrin sealant in inguinal hernia repair protects the patient from groin discomfort as far as 18 months, so mesh fixation with fibrin sealant appears to be suitable for use in open tension-free repair.[19]

Antibacterial impregation of prosthetic mesh

Carbonell et al., showed that impregation of prosthetic mesh with silver or chlorhexidine is a reasonable approach to prevent infection and does not change the character of the mesh.[13]

> ### KEY POINT
>
> *Polypropylene mesh (Polypropylene mesh = PPM) is the best and cheapest mesh available today, others are expensive materials.*

REFERENCES

1. **Halsted WS.**, (1924). Surgical papers by William Stewart Halsted. Baltimore, MD: The John Hopkins Press; 1: 271.
2. **Cumberland VH.**, (1952). A preliminary report on the use of a pre-fabricated nylon weave in the repair of ventral hernia. *Med. J. Aust.*, 1: 143.
3. **Doctor HG.**, (2006). Evaluation of various prosthetic materials and newer meshes for hernia repair, *Journal of Minimal Access Surgery*, **2**, Issue-3.
4. **Holste JL.**, (2005). Are meshes with light weight construction strong enough? *Int. Surg.*, 90: 510–512.
5. **Bringman S,** *et al.,* Three-year results of a randomized clinical trial of light weight or standard polypropylene mesh in Lichtenstein repair of primary inguinal hernia, *Br. J. Surg.*, 93: 1056–9.
6. **Debord JR, and Whitty LA.**, (2007). Biomaterials in hernia repair, Mastery of surgery, 5th edition, Lippincott Williams & Wilkins, p. 1966.
7. **Debord JR.**, (1998). The historical development of prosthetics in hernia surgery, *Surg. Clin. North Am.*, 78(6): 973.
8. **Ramshaw B.**, (2005). Laparoscopic ventral hernia repair–Managing and preventing complications. *Int. Surg.*, 90: 548–555.
9. **Divilio LT.**, (2005) Surgical adhesion development and prevention. *Int. Surg.*, 90: 56–59.
10. **Dizerega GS, Campeau JD.**, (2001). Peritoneal repair and post-surgical adhesion formation. Hum Reprod Update, 7: 547–555.
11. **Schumpelick V,** *et al.*, (2006). Light weight meshes in incisional hernia repair, *Journal of Minimal Access Surgery*, **2**, p. 117.
12. **Judge TW, Parker DM, and Dinsmore RC.**, (2007). Abdominal wall hernia repair: A comparison of sepramesh and parietex composite mesh in a rabbit hernia model, *J. Am. Coll. Surg.*, Elsevier, 33–38.
13. **Coda A, Bendavid R, Botto-Mica F,** *et al.*, (2003). Structural alterations of prosthetic meshes in humans. Hernia, 7: 29–34.
14. **Voeller G.**, (2007). Ventral abdominal hernia, Mastery of Surgery, 5th edition, Lippincott Williams & Wilkins, p. 1947.
15. **Klinge U, Klosterhalfen B, Schumpelick V., Vipro®.**, (2001). A new generation of polypropylene mesh. In: Bendavid R, Ed. abdominal wall hernias. Berlin Heidelberg: Springer-Verlag, p. 286.
16. **Franz GM.**, (2007). Complications in surgery, Lippincott Williams & Wilkins, p. 540.
17. **Carbonell** *et al.*, (2005). *Surg. Endosc.*, 19: 430.
18. **Chowbey P.**, (2004). Endoscopic repair of abdominal wall hernias, 1st edn ByWord, 57–58.
19. **Campanelli G, Pettinari D, Cavalli M, Avesani EC.**, (2006) A modified Lichtenstein hernia repair using fibrin glue, *Jour. MAS*, **2**, pp. 129–133.
20. **Earle, DB.**, (2008). Prosthetic material in inguinal hernia. *Surg. Clin. N. Am.*; 88, 188.

22

Difficulties in Hernia Surgery

"When the blood is fresh and pink and the patient is old, It is time to be active and bold, When the patient is young and the blood is dark and old, you can relax and put your knife on hold."
— **Medical Rhyme**

GENERAL RULES OF GROIN HERNIA SURGERY

- **Haemorrhage or haematoma** – Meticulous haemostasis is very important in hernia surgery.

  "The most important clotting factor is the surgeon."
  - **Anonymous**

  - A trainee or a beginner should not embark on repairing of diffuse recurrent inguinal hernia in an obese patient.
  - Do not attempt to gain mastery of all techniques of hernia repair. Be familiar and well experienced with one technique.

- Diagnosis of groin swelling is quiet perplexing and sometimes difficult. Mistakes are frequently done even by experienced surgeons. Do not depend upon preoperative diagnosis or diagnosis made by referring doctor. It is always good to make your own opinion by taking detailed history and thorough examination of the patient.

  NOTE

  Never staple in:
  - *area of lateral cutaneous nerve of thigh.*
  - *around external iliac vessels and adjacent nerves.*
  - *area below iliopubic tract.*

DIFFICULTIES IN OPEN INGUINAL HERNIA REPAIR

- Never delay the strangulated hernia operation, just take time to prepare the patient for surgery with ressuscitative measures.
- If the neck of hernia sac is torn during inguinal hernia surgery, then carefully gradually free more peritoneum from abdomen and use it as a new neck (Fig. 22.1).
- If a lipoma is found in spermatic cord then it should be excised due to following reasons:
  - It can cause inguinal hernia type symptoms.
  - It is difficult to distinguish from indirect inguinal hernia with a peritoneal sac
  - It can be responsible for a unsatisfactory result.[5]

Fig. 22.1. Tear in the neck of inguinal hernia sac.

- Lipoma, if found near the neck of sac carefully dissect it and ligate proximally, excise and check for any peritoneal tear. If tear is found, then it must be closed.
- If there is difficulty in recognizing the sac,[1] then first recognize spermatic cord by palpating the vas deferens, it is felt like a string and is followed. If you find some structure resembling the sac, open it and put the finger inside and then separate it from other structures.
- If femoral vein is torn, and:
  - If the injury is a needle prick then press with hot pack for five minutes, it will stop.
  - If the hole is big then
    a) Press with gauze for 5 minutes.
    b) Ask to arrange two bottles of blood.
    c) Apply bulldog clip.
    d) Apply tapes above and below the injury site on vein.
    e) Repair the dent with 5/0 polypropylene sutures either continuous or 1 mm apart interrupted sutures.
    f) Flush with Heparin solution.
    g) Remove clamps and tapes.
  - If the repair is not possible then pack the wound and call the vascular surgeon.

- If the cord structures and the sac are adherent and dissection is difficult then inject 2-3 ml of normal saline which will give a plane for dissection.
- Recurrence after laparoscopic hernia repair should be treated with open tension-free hernia repair and recurrence after open repair is treated with laparoscopic repair.
- Sometimes reduction is difficult due to bulk of the tissues in hernia sac, the little by little reduction with patience ultimately leads to success.
- While dealing with spermatic cord after opening the inguinal canal, lift the spermatic cord en-masse to avoid injury to cord structures. Index finger of one hand is insinuated behind the cord to meet the index finger of other hand. This avoids injurying to spermatic cord and pampiniform plexus of veins.[2]
- If the sac is adherent with omentum then one can push the sac in without its excision as some surgeons feel that it will cause less pain, however, it is not scrutinized by a randomized trial.[3]
- If the intestinal loop is injured during hernia surgery or tied during ligation or transfixation of the sac. The injured segment of intestine should be excised and end-to-end or side-to-side anastomosis is made.
- If the gangrenous loop of bowel slips inside the abdominal cavity and cannot be traced then repair the hernia and open the abdomen with another incision. Find the gangrenous loop and do the resection and anastomosis.
- Direct hernia sac is dealt in any one of the following manners:
  - The sac may be inverted in peritoneal cavity and repair is done.
  - The fascia transversalis is plicated by few sutures.
  - If the sac is narrow-necked then the sac is excised at neck.
- Direct inguinal hernia with big sac is dealt in any one of the following methods:
  - Lichtenstein's tension-free mesh repair
  - Stoppa's GPRVS method
  - Shouldice repair

DIFFICULTIES IN FEMORAL HERNIA REPAIR (Figs. 22.2A & B)

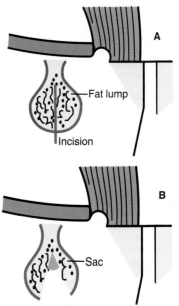

- Femoral hernia, sometimes looks like a lump of fat or lipoma. It is preperitoneal fat, dissect it slowly and you will find glistening peritoneum. Incise it and you will get lobulated omentum.
- If neck of femoral hernia is torn then gently pull it and release more peritoneum and make a new neck.
- If the content of femoral hernia sac cannot be reduced then try to dilate the femoral ring by passing little finger around the neck of the sac or dilate with the tip of blunt artery forceps.
- If it fails, cut the lacunar ligament in superomedial direction. Keep in mind the occasional (20%) presence of abnormal obturator artery. Lacunar ligament is cut with the help of hernia director and bistourey (it is a long strait narrow knife, one site is blunt and one site is sharp) to protect intestinal loops.
- If hernia sac contents are ovary and fallopian tube and gangrenous then excise, and if viable then push inside.
- If you are following low approach for femoral hernia and find a gangrenous bowel then open by high approach and close the low approach wound, and resect the bowel loop with anastomosis.

Fig. 22.2A & B. Femoral hernia sometime is like a lump of fat or lipoma, way to deal with it.

> ### NOTE
> *If the abnormal obturator artery is cut by chance then open through inguinal incision. Incise fascia transversalis and see the bleeding artery in preperitoneal space, catch it and ligate.*

DIFFICULTIES IN UMBILICAL AND PARAUMBILICAL HERNIAS REPAIR (Fig. 22.3)

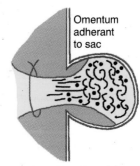

- Sometime in umbilical hernia, a large mass of omentum is adherent with sac. If blood vessels and bowel are safe then excise the mass without hesitation. If it cannot be excised due to risk of injury to intestine then let a piece of sac remain within.
- If ometum in sac is found necrotised then transfix it and excise it.

Fig. 22.3. Omentum adherent to fundus of sac.

> ### KEY POINT
> *If the mesh covers hernia prone area medially, laterally and superiorly and with good anchor line inferiorly, then results are good.*

DIFFICULTIES IN LAPAROSCOPIC REPAIR

- Urinary bladder must be emptied before the laparoscopic repair of hernia as full bladder can cause difficulty in repair and may lead to injury to bladder.

- The patient should be put in 10% Trendelenberg position, which pushes the bowel loops up and can prevent injury to the bowel.
- In TEP repair if gas escapes to peritoneal cavity due to dent in peritoneum, then pass veress needle in left upper quadrant of peritoneal cavity and remove gas to avoid interference with the dissection.
- In TEP repair if dent in peritoneum is big then either do TAPP or convert to open repair.
- In TEP repair if in the TEP repair, the indirect hernia sac is big and difficult to withdraw then either do TAPP or convert to open repair.
- If creation of pneumoperitoneum is done before inserting the first trocar then it allows easy and safe introduction of first trocar.
- If peritoneum is punctured during laparoscopic operation, then repair of peritoneum is a must either during or after the end of surgery.
- To avoid difficulties and complications identify the these landmarks before proceeding for further dissection: (i) Pubic bone; (ii) Cooper's ligament; (iii) Inferior epigastric vessels.
- Presence of very large hernia may require an additional 5 mm trocar.
- Lipoma must always be removed.
- In case of very large scrotal hernia, a scrotal incision is given to help excision of sac.[4]

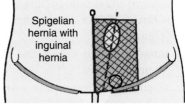

Fig. 22.4. Big mesh is applied when Spigelian hernia is found with inguinal hernia.

- Sometimes deep inguinal ring and femoral ring incision is required to reduce a large hernia.
- Post-operative seroma formation can be minimized by careful and limited dissection and proper haemostasis.
- Before finishing the procedure always do a thorough inspection to check the followings:
  - Mesh is in place.
  - Mesh is stuck firmly.
  - Look for another hernia on the same side or on the other side.
  - Look for vascular or visceral injury.
- Biological meshes are used even in contaminated fields.[20-23]
- In case of an associated Spigelian hernia use a mesh bigger than the mesh used for inguinal hernia (Fig. 22.4) so that it can well cover MPO of Fruchaud as well as Spigelian hernia site.
- Seroma is commonly formed after extensive dissection, so use abdominal binder post-operatively which causes significant reduction.[6]
- Carbondioxide burden in patients of chronic pulmonary obstructive disease and poor cardiac reserve may prove problematic so open approach and watchful waiting is better in such patients.[7]
- Bowel injury incidence is almost same in both laparoscopic and open approach in incisional hernia[8,9] but wound complications are lower in laparoscopic approach.[10]
- Mesh migration and fistula formation are avoided by "second generation" or barrier meshes.[11] as "third generation" meshes or biological meshes are used in contaminated and infected fields.[12-15]
- Intraabdominal patients is measured by some worker up to 27 N/cm. Marlex has a tensile strength of 59 N/cm, Atrium mesh 56 N/cm, Vipro (light weight mesh) 16 N/cm.[16-19]

KEY POINT

In TEP repair, the camera should be placed such that it should not cause pressure on peritoneum as it may penetrate peritoneal cavity.

REFERENCES

1. **Kirk RM.**, (2000). General surgical operation, 8th edition, p. 122.
2. **Brunicardi, FC.**, (2005). Schwartz's principles of surgery, 8th edition, p. 1369.
3. **Smegerg, SGG Bromme AEA,** *et al.* (1984) Ligation of hernia sac? *Surg. Cl. N Am.*, 64: 299.
4. **Dulucq JL.**, (2005). Tips and techniques in laparoscopic surgery, pp. 171–182.
5. **Lilly MC, Arregui ME.**, (2002). Lipomas of cord and round ligament, *Ann. Surg.*, 235: 586.
6. **LeBlanc KA.** (2004). Laparoscopic incisional and ventral herniarepair: complications–how to avoid and handle. *Hernia*; 8: 323–31.
7. **Henny CP, Hofland J.** (2005). Laparoscopic surgery: pitfalls due to anesthesia, positioning, and pneumoperitoneum. *Surg Endosc*; 19:1163–71.
8. **Itani KMF, Neumayer L,** *et al.* (2004). Repair of ventral incisional hernia: design of a randomized trial to compare open & laparoscopic surgical techniques. *Am J Surg.;* 188: 22S–9S.
9. **Feldman LS, Wexler MJ, Fraser SA.** (2007). Laparoscopic hernia repair. What's new ACS surgery. Available at: http://www.medscape.com/viewarticle/506634. Accessed November, 2007.
10. **Olmi S, Scaini A, Cesana GC,** *et al.* (2001). Laparoscopic versus open incisional hernia repair. *Surg Endosc;* 21:555–9.
11. **Ott V, Groebli Y, Schneider R.** (2005). Later intestinal fistula formation after incisional hernia using intraperitoneal mesh. *Hernia*; 9(1): 103–4.
12. **Helton WS, Fisichella PM, Berger R,** *et al.* Short-term outcomes with small intestinal submucosa for ventral abdominal hernia. Arch Surg.: 140(6): 549–60 [discussion: 560–2].
13. **Catena F, Ansaloni L, Gazzotti F,** *et al.* (2007). Use of procine dermal collagen graft (Permacol) for hernia repair in contaminated fields. Hernia: 22(1): 57–60.
14. **Schuster R, Singh J,** *et al.* (2006). The use of acellular dermal matrix for contaimined abdominal wall defects: Wound status predicts success. *Am J Surg.*; 192(5): 594–7.
15. **Diaz JJ Jr, Guy J, Berkes MB,** *et al.* (2006). Acellular dermal allograft for ventral hernia repair in the compromised surgical field. *Am Surg.*; 72(12): 1181–7 [discussion: 11887–8]
16. **Cobb WS, Burns JM, Kercher KW,** *et al.* (2005). Normal intraabdominal pressure in healthy adults. *J Surg Res.* 129(2):231–5.
17. **Welty G, Klinge U, Klosterhalfen B,** *et al.* (2001). Functional impairment and complaints following incisional hernia repair with different polypropylene meshes. *Hernia*; 5(3): 113–8.
18. **Binnebosel M, Rosch R, Junge K,** *et al.* (2007). Biomechanical analyses of overlap and mesh dislocation in an incisional hernia model in vitro. *Surgery*; 142(3): 365–71.
19. **Cobb WS, Burns JM, Peindl RD,** *et al.* (2006). Textile analysis of heavy weight, mid-weight, and light weight polypropylene mesh in a porcine ventral model. *J. Surg. Res.*; 136(1): 1–7.
20. **Kim H, Bruen K, Vargo D.** (2006) Acellular Dermal matrix in the management of high-risk abdominal wall defects. *Am. J. Surg.*; 192(6): 705–9.
21. **Patton JH Jr, Berry S, Kralovich KA.** (2007) Use of human acellular dermal matrix in complex and contaminated abdominal wall reconstructions. *Am. J. Surg.*; 193(3): 360–3 [discussion: 3].
22. **Ansaloni L, Catena F, Gagliardi S.,** *et al.* (2007) Hernia repair with porcine small-intestinal submucosa. *Hernia*; 11(4): 321–6.
23. **Gagliardi S, Ansaloni L, Catena F,** *et al.* (2007) Hernioplasty with Surgisis Inguinal Hernia Matrix (IHM) trade mark. *Surg Technol Int*; 16:128–33.

23 Important Things to Remember

"As long as the abdomen is open you control it. If closed it controls you."
— Moshe Schein
"Somebody's leak is a curiosity – one's own leak is a calamity."
— Moshe Schein
"Complications are made in operation theatre."
— Anonymous

- The most common hernia in the human body is inguinal hernia.
- Most common inguinal hernia is on the right side.
- Types of indirect inguinal hernia:
  - Bubuocele, limited to inguinal canal.
  - Funicular, limited to spermatic cord and separated from testis.
  - Complete (inguinoscrotal), involving inguinal region and scrotum.
- Direct inguinal hernia is common in old age.
- Direct inguinal hernia occurs in 35% of all inguinal hernias.
- Direct inguinal hernia is always acquired.
- Direct inguinal hernia never occurs in females.
- Hernia sac lies posteromedial to the spermatic cord in direct inguinal hernia whereas it lies anterolateral to spermatic cord in indirect inguinal hernia.
- Most common hernia to strangulate is femoral hernia, due to its narrow neck.
- Inguinal hernia is 10 times more common than femoral hernia.
- Femoral hernia is 10 times more likely to strangulate than inguinal hernia.
- Rare hernia to strangulate is direct inguinal hernia due to its wide neck or no neck.
- In order of frequency, the constricting agents in inguinal hernia are:
  - Neck of the sac
  - Deep inguinal ring
  - External inguinal ring
  - Adhesions within the sac
- Epiplocele contains omentum.
- Enterocele contains small intestine but occasionally may contain colon.
- Littre's hernia contains Meckel's diverticulum.
- Richter's hernia contains a part of circumference of intestine.
- Incarcerated hernia is synonymous with obstructed hernia. It is an irreducible hernia containing intestine obstructed with faeces.
- Maydl's hernia contains loops of intestine present in the sac in form of "W".
- In sliding hernia, posterior peritoneum slides down and forms the posterior wall of hernia sac associated with caecum on the right side and sigmoid colon on left side.

- In interstitial hernia, the sac lies between different layers of anterior abdominal wall. Interstitial hernia cannot develop easily between internal oblique and transversus abdominis muscles due to formation of conjoint tendon (Fig. 23.1).

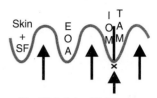

- de Laugier's femoral hernia develops through Gimbernat's ligament.
- In Cloquet's femoral hernia, the sac lies deep to fascia covering pectineus muscle.

Fig. 23.1. Interstitial hernia cannot develop between internal oblique and transversus abdominis muscles.

- Spigelian hernia occurs at arcuate line and under the internal oblique muscle.
- Obturator hernia occurs six times more in females than males.
- In infants, deep and superficial inguinal rings are superimposed.
- Inguinal canal in males transmits spermatic cord, ilioinguinal nerve and genital branch of genitofemoral nerve. In females, it transmits round ligament of uterus, ilio-inguinal nerve and genital branch of genitofemoral nerve.
- Early recurrence occurs due to technical reasons and late recurrence occurs due to tissue failure.
- Most of the incisional hernias start in the immediate post-operative period due to partial disruption of deeper layers in the wound.
- Recurrence rate of incisional hernia after open repair is 30-40% and after laparoscopic repair is 10%.
- In direct inguinal hernia the dissection should cross the midline in laparoscopic repair to put the mesh properly without folding to avoid recurrence.
- Mesh must be examined before finishing the laparoscopic repair of inguinal hernia to see that there is no folding of mesh which may lead to recurrence.

DIAGNOSTIC SIGNS OF UNCOMPLICATED INGUINAL HERNIA

- Hernia has two characteristic signs:
  - Expansile impulse on coughing
  - Reducibility
- Common causes of hernia are:
  - Straining on micturition
  - Chronic constipation
  - Chronic cough
  - Obesity
- Hernia without neck are:
  - Direct inguinal hernia
  - Incisional hernia
- The complete diagnosis of inguinal hernia is done in following manner:
  - Right sided, indirect, incomplete, uncomplicated, inguinal enterocele.
- Impulse on coughing is an important sign of a hernia. Impulse on coughing is absent in the following hernias:
  - Strangulated hernia
  - Obstructed hernia
  - Irreducible hernia

NATURAL HISTORY OF HERNIA

History of one of the common causes
↓
Reducible hernia
↓
Irreducible hernia
↓
Obstructed hernia
↓
Strangulated hernia

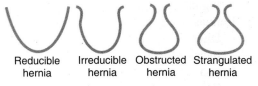

| Reducible hernia | Irreducible hernia | Obstructed hernia | Strangulated hernia |

Fig. 23.2. Natural history of hernia.

- Stranulgation occurs commonly in a narrow-necked hernia.
- Strangulated hernia requires urgent surgery.

> *Risk factors in an adult patient with groin hernia*
>
> - Old age
> - Short duration
> - Female hernia
> - Co-existing medical disease[1]
>
> *Risk factors in a child with groin hernia*
>
> - Very young patient
> - Male sex
> - Short duration
> - Right-sided hernia[2]

- A Richter's hernia is commonly seen in:
  - Femoral hernia
  - Obturator hernia
- Common irreducible hernias are:
  - Femoral hernia
  - Umbilical hernia
- Clinical features of acute intestinal obstruction are:
  - Pain in abdomen
  - Vomiting
  - Abdominal distension
  - Absolute constipation
- Strangulated hernia without intestinal obstruction (Fig. 23.3) are:
  - Omentocele
  - Richter's hernia
  - Littre's hernia

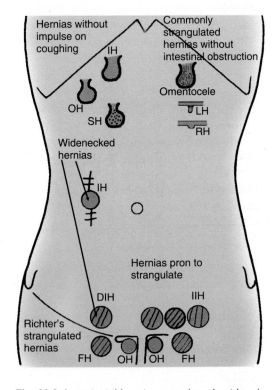

Fig. 23.3. Important things to remember about hernias.
IH = Irreducible hernia, SH = Strangularted hernia,
RH = Richters hernia

- Hernia prone to strangulate are:
  - Femoral hernia
  - Obturator hernia
  - Inguinal hernia
- Hernias without neck or the hernias with very wide neck are:
  - Direct hernia
  - Incisional hernia
- Hernia without a sac is:
  - Epigastric hernia
- Male to female ratio of inguinal hernia is 10 : 1.
- Lifetime prevalence is 25% in men and 2% in females.
- Two-thirds of inguinal hernia are indirect inguinal hernia.
- Two-thirds of recurrent hernia are direct inguinal hernia.
- Incidence of incarceration is 10% in case of inguinal hernia.
- Recurrence rate is less than 1%.
- Laparoscopic repair of inguinal hernia is best for:
  - Recurrent hernia
  - Bilateral hernia
  - If laparoscopy is done for any other cause
  - Obese patient
  - Individual with a unilateral hernia and for whom a rapid recovery is critical, i.e. athletes and labourers.
- Open tension-free repair of inguinal hernia is best for uncomplicated primary unilateral inguinal hernia.
- Prosthetic mesh must be large enough to cover MPO properly, atleast 2 cm beyond pubic tubercle and all other sides to avoid recurrence.[3]
  - Femoral hernia is very much prone to strangulation.
- A femoral hernia is rare in:
  - Males.
  - Nulliparous women.
- An inguinal hernia can be differentiated from a femoral hernia by finding the relation of neck of the sac to the medial part of inguinal ligament and pubic tubercle. The neck of the sac in inguinal hernia is medial and above pubic tubercle while in femoral hernia it is lateral and below.

GPRVS is suitable for:

- Elderly patients with bilateral hernia
- Recurrent hernia
- Large hernia
- Hernia associated with collagen disorder

- Recurrence occurs more rapidly than initial hernia development.[7]
- Quantitative experience after complition of residency gives confidence in herniorraphies[8,9]
- Laparoscopic herniorraphy has advantages over open repair ie low rate of infection, short hospital stay, less post operative pain, ileus and other complications.[10-14]

MESH HERNIOPLASTY

- Light weight macroporous polypropylene mesh is preferred in tension-free repair.
- The use of tacks and staples should be minimized.
- Mesh should cover at least 2 cm medial to pubic tubercle and more than 4 cm lateral to deep inguinal ring.
- The mesh must be lax after fixation and not tight like a tent.
- ePTFE mesh is preferred in intraperitneal repair or a macroporous PPM mesh. The antiadhesion layer is used to avoid viseral adhesions.
- Extraperitoneal retromuscular light weight PPM is preferred for ventral hernia repair.
- Light weight macroporous mesh should be anchored with absorbable sutures.
- The use of biological mesh is satisfying in the presence of infection.[4,5,6]

KEY POINT

Weakness of transversalis fascia and aponeurosis is the major cause of groin hernias.

REFERENCES

1. **Brunicardi FC.**, (2005). Schwartz's principles of surgery, 8th edition, p. 1355.
2. **Rai S, Chandra SS, Smile SR.**, (1998). A study of risk of strangulation and obstruction in groin hernia. *Aust. NZ J. Surg.*, 68: 650.
3. **Kirk RM.**, (2000). General surgical operations, 4th edition, p. 126.
4. **Bendavid R.**, (2004). The unified theory of hernia formation. Hernia, 8: 171.
5. **Fitzgibbons RJ, Greenburg AG, Eds.**, (2002). Nyhus and Condon's hernia, 5th edition Philadelphia: Lippincott Williams & Wilkins.
6. **Schumpelick V, Nyhus LM, Eds.**, (2004). Meshes: benefits and risks. Heidelberg: Springer-Verlag.
7. **Park AE, Roth JS, Kavic SM.** (2006). Abdominal wall hernia. *Curr Probl Surg.*; 43:321–75.
8. **Park A, Kavic SM, Lee TH,** *et al.* (2007). Minimally invasive surgery: the evolution of fellowship. *Surgery*; 142: 505–13.
9. **Tichansky DS, Taddeucci RJ, Harper J,** *et al.* (2007). Minimally invasive surgery fellows would perform a wider variety of cases in their "ideal" fellowship. Surg. Endosc [serial online]. Available at: http://www.springerlink.com/content/0466p26276411390/.
10. **Earle D, Seymour N, Fellinger E,** *et al.* (2006). Laparoscopic versus open incisional hernia repair. A single-institution analysis of hospital resource utilization for 884 consecutive cases. *Surg. Endosc.*; 20:71–5.
11. **Beldi G, Ipaktchi R, Wagner M,** *et al.* (2006). Laparoscopic ventral hernia repair is safe and cost effective. *Surg Endosc.* 20:92–5.
12. **Sains PS, Tilney HS, Purkayashtha S,** *et al.* (2006). Outcomes following laparoscopic versus open repair of incisional hernia. *World J. Surg.*, 30: 2556-64.
13. **Stickel M, Rentsch M, Clevert D-A,** *et al.* (2007). Laparoscopic mesh repair of incisional hernia: an alternative to the conventional open repair? *Hernia*; 11:217–22.
14. **Halm JA, de Wall LL, Steyerberg EW,** *et al.* (2007). Intraperitoneal polypropylene mesh hernia repair complicates subsequent abdominal surgery. *World J Surg;* 31: 423–9.

24 Recent Advances and Modern Trends in Hernia Surgery

"Medical research is only justified if there is a reasonable likelihood that the populations in which the research is carried out stand to benefit from the result of the research."
— **World Medical Association, Declaration Of Helsinki, 2000**

> Recently molecular biological investigations have proven the theory of disturbed composition of the extracellular matrix in patients with recurrent hernia. In particular, there is a decreased ratio of collagens of types I and III.[1]

• Hernia repair surgery has changed a lot during the last two decades.

GASLESS LAPAROSCOPY (Fig. 24.1)

• In 1991, a Japanese team led by Nagai performed Laparoscopic Cholecystectomy without pneumoperitoneum.[2]
• In this technique, gas insufflation is not used, instead the abdominal wall is lifted up with suspension device. The absence of carbon insufflation helps in the following ways:
    – It reduces the risks and complications of insufflation. This increases the safety of laparoscopic surgery.
    – It increases the indications of laparoscopic surgery by performing more complicated procedures.
    – Visualization is uninterrupted due to the absence of gas leaks and gas reduction due to suction application.

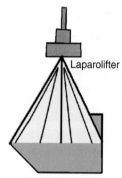

Laparolifter

Fig. 24.1. Gasless laparoscopy.

High Frequency Ultrasonography and Colour Doppler Study

• It is nowadays an important method of investigation of hernia. It helps in diagnosing an occult contralateral inguinal hernia in children and infants. It can easily and accurately detect an occult inguinal hernia before the surgery.

Prosthesis

• **Fibrin glue**
    – It is nowadays used by some workers[3] for prosthetic mesh and plug fixation to avoid migration of mesh, recurrence, inguinodynia and post-operative morbidity.

- **Light weight self-gripping meshes**
  - Some surgeons are using light weight self-gripping meshes with absorbable properties to reduce post-operative complications.[4 & 5]
- **Macroporous compound meshes**
  - The new macroporous compound meshes present both the successful reduction of the overall foreign body amount and the preservation of mesh elasticity after the scar tissue ingrowth, due to very limited shrinking and reduced bridging effect.[6]

PEER (PERCUTANEOUS ENDOSCOPIC EXTERNAL-RING REPAIR) HERNIOPLASTY[7]

This procedure is in early evaluation stages, but results are promising. An incision of 2.5 cm is made over external inguinal ring. After cutting the external oblique aponeurosis from external inguinal ring, index finger is inserted into the inguinal canal. Later on the finger is replaced by the endoscopic inguinal canal retractor, which keeps a 30 degree 5 mm telescope.

It is a repair with minimum pain done under local anaesthesia.

Laparoscopic and Open Hernia Repair

- TEP or TAPP – The TEP technique is getting more and more popular as compared to TAPP due to less complications.
- Metaanalysis of randomized controlled trials has shown that:
  - Laparoscopic repair of inguinal hernia has post-operative discomfort and a fast return to normal activity than open mesh repair.
  - Laparoscopic repair of inguinal hernia carries risk of serious bowel, bladder or vascular injuries and is more difficult to learn than open repair.

> - NICE (National Institute of Clinical Excellence) guidelines recommend that laparoscopic hernia repair should be reserved for recurrent and bilateral inguinal hernia. Open tension-free repair is the procedure of choice for primary unilateral inguinal hernia.

ROBOTIC HERNIA SURGERY (Fig. 24.2)

Davies in 2000 stated "Surgical robot is powered, computer controlled manipulator with artificial sensing that can be reprogrammed to move and position tools to carry out a wide range of surgical tasks."

Today surgery is under transformation due to advancing technology.

The word "Robot" derives from the Czech word "*Roboto*" meaning "Compulsory labor". The work was first time used by Karel Capek, a Czech writer. Robot is nowadays used maximum in minimal invasive surgery including laparoscopic surgery in medical field. It is a state of the art in medical field.[7]

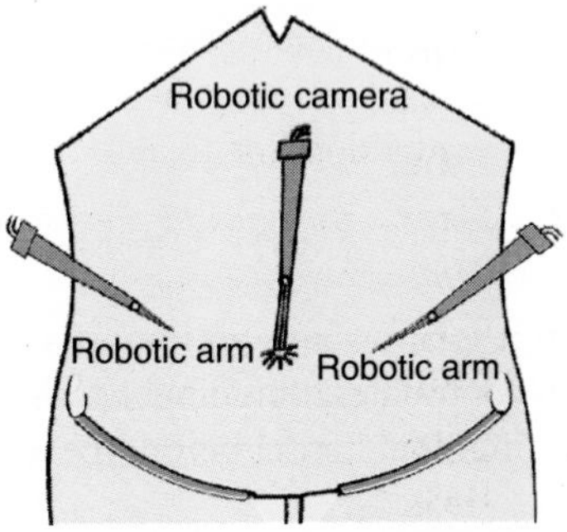

Fig. 24.2. Robotic hernia surgery.

Professor Noel Sharkey[8] states, "today there are 40,000 professionals and 3.5 million personal robots, in use. The most interesting are the surgical robots, and this segment is growing very rapidly specially for use in by passe surgery and removal of prostate. The hernia is not far behind, it will catch with other surgical procedures."

Use of Robotic Surgery

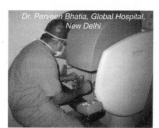

Fig. 24.3. da Vinci robotic machine.

Presently, the robotic surgery is being used in the following areas:
*   Image-guided procedures like biopsy and brain surgery.
*   Computer-assisted laparoscopic surgery.
*   Robotic Tele surgery – It is a Master-Slave Unit. Surgeon controls the procedure from master unit and robotic arm (slave unit) controls movement of instruments.
*   True robotic surgery is used in orthopedics.
*   Robotic surgery is used in cardiac, urologic and paediatric surgeries.
*   Robotic repair of indirect inguinal hernia is started by some herniologists. Long term follow-up is required to prove its worth in hernia surgery.

Advantages of Robotic Surgery (Fig. 24.3)

*   Wrist articulation – additional wrist movement can enhance surgical capability.
*   Hand-held instrument shaking is eliminated.
*   Surgeon has complete control of instrument.
*   Three-dimensional visual field created by robotic surgery camera gives better image.

Shortcomings of Robotic Surgery

*   At present, the size of robot and machine is big. Nanotechnology is helping to miniature robots.
*   No tactile feedback.
*   Camera is static and cannot be moved from port to port.

KEY POINT

Surgical research benefits everybody. It advances the medicine, the patient has better chance of cure and surgeon keeps awareness.

REFERENCES

1. **Jansen PL, Merten Pr. P, Klinge U, Schumpelick V.**, (2004). The biology of hernia formation. *Surgery*, 136: 1–4.
2. **Edmund KM, and Claude HO Jr., TSO.**, (2007). The sages manual, 2nd edition, p. 33.
3. **Campanelli G,** *et al.,* (2006). A modified Lichtenstein hernia repair using fibrin glue, *Journal of Minimum Access Surgery*, **2**, 3, 129–133.
4. **Cucshieri A,** *et al.,* (2002). Essential Surgical Practice, 4th edition, p. 176.
5. **Philippe Chastan.**, (2006). Tension-free open inguinal hernia repair using an innovative self-gripping semi-resolvable mesh, *Journal of Minimal Access Surgery*, **2**, 3, 139.
6. **Basoglu M, Yildirgam MI, Yilmaz I, Balik A, Celebi F, Atamanalp SS,** *et al.,* (2004). Late complications of incisional hernias following prosthetic mesh repair. *Acta Chir. Belog.*, 104: 425.
7. **Andreas Kirkopolus,** *et al.,* (2007). Robotics in laparoscopic and thoracoscopic surgery, *The SAGES Manual*, 2nd edition, 95–103.
8. **Noel S.**, (2008). Robots are dumb machines and cannot think for themselves, Economic Times, New Delhi, 15 March, p. 22.

25 Arguments, Controversies and Discussions in Hernia Surgery

The surgical community is divided into opponents and supporters of laparoscopic hernia surgery. Following controversies are important in today's inguinal hernia repair (Fig. 25.1):

* Laparoscopic or open tension-free hernia repair
* TAPP or TEP
* Mesh fixation or free mesh
* Contralateral area should be operated or not
* Metachronous hernia
* Femoral hernia occurring after inguinal hernia repair
* Learning curve for the beginner

Schumpelick feels that study at 14th Veterans Affairs Medical Centers (randomized 2000 patients, laparoscopic hernia repair or Lichtenstein open tension-free mesh repair for primary or first time recurrent inguinal hernias) is an eye opener as it showed, based on the results, open Lichtenstein's repair was superior to laparoscopic repair.[2]

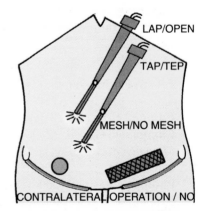

Fig. 25.1. Main areas of controversies.

(I) LAPAROSCOPIC OR OPEN HERNIA REPAIR

* Various large randomized controlled trials have confirmed that laparoscopic hernia repair has the following advantages:
  – Less painful

– Faster recovery
– Lower recurrence rate in recurrent hernia rapair
- Laparoscopic hernia repair has the following disadvantages:
  – More costly
  – Longer operation period
  – Serious complications
  – Longer learning curve
- Several studies have shown the benefits of laparoscopic herniorrhaphy over open tension-free mesh repairs.[3]

Keeping all these advantages and disadvantages in mind most of surgeons agree to the following criteria:
- Laparoscopic inguinal hernia repair is for:
  – Recurrent hernia
  – Bilateral hernia
  – Hernia repair if some other laparoscopic surgery is to be done
- Open tension-free hernia repair is for:
  – Uncomplicated unilateral reducible hernia

- Lichtenstein claims that laparoscopic hernia repair cannot equal the safety, simplicity, and cost-effectiveness of open tension-free hernioplasty, nor can it surpass its post-operative durability.[4]
- Rutkow blames the instrument manufacturers for undue publicity of laparoscopic technique over open hernia repair by "socio-economic tyranny of surgical technology".[5]
- The ultimate indicator of success of a hernia surgeon is rate of recurrence.[6]

(II) TAPP OR TEP

TEP should be used in those patients who have no previous lower abdominal peritoneal operation and TAPP should be preferred in those patients[7] who have undergone previous lower abdominal peritoneal operation.

Advantages of TEP

- Dissection is easy and safe.
- It prevents bowel and vascular injuries.
- No intraperitoneal adhesion.

Disadvantages of TEP

- Visualization of anatomical landmarks is difficult.
- If there is a peritoneal tear then it has to be converted to TAPP or open.

(III) MESH FIXATION OR FREE MESH

According to the Pascals hydrostatic principle, "pressure of a fluid is evenly distributed across the wall of its container". Intra-abdominal pressure will be evenly distributed across a mesh placed between the high pressure region (intra-abdominal), and the hernia orifice. Distribution of intra-abdominal pressure over a wide area should be adequate to hold the mesh in place. This principle has led some to advocate the placement of mesh without fixation by staples or tacks in order to lessen the risk of nerve injury.[8]

Debate is on that mesh fixation may lead to neuralgia or chronic pain and on the other side non-fixation of mesh leads to mesh migration, mesh shrinkage and rolling which lead to recurrence.[9]

To avoid the above controversy, it is safe to:
- Use a big mesh (15 cm × 12 cm) size.
- Carefully do fixation of mesh. Do not use may staples or tacks.

(IV) CONTRALATERAL HERNIA

Contralateral Hernia should be Operated Routinely or Not in Children.[10, 11] The contralateral side is screened with high resolution ultrasound to diagnose hernia on the other side. If patency is found in processus vaginalis and there is a concealed hernia then only contralateral side is operated.
- Processus vaginalis is patent in 100% cases within one week after birth.
- Processus vaginalis is patent, 1 week to 2 years of age in 25% cases.
- All patients of patent processus vaginalis do not develop hernia.
- 20% cases develop hernia on contralateral side.

Diagnosis of Contralateral Inguinal Hernia

It can be accurately done by:
- High frequency ultrasonography
- Diagnostic laparoscopy
- Herniography

Contralateral inguinal hernia exploration in children with unilateral inguinal hernia is now taken differently in the evidence-based medicine era. Exploration should be done if it is proved that the other side has an occult hernia.

If the contralateral inguinal hernia is diagnosed at the time or before herniorrhaphy for unilateral hernia repair then, bilateral surgery can be done at the same time. It has the following advantages:
- It avoids second surgery.
- It avoids unnecessary TEP repair on contralateral side. Some surgeons are concerned about unnecessary TEP repair of contralateral side as only 20% will get hernia on contralateral side in their lifetime.

(V) METACHRONOUS INGUINAL HERNIA

The inguinal hernia which occurs at different times and not simultaneously in bilateral inguinal hernia is called metachronous inguinal hernia. Nowadays, the metachronous inguinal hernia is operated in two phases, wait till the hernia develops.

(VI) FEMORAL HERNIA OCCURRING AFTER INGUINAL OPERATION[12]

- When inguinal hernia operation involves the approximation of transversalis fascia and conjoint tendon to inguinal ligament then there is tension on fascia transversalis and inguinal ligament is also pulled up and this causes weakness of the tissues of femoral canal leading to femoral hernia.

- The femoral hernia was present earlier and was missed during first operation.
- If during inguinal hernia operation, the preperitoneal space is explored, then a cone-shaped defect (femoral cone) results over femoral ring and preperitoneal fat enters during rise of intra-abdominal pressure and femoral hernia results.

(VII) LEARNING CURVE FOR BEGINNERS

The learning curve is not technique oriented, but it is individual oriented, as different individuals have different skills and devotion to learn. Some require 50 operations as cut-off level while others require 250 operations. Neumayer[13] says that learning curve for laparoscopic hernia repair may be as high as 250 operations which is quite a big number.

- In incisional hernia sublay mesh is most physiological method, most effective and most advantageous (15-17).
- Many patient related risk factors have been implicated in the development of incisional hernias but no single factor is so regularly associated that it may be declared as serving a truely etiological role (18-21).
- Widening defect in incisional hernia causes abdominal wall physiology derangements so surgical approaches also shifted from primary suture repair to mesh repairs (22-27).
- Recurrent ventral incisional hernia repair is a unique and difficult problem. Therefore various techniques were developed. Understanding and restoration of structural and functional anatomy is necessary for successful repair. (28-30).

NOTE

Laparoscopic hernia repair can be performed successfully in clinical practice even by surgeons in training. Precondition for the success is a strictly standardized operation technique and a well-structured evaluation programme.[14]

KEY POINT

"The strategy of repair of inguinal hernia depends upon circumstances, location of hernia, size of hernia, age of the patient, general condition of the patient and recurrence status."

REFERENCES

1. **Matt Ritter E,** *et al.,* Inguinal hernia repair, controversies in laparoscopic surgery, p. 401.
2. **Schumpelick V, Klinge U.,** (2003). Prosthetic implants for hernia repair, *BJS.,* 90:1457–1458.
3. **Mc Cormack K, Scott N, GOP, Ross S, Grant A.,** (2003). EU hernia trialists collaboration laparoscopic technique versus open technique for inguinal hernia repair. *Cochrane Database, Syst. Rev.,* 1: CD001785.
4. **Lichtenstein IL, Shulman AG, Amid PK.,** (1991). Lap hernioplasty, *Arch. Surg.,* 126: 1449.
5. **Rutkow IM.,** (1992). Laparoscopic hernia repair: The socioeconomic tyranny of surgical technology, *Arch. Surg.,* 127: 1271.
6. **Brooks DC.,** (1998). Minimal invasive surgery, p. 83–84.
7. **Ahmad Assalia** *et al.,* (2006). Controversies in laparoscopic surgery, p. 406–407.

8. **Rattner D, NOORD MV.**, (2007). Totally extraperitoneal inguinal hernia repair, Mastery of surgery, 5th edition, Lippincott Williams & Wilkins, pp. 1905–1911.

9. **Hume R, Bour J.**, (1996). Mesh migration following laparoscopic inguinal hernia repair. *J. Laparoscop. Surg.*, 6: 333–335.

10. **Chen KC, Chu CC, Chou Ty**, *et al.*, (1999). Ultrasonography for inguinal hernias in boys *J. Pedtr. Surg.*, 34: 1890.

11. **Erez I, Rathause V,** *et al.*, (2002). Preoperative ultrasound and intra-operative findings of inguinal hernias in children: A prospective study of 642 children, *J. Paed. Surg.*, 37: 865.

12. **Bendavid R.**, (2002). Femoral pseudo-hernia, *Hernia* 6: 141.

13. **Neumeyer L, Giobbie–Hurder A, Jonasson O, Fitzgibbons R, Dullop D, Gibbs D, Reda D, Henderson W.**, (2004). Open mesh versus laparoscopic mesh repair of inguinal hernia. *N. Engl. J. Med.*, 350: 1819–1827.

14. **Bittner R, Leibl B, Jager C, Kraft B, Ulrich M, Schwartz J.**, (2006). TAPP-stuttgart technique and result of a large single center series, *J. Min. Acce. Surg.*, **2**, 155–159.

15. **Novitsky YW, Porter JR, Ruicho ZC,** *et al.* (2006) Open preperitoneal retrofascial mesh repair for multiply recurrent ventral incisional hernias. *J Am Coll surg.*; 203(3): 283–9.

16. **Lomanto D, Iyer SG, Shabbir A,** *et al.* (2006) Laparoscopic versus open ventral hernia mesh repair: a prospective study. *Surg Endosc*; 20(7): 1030–5.

17. **Kurzer M, Kark A, Selouk S,** *et al.* (2008). Open mesh repair of incisional hernia using a sublay technique: long-term follow-up. *World J Surg.* 32(1): 31–6.

18. **Millikan KW.** (2003). Incisional hernia repair. *Surg Clin North Am.* 83: 1223-34.

19. **Sorenson LT,** *et al.* (2005). Smoking is a risk factor for incisional hernia. *Arch Surg.*; 140(2): 119–23.

20. **Reffetto JD, Cheung Y, Fisher JB,** *et al.* (2003). Incision and abdominal wall hernias in patients with aneurysm or occlusive aortic disease. *J Vasc Surg.*; 37: 1150–4.

21. **Condon RE.** Ventral abdominal hernia. (2001) In: Baker RJ, Fischer JE, editors. Mastery of surgery. 4th edition. Philadelphia: Lippincott Williams & Wilkins.

22. **Grevious MA, Cohen M, Shah SR,** (2006). Structural and functional anatomy of the abdominal wall. *Clin Plast Surg.*; 33: 169–79.

23. **Nguyen V, Shestak KC.** (2006) Separation of anatomic components method of abdominal wall reconstruction: clinical outcome analysis and an update of surgical modifications using the technique. *Clin Plat Surg.*; 33:247–57.

24. **Sauerland S, Schmedt CG, Lein S,** *et al.* (2005). Primary incisional hernia repair with or without polypropylene mesh: a report on 384 patients. *Lang. Arch Surg.*; 33: 247–57.

25. **Al-Salamah SM, Hussain MI, Khalid K,** *et al.* (2006). Suture vs mesh repair for incisional hernia Saudi *Med J.* 27(5): 652–6.

26. **Grevious MA, Cohen M,** *et al.* (1999). Incisional hernia. *J Am Coll Surg*; 189(6): 635–7.

27. **Cobb WS, Kercher KW, Heniford BT.** (2005). The argument for lightweight polypropylene mesh in hernia repair. *Surg. Innov* 12(1): T1–7.

28. **Butler CE, Langstein HN, Kornowitz SJ. Pelvic,** (2005). Abdominal, and chest wall reconstruction with Alloderm in patients at increased risk for mesh-related complications. *Plast Reconstr. Surg.* 116:1263–75.

29. **Espinosa-de-los-Monteros A, de la torre JI, Marrero I,** *et al.* (2007). Utilization of human cadaveric acellular dermis for abdominal hernia reconstruction. *Ann Plast Surg.*; 58: 264–7.

26 Surgical Hernia Audit and Hernia Registers

"The recognition of the existing problem is the first step in its solution"
— **M. Fischer**

"Surgery without audit is like playing cricket without keeping the score"
— **H. B. Devlin**
Surgeon, The North Tees
General Hospitals, England

Clinical audits are the best source of feedback. So far, in India the clinical audit for hernia is not a common thing. If we wish to improve upon the incidence of recurrence, post-operative discomforts and complications, we have to streamline the post-operative feedback in the name of clinical audit and registers.

AUDIT

Audit is a fundamental part of surgical practice in UK.[1] Local audit can be improved by applying the guidelines given by national audit and projects etc.[2]

"Clinically-led initiative which seeks to improve the quality and outcome of patient care through structured peer review, whereby clinicians examine their practice and results against acquired standards and modify their practice where indicated.[3]"

REGISTER

"It is the prospective recording of information concerning diagnosis and operations of invidiual patient followup-over time beyond the mere coding according to official classifications.[4]"

AIMS (Fig. 26.1)

- To increase the post-operative care of hernia patients.
- To increase the QOL (quality of life) after hernia surgery.
- To reduce the cost of hernia operation with better care.
- New operative techniques can be studied and assessed for hernia surgery.
- A plan and policy can be made for hernia surgery.

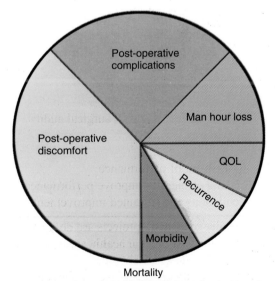

Fig. 26.1. Main areas of help from surgical hernia audit, as per incidence.

Surgical audit keeps a control on hernia surgery operation standards. If they are falling then they are improved or sometimes even the policy is changed.

The main areas of help are:
- Post-operative discomforts
- Post-operative complications
- Morbidity
- Mortality
- Post-operative QOL
- Return to work and manhour loss
- Recurrence rate

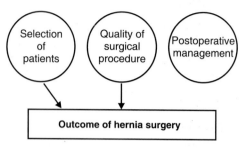

Fig. 26.2. Factors for outcome of hernia surgery.

Whether the hernia surgery procedure was correct and effective can be judged by the outcome. The outcome of hernia surgery depends upon:
- Selection of patients
- Quality of surgical procedure
- Post-operative treatment, antibiotic policy, and follow-up programme
- Associated ailments

An **audit cycle** if properly completed only then the outcome of hernia surgery will improve.

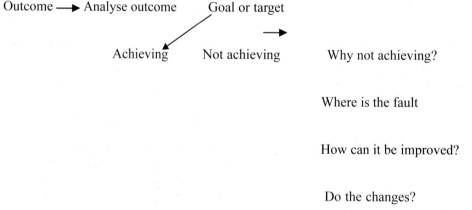

There are five stages of surgical audit:
- Preparation for audit
- Selection of criteria
- Assessment of performance
- Making changes to improve performance
- Continuous and sustained improvement

- In India some audit projects are doing a good job.[5-6]
- Given the pressure, our healthcare systems economic evaluations are crucial if we are to allocate scarce resources efficiently.[7]
- Ask yourself that your line of surgical treatment is giving desired results or not. Can you justify yourself to your patients and to your peers. Do not hesitate to ask for help or opinion from senior colleagues.

The benefits of surgical hernia audit and hernia registers are many for example Robertson and colleagues demonstrated that isolation of incision away from the hernia repair through an abdominoplasty approach is associated with lower complication and recurence rates. It was particularly helpful in obese patients and patients with multiple or recurrent hernias.[8,9]

KEY POINT

If results fall short of the criteria chosen, some changes in the care must be proposed.

RESOURCES

- **Cochrane library**: www.update-software.co,/clibhome/clib.ltm.
- **National Institute of Clinical Excellence (NICE)**: www.nice.org.uk
- **Royal College of Surgeons of England:** Clinical effectiveness unit: www.reseng.ac.uk/ ccu/ default.asp

REFERENCES

1. **Brown CJ, Emberton M.**, (2006). Surgical audit and the evaluation of surgery, *Surgery International*, **43,** p. 276.
2. **Thomas K, Emberton M.**, (2000). Modern surgical audit, *Surgery,* 18(IU): 250–2.
3. **Riodare** *et al.,* (1998). Audit of patient's outcomes after herniorrhaphies, *Surg. Clin. North Am.*, **78,** 6, 1129–39.
4. **Nilsson** *et al.*, (1998). Hernia registers and specialization, *Surg. Clin. North Am.*, **78,** 6, 1141–55.
5. **Surgical Audit 2000.**, Department of surgery, ESI Hospital Basaidarapur, New Delhi–110015.
6. **Surgical Audit.**, Department of general surgery, Christian Medical College, Vellore, Tamil Nadu.
7. **Helen E Campbell.**, (2006). Health economics and surgical care, *Surgery International*, **43,** 271.
8. **Shell DH.**, *et al.*, (2008). Open repair of ventral incisional hernias. *Surg. Clin. N. Am.*, 88, 70.
9. **Robertson JD, de la Torre JI, Gardner PM,** *et al.*, (2003). Abdominoplasty repair for abdominal wall hernias. *Ann Plast Surg.*; 51: 10–6.

27

Medicolegal Aspects of Hernia and Ethics

"I swear by Apollo physician, by Asclepius, by Health, by Panacea and by all god and goddesses, making them my witness, I will carry out, according to my ability and judgement, but never with view of injury or wrong doing.... I will keep pure and holy both my life and art...""
— **Hippocratic Oath**

"Thou shall be free from envy, not cause anothers death, and pray for the welfare of all creatures. Day in and day out, thou shall be engaged in the relief of patients, thou shall not desert thy patients."
— **Sushruta**

"Not for the self, not for the fulfillment of my any worldly material desire or gain, but solely for the good of humanity, I will treat my patients and excel all...."
— **Charack Oath**

"Doctors must tell patients any facts necessary for them to decide whether they want the operation. Exactly how much the doctor should tell is a matter of discretion, but real and forseeable risks should be disclosed" (National Consumer Council, 1983)[1].

INFORMED CONSENT (Figs. 27.1, 27.2 & 27.3)

It's surgeon's responsibility to take the consent from the patient. The consent should be "informed written consent".

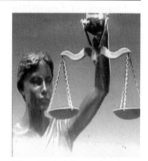

Fig. 27.1. Informed written consent is must before hernia surgery.

- Patient must be given proper, accurate and sufficient information about the following matters:
  - What type of hernia he or she is suffering from?
  - What type of surgery is proposed for his or her hernia?
  - Prognosis of hernia surgery.
  - Side effects and untoward effects of surgery.
  - Consequences of refusal for surgery.
- Patient must be an adult of sound mental state. In case of a child, parent's informed written consent is taken. In case of mental unstable person, a close relative or health authority can act on behalf of patient in giving written consent.
- It is always better if a nurse accompanies you during the session of informed consent.
- Get a second opinion in case of re-recurrence of a hernia about further plan of surgery if you are not experienced with treating re-recurrence of hernia.
- Be informed about new procedures of hernia repair but do not use unless they are properly tried and discussed at international platform.
- Informed written consent for conversion of laparoscopic repair to open repair must be taken explained.

For hernia surgery a number of operative techniques are available and thus each case becomes unique. In spite of so much developments and advancement in hernia surgery, new techniques and new prosthetic materials are being searched continuously for best technique and best prosthetic material.

> *Some of the following developments have changed the scene of hernia surgery today than 30 years back:*
>
> - Laparoscopic surgery
> - Prosthetic repair of hernia
> - Day case hernia surgery or "Come and Go" hernia surgery
> - Newer variety of prosthetic materials are in use i.e. non-adhesive meshes

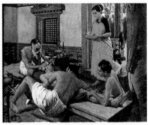

Fig. 27.2. Sushruta, father of Indian surgery.

- Hernia surgery is the one field where surgeon's dedication, conscience and moral plays a great part.
- Selection of patient is surgeon's job and there is no legal binding on it.
- No hernia operation is a minor operation, however, small and uncomplicated. All must be done with the same dedication and painstaking efforts. There is no place of hurry in this regard.
- Surgeon is not liable for any known complication such as post-operative infection or recurrence.
- Recurrence is not a negligence but it must be explained that every procedure of hernia repair has a recurrence rate.

   History of medical ailments such diabetes, heart disease, hypertension, asthma, allergy to drugs and history of drugs such as aspirin or clopidogrel must be recorded in case sheet.
- Documentation and detailed informed consent is important.
- The surgeon must always explain the procedure he is selecting for his patient and its complications and prognosis. Best is to make a note of it in consent and in clinical notes in case sheet.
- Consent for orchidectomy in Kuntz's operation must be taken from the patient in detail.
- Some patients have chronic groin pain for 1 to 2 years after hernia operation. So all patients must be explained that they may have chronic groin pain.
- In case of strangulated hernia one must explain the risks involved. It must be in writing in case notes.
- Documentation of the information given to the patient about his condition must be noted in case notes. It must be explained to the patient in the language he or she understands or a translator is kept during conversation.
- Type of anaesthesia and its details must be explained to the patient by the anaesthestist and not by the surgeon.

NEGLIGENCE

Common allegations of negligence for a surgeon for hernia are:
- **Leaving gauze or instrument or part of instrument inside the wound**
    - It is the whole responsibility of operating surgeon to ensure that nothing is left in the wound.
- **Operating on wrong side**
    - Always ensure on the operation table that you are operating on correct side.

- **Damage to a structure during surgery**
  - It is not an act of negligence. Patient has given a consent for known accidental damage to a structure.

MEETING WITH THE PATIENT

A surgeon must know how to communicate with patient and his relatives. Following topics are to be dealt with patient:

- **Tell the truth**
  - Tell the diagnosis and the treatment you are going to give. Tell about the prognosis.
- **Tell the patient and close relatives**
  - Patient has right to know about his sickness. Tell him what has happened with him and allow him to ask questions.
- **Risk of the treatment**
  - All the surgical procedures are associated with some risk. Patient should be explained about the risks and gains associated with the hernia repair. The surgeon should not involve himself in risk taking. Risk taking should be patient's responsibility.[2] The different hernia repair procedures have different risks and different gains.

Always talk with patient and close relatives in a separate quite room and not in a gallery or a corridor.

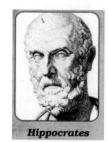

Hippocrates

Fig. 27.3. Father of modern medicine.

No lose philosophy of Pascal in hernia surgery[3]

When we operate on a recurrent hernia which is strangulated in an obese elderly patient, no lose philosophy is helpful. While telling about the prognosis of the operation to the patient and the relatives we must tell the truth and the possible serious complications. If they accept the responsibility and unfortunately complications happen then the surgeon is not blamed and if the patient survives without serious complications then nothing is lost.

Reassuring the Patient

Reassurance reduces the auxiety of the patient[4] in complicated and recurrent cases of hernia, specially huge recurrent incisional hernia.

Make your decision without involving the anxiety and fear of the patient, and take a right decision to select the correct hernia repair procedure.

Tell him clearly about the dangers and prognosis without giving irrelevant information and without making him more anxious. It is an art and one has to learn it.

Reassurance is more helpful if it is done in the presence of a close relative.

ETHICS OF A SURGEON IN HERNIA SURGERY

- Maintain the professional standard.[5]
- Confidentials of the patient is to be maintained.
- Second opinion if required or referral to the specialised hernia centre is required must be done without any thought of monetary profit.

- Knowledge of new discoveries and techniques are required.
- Do the hernia repair of which you have sufficient experience.
- One must know time to time about hernia treatment recommendations from various international societies and associations of hernia for the treatment, for example now a days surgeon are asking whether watchful waiting for minimaly symptomatic hernias is better than immediate surgery, a trial is performed in Glasgow in the United Kingdom.[11]

KEY POINT

Surgical ethics and surgical interventions are like hand in glove.

REFERENCES

1. **National Consumer Council.**, Patient's rights. HMSO, London.
2. **Mc Neil BJ.**, On the elicitation of preferenses for alternative therapies.
3. **Galbraith S.**, (1978). The 'no-lose' philosophy in medicine, *Journal of Medical Ethics*, 4: 61–3.
4. **Mc Latchie GR.**, (1994). The surgical patient, *Oxford Handbook of Clinical Surgery*, 2–11.
5. **General Medical Council.**, (1989). Advice on standards of professional conduct and on medical ethics. In Professional Conduct and Discipline: Fitness to Practice, pp. 18–28.
6. **www.bma.org.uk** for general information.
7. **Wear S.**, (1998). Informed consent georgetown, University Press, Washington DC, USA.
8. **British Medical Association**, (2003). Medical ethics today. *BMJ Books*, London.
9. **Royal College of Surgeon of England,** (1996). Code of practice for the surgical management of Jehovah's witness. Royal College of Surgeons, London.
10. **Warwick HMC, Salkovskis PM.**, (1985). Reassurance, *British Medical Journal*, 290: 1028.
11. **Turaga K., Fitzgibbons RJ.,** *et al.*, (2008). Inguinal hernia: should we repair? *Surg. Clin. N. Am.*; 88, 132.

28

Statistics of Hernia

"Personal statistics are at the bottom of all unsound teachings; they are either too good to be true or too true to be good."
— **William Heneage Ogilvie (1887-1971)**

The world *statistics* derives from Latin for "state", indicates the historical importance of governmental gathering of data[1].

Statistics: "It is the science of assembling and interpreting numerical data."

Broadly, statistics has the following stages:

Organization of data
↓
Interpretation of data
↓
Summarization of data
↓
Communication of final result of research

> In surgical research, even simple collection of data and interpretation can be a good thing for both society and medicine. It is good to collect your own data of hernia surgery. It can be then compared with other standard research work. This will give an idea of the standard of your surgical technique.

Any hernia research has to be statistically analyzed, as surgery has become now evidence-based. (Figs. 28.1 & 28.2).

- 5% of Indian population will suffer from abdominal wall hernia in their lifetime.
- One in five men will get hernia in his lifetime.
- One in 50 women will get hernia in her lifetime.
- In females, inguinal hernia is five times more common than femoral hernia but femoral hernia is more common in females than in males.
- As an approximate calculation, 15-20% operations in any hospital are hernia operations.
    - External abdominal hernia is the most common hernia.
    - 73% cases of hernia are inguinal hernia.
    - Femoral hernia accounts for 17%.
- 12% inguinal hernias incarcerate.
- 50% incarcerated inguinal hernias occur in the first six months of life.
    - Incarcerated inguinal hernia in infants is more common in girls.
- 80% of incarcerated inguinal hernias in children and infants are managed by conservative treatment.

- Male to female ratio of inguinal hernia in adults is 12 : 1.
- Inguinal hernia occurs most in the sixth decade.
- 55% inguinal hernias occur at the right side.
- 65% inguinal hernias are indirect.
- Bilateral inguinal hernias are 12%.
- Bilateral inguinal hernias are four times more common in direct than in indirect form.
- 15-30% adult males have patent processus vaginalis without clinically apparent hernia.
- 60% infant of operated inguinal hernias have contralateral patent processus vaginalis.
- 20% individuals will develop contralateral hernias in their lifetime.
- Inguinal hernia is 10 times more common than femoral hernia.
- Femoral hernia is 10 times more likely to strangulate than inguinal hernia.
- Recurrence rate varies between 0.2% to 15% depending upon the technique used in hernia surgery.
- 50% recurrence is apparent in first 2 years.

Doll and Hill in 1956 did a landmark study in carcinoma of lung.[2] It was a cohort study (long study of several years with large number of cases).
  - Randomised study means the study of two randomly allocated treatment.
  - Randomised controlled trials include control group also with no treatment.

Nowadays **randomized studies** are done by using coins, dice for toss. Random allocation is the best method of assigning subjects to the treatment.

"Blind study" is either single (only one, investigator or subject is blind) or double (both the investigator and the subject are blind) blind. Blind studies avoid assessment bias.

Mean

Sum of the values divided by the number of values.

Median

The value that divides the distribution in half.

Mode

The value which occurs most often.

Range

The difference between the highest and the lowest values.
- Autopsies have found 0.5-10% of general population suffers with epigastric hernia.
- Male to female ratio for epigastric hernia is 4 : 1.
- 75% epigastric hernias are asymptomatic.
- Umbilical and paraumbilical hernias are 8.5%.
- Incidence of infantile umbilical hernia is the third most common surgical disorder in children.
- Black and Asian infants have eight times higher incidence of infantile umbilical hernia than Caucasian infants.

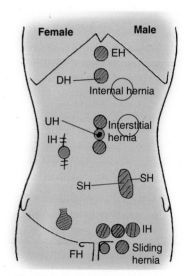

Fig. 28.1. Sexwise distribution of hernias.

- 90% infantile umbilical hernias disappear by the age of two years.
- Paraumbilical hernias are five times more common in female than males.
- Adult umbilical hernia occurs 90% in females, almost all are obese.
- 3-5% full term babies are born with clinical inguinal hernia.
- 80% infantile hernias occur in boys.
- 33% infantile hernias occur and present in the first six months of life.
- 55% congenital inguinal hernias are on right side.
- In 90% infants with inguinal hernia there is associated undescended testis.
- 60% of interstitial hernias are inter-muscular variety.
- 20% of interstitial hernias are preperitoneal hernias.
- 20% of interstitial hernias are of superficial type.
- Total 1000 cases of Spigelian hernias are reported so far in the world literature.

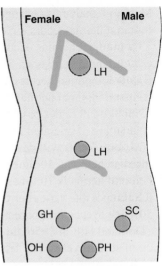

Fig. 28.2. Sexwise distribution of rare hernias.
LH = Lumbar hernia,
OH = Obturator hernia,
SC = Sciatic hernia

Collection of reviews are available. The Cochrane Collaboration brings together evidence-based medical information[3] (Cochrane, Archibald Leman, 1909-1988, Director of Medical Research Council Epidemiology Unit, Cardiff, Wales and President of Community Medicine, Royal College of Physicians of London, England).

One of the purposes of statistical study for a surgeon is to find the evidence that whether his method of treatment is upto the mark and gives expected results or he has to improve upon by more training, more concentration and more exposure so that he can give better results.

The evidence-based surgery for hernia is based on relevant data and gives us an opportunity to improve the surgical treatment of hernia.

Only 53 documented cases of sciatic hernia are reported.[6]

Only 20% patients of chronic groin pain were found to have the normal pattern of distribution of iliohypogastric and ilioinguinal nerves and only 40% having symmetrical pattern.[7]

KEY POINT

The conscientious, explicit and judicious use of current best evidence in making decision about the care of individual patients.

Prof. David Sackett[4]

REFERENCES

1. **Hemadi S, and Stand Field N.**, (2006). Statistics and computing in surgery, *Surgery International*, **43**, 6, p. 279.
2. **Doll R, Hill AB.**, (1950). Smoking and carcinoma lung, BMJ, II: 739–748.
3. **Russell RCG**, *et al.*, (2004). Bailey and Love's short practice of Surgery, 24th edition, p. 246.
4. **Sackett DL, Richardson W, Haynes RB.**, (1997). Evidence based medicine: How to practice and teach EBM, Edinburgh: Churchill Livingstone.
4. **Moher D, Cooke DJ, Eastwood S,** *et al.,* (1999). Improving the quality of reports of meta-analyses of randomized controlled trials. The QUORUM statement. *Lancet.* 354: 1896–1900.
5. **Gardner MJ, Altman DG.**, (1989). Statistics with-confidence, BMJ Publishing Group. London.
6. **Salameh JR.**, (2008). Primary and unusual abdominal wall hernias. *Surg. Clin. N. Am.*; 88, 58
7. **Ferzli GS.,** *et al.*, (2008). post herniorrhaphy groin pain and how to avoid it, *Surg. Clin. N. Am.*; 88, 203–204.

29

Information Patients Need from Surgeon

"One should advise surgery only if there is a reasonable chance of success."
— **Theodor Billroth (1829-1894)**

Q: What is hernia?

A: Hernia is a protrusion of body organ through a weak area (Fig. 29.1) or a natural orifice through which it does not pass ordinarily. Usually when we use the term hernia, we mean abdominal wall hernia. It occurs due to a weakness in abdominal wall. It may be congenital (by birth) or acquired. Swelling or a bulge is noticed when patient strains or stands. Some hernias cause pain and some do not cause any pain. First sign may be a bulge. You may have discomfort or dragging pain.

Q: Why operation is required?

A: Hernia never gets cured itself. It causes pain and discomfort. It can cause dangerous complications such as intestinal obstruction, strangulation (hampering of blood supply) and gangrene (tissue death) which are life-threatening conditions.

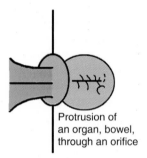

Protrusion of an organ, bowel, through an orifice

Fig. 29.1. Hernia.

Natural history of hernia is that it progressively enlarges and weakens the abdominal wall. Delay in operation can cause the following problems:

• Gradual enlargement of hernia causing more and more discomfort
• Chances of complications increase with time
• Risk of recurrence after operation is more if the hernia is large.

Q: What is the cause of hernia?

A: The most common hernia is abdominal wall hernia. The cause is straining which increases the pressure inside the abdominal cavity.

The common causes are:

• Straining while defecating as in chronic constipation
• Excessive coughing.
• Over strenuous exercises.
• Smoking causes coughing and deficiency of collagen tissue which causes weakness of abdominal wall.

Q: What is the operation for hernia?

A: Hernia operation is done with two aims:

• To replace the protruded organ back to the abdominal cavity.
• To repair the weak area of abdominal wall through which protrusion occurs.

Usually the hernia operation is performed by either of the two following techniques:
*   Open tension-free hernia repair: A prosthesis such as polypropylene mesh is introduced from outside to cover the defect. Open operation may be done under local anaesthesia.
*   Laparoscopic hernia repair: A prosthesis such as polypropylene mesh is used to cover the defect through abdominal cavity. Laparoscopic hernia repair is done under general anaesthesia.

    Nowadays local anaesthesia used is long acting, so the effect lasts for 4 to 6 hours. The patient walks out of operation theatre and is soon discharged.

Q: **Which anaesthesia will be given?**
A: It is performed under:
*   General anaesthesia
*   Epidural anaesthesia
*   Spinal anaesthesia

Even it can be performed under local anaethesia if the general condition of the patient does not permit other anaesthesia.

Q: **What are the post-operative advice?**
A: Patient will be discharged on the next day or after two days:
*   Laughing, walking and coughing may be uncomfortable for a few days.
*   Straining is avoided for one week.
*   Lifting of objects and strenuous exercises are not allowed for six weeks.

Q: **What are long term effects?**
A: It gives complete cure.
Risk of recurrence is 1% or below. It is generally brought out by overexertion.

Q: **What are various types of hernias?**
A: There are several types of hernias. Common[1] hernias are (Fig. 29.2):
*   Inguinal
*   Femoral
*   Umbilical

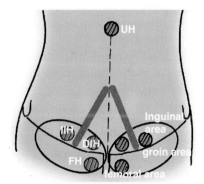

INGUINAL HERNIA

It is the commonest hernia. It is more common in men.

A loop of intestine descends down through the canal, through which the testis descends in the scrotum at birth.

FEMORAL HERNIA

Fig. 29.2. Various regions of common hernia in abdominal wall.

It is more common in women. The loop of intestine descends down to the thigh through a canal which passes blood vessels to the thigh. It causes a bulge in groin and upper part of thigh.

UMBILICAL HERNIA

It is common in both sexes. The loop of intestine passes out and protrudes through the weak area of abdominal wall at the naval and makes a bulge under skin.

Q: **How long I should avoid lifting heavy weight after my hernia operation?**
A: Standard advice is six weeks but self-assessment with pain is an excellent guide.

Q: **What if, I use truss for my hernia and decline the operation?**
A: Truss is used for the following purposes:[2]
  - To maintain the reduction of hernia.
  - To prevent enlargement.
    Truss or corset may give you relief but it will not cure the hernia, on contrary it may precipitate strangulation and may prove dangerous if applied wrongly.[3]

Q: **When can I return to work after hernia operation?**
A: Most of the patients return to work 8 - 10 days after hernia operation and do the normal activities.

Q: **How much time the operation takes?**
A: Most of the hernia operations take 40 - 45 minutes.

Q: **What are the contents of groin hernia?**
A: It usually contains fat, fluid or loop of intestine or omentum. Sometimes it may contain ovary, urinary bladder or even appendix.

Q. **What is the age of hernia surgery?**
A: Age is no bar for hernia operation as hernia can occur at any age, even to newborns.

Q: **If I do not agree for hernia operation then what harm it can cause?**
A: Uusally hernia is a reducible bulge and goes back to abdomen on lying or on manipulation. Hernia can lead to the following complications:

Reducible   Irreducible   Obstructed   Strangulated
hernia   hernia   hernia   hernia

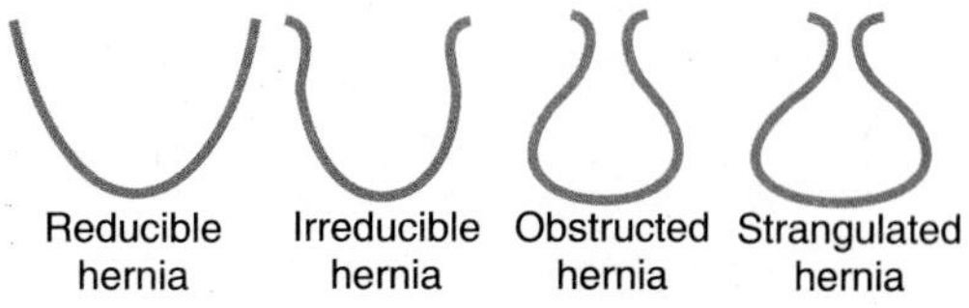

Fig.29.2A. Natural history of hernia.

  - Irreducibility – Hernia cannot be pushed back into the abdomen.
  - Obstruction – Intenstine in hernia is blocked.
  - Incarceration – hernia is painful and not reducible.
  - Strangulation – Pain, vomiting and inability to pass flatus and stool develops. Blood supply of the intestine is cut off. The intestine loop dies. It is a dangerous and life-threatening condition.

Q: **What are the improvements in hernia surgery?**
A: Nowadays the following improvements have occurred because of improved techniques of surgery and anaesthesia.
  - Shorter hospital stay, as nowadays most of the hernia surgery can be done as a day care surgery.
  - Morbidity is reduced.
  - Recurrence rate is reduced after the mesh prosthesis came in use. Usually the recurrence is less than 1% after mesh hernioplasty.
  - Early return to work.
  - The patient is able to walk soon after operation.
  - Post-operative pain is not a big problem.
  - No post-operative vomiting or respiratory problem.

Q: **Why nowadays the prosthetic mesh is used in hernia repair?**
A: The prosthetic mesh is a non-absorabable material. It is used to restore the anatomy of the area without producing tension on the suture line.

Mesh provides the following benefits:
- Low recurrence rate due to tension-free repair.
- It is an anatomical repair.
- Early and better strength.
- Long term reinforcement.

Q: What information should I give to the doctor about my body for operation?

A: Following informations are essential about the individual going for surgery:
- History of operation, anaesthesia, drug allergy, hepatitis B/C, HIV.
- Past history of diabetes, hypertension, heart disease, asthma, DVT (deep vein thrombosis) and bleeding tendencies.
- List of medication including blood thinners such as aspirin, clopidogrel and warfarin.
- Smoking as it increases the risks of surgery and it delays healing also.
- Alcohol, as excess of alcohol may increase the risks of surgery.

Q: What care should be taken after surgery?

A : When you will be discharged after operation:
- Some medicines are advised for pain and if you do not feel pain you may omit pain killer drug. Antibiotics are not given routinely.
- A waterproof dressing will be applied over the operated area so that you can take bath directly over the dressing, but do not rub the dressing.
- Surgeon will encourage you to be mobile as much as possible.
- Get up slowly and walk slowly.
- You may be given mild laxative to avoid straining at the time of passing stool.
- When you cough or sneeze or laugh then put your hand over the operation site to give support, it will reduce the discomfort and pain.
- Wound site may feel thickened and often a ridge is palpable at the operation site. This will become normal after a few weeks or months.
- You should avoid driving for one week or 10 days as sudden application of break may cause discomfort and pain.[4]
- Heavy weight lifting is not encouraged for 4-6 weeks.

Q: I am 80 years old. Am I too old for hernia surgery?

A: No, nowadays with safer surgery and safer anaethesia techniques age is no bar for hernia surgery.

Q: I do not have a 'bulge' so how can I be sure that I have hernia or not?

A: Bulge is a common symptom of hernia but all bulges are not hernias and not all hernias have bulges. Show to some surgeon or hernia specialist.

Q: My doctor says that as my hernia is not painful and it does not hurt so I should just leave it as it is?

A: Hernias only get worse day-by-day. If it is untreated, then it will develop complications. If a hernia is diagnosed then it should be operated.

Q: Can a hernia affect erection?

A: Painful hernias may cause erectile dysfunction.

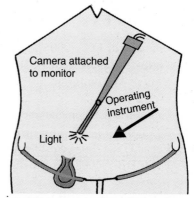

Fig. 29.3. Laparoscopic hernia surgery.

Q: Is key hole surgery is the best method of surgery for hernia?

A: Key hole (laparoscopic) surgery is an advancement in hernia treatment. Key hole surgery requires general anaesthesia and "tension-free" hernia repair is done under local anaesthesia. General anaesthesia has some complications and, therefore, we prefer to do hernia surgery under local ananesthesia (Fig. 29.3).

Q: How much weight can I lift after my hernia operation?

A: After groin hernia operation it is recommended not to lift more than 5 kg weight (approximately the laptop bag for the first week then not more than 10 kg after six weeks).

Q: When can I resume sexual intercourse after my hernia surgery?

A: A good hernia repair will have no problem with daily routine activities. Intercourse is advised with care in first week after operation. Intercourse in "missionary position" is to be avoided for one week after operation. "Woman superior" can be substituted during this period.[5]

Q: What exercise I should do to avoid hernia?

A: Head raising and leg raising exercises improve the strength and tone of muscles of abdomen and thus prevent developement of abdominal wall hernia.

Q: What is post hernia operation chronic groin pain?

A: Pain that persists after the normal healing process has occured–typically 3 months after hernia surgery.[6]

Q: What are the various sizes and densities of various prosthetic meshes?

A: Sizes and densities of various prosthetic meshes are as following[7,8]:

Size	Density
• Heavy weight > 90 g/m2	• Very large pore > 2000 μm
• Median weight 50-90 g/m2	• Large pore 1000-2000 μm
• Light weight 35-50 g/m2	• Medium pore 600-1000 μm
• Ultra light weight < 35 gm2	• Small pore 100-600 μm
	• Micro porous < 100 μm

KEY POINT

Be open, informative, honest and caring to patient. Detailed consent and documentation are most important tools of a surgeon.

REFERENCES

1. **Brunicardi FC.,** (2005). Schwartz's principles of surgery, 8th edition, p. 1366.
2. **Philip T Hagen.,** (2001). Hernia, Mayo clinic guide to self care, p. 75.
3. **Robert M Youngson.,** (1993). The surgery book, pp. 282–85.
4. **Welsh CI,** *et al.,* (1980). Advice about driving after herniorrhaphy. *Br. Med. Jour.,* 1: 1133–4.
5. **Condon RE.,** Iliopubic tract repair of inguinal hernia, The Anterior (Inguinal Canal) Approach, Chapter 72, p. 17, http:\\\www.masteryofsurgery.com.
6. **Ferzli GS.,** (2008). Post herniorrhaphy groin pain and how to avoid it. *S. Clin. N. Am.;* 88, 203.
7. **Earle DB.;** (2008). Prosthetic material in inguinal hernia repair: How do I choose? *Surg. Clin. N. Am.;* 88, 179.
8. **Schumpelick V,** *et al.,* (2006). Light weight meshes in incisional hernia repair. *JMAS.;* 3:117–23.

30 Famous International Hernia Centers and Clinics

"Good surgery is 75% decision making and only 25% manual dexterity."
— **Spencer F.C. , 1979**
American Surgeon[1]

In this era of superspeciality, various clinics and hospitals have devoted themselves only for hernia care. Following are famous hernia clinics and centres:

- Shouldice Hernia Center
- Lichtenstein Hernia Institute
- British Hernia Center
- Sydney Hernia Center and Melbourne Hernia Clinic
- Rutkow Robbin's Hernia Center
- Kugel Hernia Center

Shouldice Hernia Center

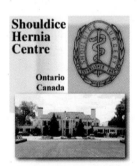

Shouldice Hospital
7750 Bayview Avenue
Thornhill, Ontario, Canada L3T 4A3
Tel: (905)889-1125 Fax: (905)889-4216 Toll Free: 1-800-291-7750

Dr Edward Earle Shouldice passed his medical degree in 1916 from University of Toronto, Canada. He worked in army as a Major during World War II. He noticed that a lot of young men were made medically unfit to join army due to the presence of groin hernias. He developed his surgical technique of hernia operation. He then operated persons who were willing to join army but suffering with groin hernias. All of them became fit and later joined the army.

In July 1945, Dr Shouldice opened "Shouldice Hospital" at Church St. in Toronto.

In 1953, he purchased a country estate in Thornhill and second hospital was opened. The hospital is now 55 years old and about 300,000 operations for various groin hernias have been done so far. 10 surgeons now operate 5000 to 7000 cases every year.

The Shouldice operation nowadays is called "Shouldice technique" or "Canadian method" or "Toronto method".

The recurrence rate after hernia operation is less than 1%.
Most of the Shouldice operations are performed under local anaesthesia and sedation.
Shouldice Hospital has 5 operation theaters and 89 beds.

Harward Business School teaches its students about Shouldice Hospital as a case report "Example of Excellence".

Now the Shouldice Clinic is run by Byrnes Shouldice, son of Dr Edward Earle Shouldice. Byrnes is also a hernia surgeon. Shouldice hernia clinic is a hernia factory where 10 to 12 surgeons operate. Hospital is specially designed for hernia operations. Rooms have no telephones or televisions. Meals are not served in room but served in dining hall. Patient has to walk to the dining hall to avoid the problems of inactivity. So pneumonia and leg clots are prevented.

Lichtenstein Hernia Institute

Hernia Institute-South Jersey
(856) 428-4434
1935 Marlton Pike E, Cherry Hill

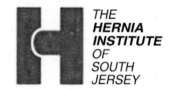

THE
HERNIA
INSTITUTE
OF
SOUTH
JERSEY

The institute was established in 1984. The Lichtenstein Hernia Institute is exclusively devoted to surgery of abdominal wall hernias. It is devoted to surgery, teaching and research of abdominal wall hernias.

"This institute deals with abdominal wall hernias such as inguinal hernia, femoral hernia, umbilical hernia and ventral hernia. This institute originated the Gold standard hernia operation method, "Tension-free mesh hernioplasty".

The principle of *"Tension-free mesh hernioplasty"* is explained as hernia is a tear in the abdominal wall musculature. The stitching of this tear creates distortion of muscle fibres and undue strain and tension is created along the suture line. It causes pain and has longer recovery period. It also leads to recurrence. The *"Tension-free"* repair is accomplished by covering the opening of hernia and weak area of musculature with a patch of mesh. Mesh becomes a part of body in 2-3 weeks.

This operation is performed under local anaesthesia as a day care surgery.

Sydney Hernia Center and Melbourne Hernia Clinic

Suite 551,
Spring Street,
Bondi Junction,
Sydney, Australia

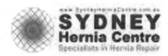

Melbourne Hernia Clinic is the first specialized hernia center in Australia. The clinic was established 20 years ago.

Mr. Maurice Brygel is the founder of both the Sydney Hernia Center and Melbourne Hernia Clinic.

Most of the abdominal hernias are operated here as day surgery under local anaesthesia.

British Hernia Center

87 Watford Way, Hendon, London NW4 4RS U.K.

"This center of excellence for hernia surgery does more tension-free hernia repairs than any hospital in the World".

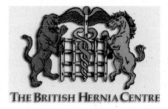

The Rutkow Robbins Hernia Center

222, SCHANCK ROAD,
Suite 100,
FREE HOLD
NEW JERSEY, USA

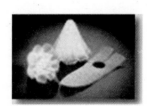

Dr Ira, M. Rutkow and Dr Alan W. Robbin developed this center for hernia surgery. ***Rutkow and Robbin have developed "Mesh Plug" technique for inguinal hernia*** but hernia is operated by other methods also at this center.

Kugel Hernia Center

Hernia Treatment Center,
NW, 205 Lilly Road,
Suite D,
Olympia WA 98532
USA

Robert D. Kugel developed pre-peritoneal mesh patch technique. This center operates various abdominal wall hernias with various other methods also.

KEY POINT

"You must use the new treatment whilst it still has the power to cure"

–Voltaire
French Philosopher

REFERENCE

Spencer FC., Competence and compassion, two qualities of surgical excellence, *Bulletin of American College of Surgeon*, 64: 15–22.

31

Frequently Asked Questions (FAQs)

"The trouble with doctors is not that they don't know enough but that they don't see enough."
— **Sir Dominic Corrigan (1802-1880)**

Q: **What is 'Malgaigne's Bulge"?**

A: The men with poor abdominal musculature show elongated bulges specially in flanks on straining. It is called "Malgaigne's Bulge" after Joseph Francois Malgaigne, 1806-1865, Professor of Surgery, Paris, France. "Malgaigne's Bulges" are diagnostic of poor abdominal musculature. Sometimes these are confused with inguinal hernia. The persons with Malgaigne's bulge are prone to develop direct inguinal hernia.

Q: **How smoking predisposes to direct inguinal hernia?**

A: Smoking causes collagen deficiency in tissues, which results in weakness of tissues making them susceptible to give way to intra-abdominal pressure leading to hernia.

Q: **Which direct inguinal hernia strangulates?**

A: Prevesical hernia strangulates. It is also called Funicular direct inguinal hernia or Ogilvie hernia. It is a narrow-necked hernia.

Q: **What is a "Hernia en W"?**

A: It is also called "Maydl's hernia". It is a rare hernia. The hernia loop of intestine becomes 'W' in shape. The strangulated loop of 'W' lies in abdomen and the loop, which lies in the sac is not strangulated. So there is no local signs of strangulation in hernia.

During operation sometimes the hernia is reduced without checking the gangrenous loop then it requires laparotomy again.

It is named after Karl Maydl, 1853-1903, Professor of Surgery, Prague, the Czech Republic.

Q: **What is Hoguet's maneuver?**

A: It is a maneuver in hernioplasty to convert a direct inguinal hernia sac to an indirect hernia, by withdrawing the contents from behind the inferior epigastric vessels (Figs. 31.1A & B).

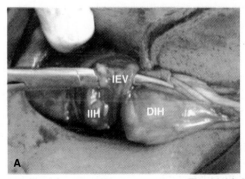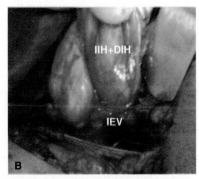

Fig. 31.1A & B. Hoguet's maneuver.

Q: What are the two most important features of inguinoscrotal hernia?
A: • Expansile impulse on coughing.
   • Cannot get above the swelling (differentiates from hydrocele, however large it is).

Q: Name structures which are more wide than long.
A: • Pituitary gland
   • Pons
   • Caecum
   • Femoral canal
   • Prostate gland

Q: If a patient requires both prostatectomy and herniorrhaphy then how you would proceed?
A: Both the prostatectomy and herniorrhaphy can be performed at the same time, if required. But prostatectomy should be done only if one operation is to be done at a time. If herniorrhaphy is done earlier then retention of urine and straining at micturition may cause recurrence of hernia.

Q: Which type of recurrent inguinal hernia occurs after inguinal hernia repair?
A: Direct inguinal hernia usually occurs.

Q: How you would treat strangulated inguinal hernia in an infant?
A: Conservative treatment. Sedation and hanging feet up on a Balkan beam usually relieves the strangulation in 80% of cases and 20% of cases require operation.

Q: What is the preferred operation for strangulated femoral hernia?
A: MeEvedy operation.

Q: What is classical Halsted Operation?
A: It includes the following features:
   • Lateral mobilization of spermatic cord.
   • Bassini's repair of inguinal canal.
   • Spermatic cord is placed in subcutaneous space superficial to external oblique aponeurosis.

Q: What is "Phantom hernia"?
A: It occurs due to damage of nerve supply to muscle. It occurs in post-polio case. It commonly recurs in lumbar region (Fig. 31.2).

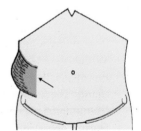

Fig. 31.2. Phantom hernia.

Q: What is parastomal hernia?
A: It protrudes through the stoma.

Q: What is "Giant inguinal hernia"?
A: Inguinal hernia which reaches below mid level of the thigh when the patient stands. Sometimes giant hernia contains most of intestine and even stomach (Fig. 31.3).

Q: What is "Sports hernia"?
A: Undiagnosed chronic groin pain associated with groin hernia in an athelete.

Q: What are the types of parastomal hernia?
A: It is a post-operative hernia related to the stoma of bowel. According to Devlin's classification, it is of the following four varieties:
   • **Subcutaneous hernia** – Bowel loops lie along side of bowel of stoma in subcutaneous tissue.
   • **Interstitial hernia** – Bowel protrudes in intermuscular plane.

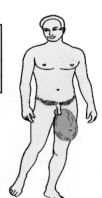

Fig. 31.3. Giant inguinal hernia.

- **Intrastomal hernia** – Bowel herniates along the bowel loop of stoma.
- **Perstomal hernia** – Prolapse of stoma associated with bowel loops.

Q: **What treatments are available for parastomal hernia?**

A: • Relocation of ostomy with repair of the defect.
- Special polypropylene prostheses are available with a ring mounted in the centre.

Q: **Who is known as the "father of hernia surgery"?**

A: Edoardo Bassini.

Q: **What is Lytle's technique?**

A: Narrowing of deep inguinal ring by placing interrupted sutures in deep inguinal ring medial to spermatic cord.

Q: **What is "Canal of Nuck"?**

A: Canal of Nuck is a persistent processus vaginalis peritonei after birth in females. It is named after Anton Nuck, 1650-1692, Professor of Anatomy and Medicine, Leiden, the Netherlands.

Q: **Which hernias are prone to get strangulated?**

A: • Femoral
- Obturator
- Paraumbilical
- Inguinal

Q: **Which type of gangrene develops in strangulated hernia?**

A: Wet type of gangrene.

Q: **What do you mean by "Groin" hernia[1]?**

A: A groin hernia refers to (Fig. 31.4):
- Direct inguinal hernia
- Indirect inguinal hernia
- Femoral hernia

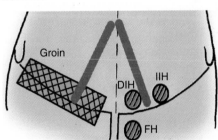

Fig. 31.4. Groin hernias.

Q: **Where is Shouldice hernia clinic?**

A: Toronto, Canada.

Q: **Which hernias do not have neck?**

A: • Direct inguinal hernia
- Incisional hernia

Q: **Which hernia has no sac?**

A: Epigastric hernia has no sac. It is a protrusion of extraperitoneal fat through linea alba.

Q: **What are the causes of inflamed hernia?**

A: Inflammation of sac occurs in hernia containing:
- Appendicitis
- Meckel's diverticulitis
- Salpingitis
- Ill-fitted truss

Q: **Why hernia is most common in inguinal area?**

A: • It is a junction between trunk and lower limb. It causes weakness.
- This area is weak due to the presence of
  - Superficial inguinal ring
  - Spermatic cord

– Deep inguinal ring
– Inguinal canal

Q: **What is "Shoe lace repair"?**

A: It is an operation for incisional hernia. A new linea alba is constructed in the midline, with non-absorbable suture, after excision of scar. This unites both the rectus sheaths (Fig. 31.5).

Q: **How does the operation for strangulated inguinal hernia differ from uncomplicated inguinal hernia operation?**

A: In strangulated hernia:
* Sac is opened first.
* Toxic fluid is removed.
* Then the inguinal canal is opened and constriction is relieved.
* The constriction of deep inguinal ring is cut laterally and not medially to avoid injury to inferior epigastric vessels.

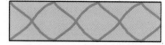

Fig. 31.5. Shoe lace repair of incisional hernia.

Q: **What is "Enthesopathy"?**

A: It is the inflammation on insertion of ligament or tendon. "Enthesis" means insertion. It is one of the causes of chronic groin pain.

Q: **What is "Gilmore Groin"?**

A: It is also called "groin disruption". It is seen in sport persons. It is the disruption of fascia transversalis and is a cause of chronic groin pain in sport persons.

Q: **What happens to polypropylene mesh in body after hernioplasty? Or**
   What is the fate of polypropylene mesh after hernioplasty?

A: With healing process, the fibroblast and capillaries grow over the mesh and gradually the polypropylene mesh converts into a thick fibrous sheath.

Q: **Which hernias are prone to left side?**

A: • Direct inguinal hernia
   • Sliding hernia

Q: **How to deal with sliding inguinal hernia?**

A: • Do not open sac.
   • Do not separate the contents of sac.
   • Reduce the sac with contents in total.
   • Repair the inguinal canal.

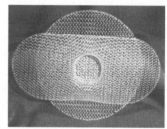

Fig. 31.5A. Polypropylene Hernia System.

Q: **What is PHS?**

A: PHS means Polypropylene Hernia System.
   * It is devised by Arthur I Gilbert, Miami Clinic Hernia, USA.
   * It is made up of two components with a connector:
     – Outer circular mesh
     – Inner rectangular mesh
   * The recurrence rate is 0.1% or less.

Q: **Why early operation is indicated in congenital inguinal hernia in infants?**

A: Due to high incidence of strangulation.

Q: **What is the difference between operation of congenital inguinal hernia in infants and older children?**

A: In infants both deep and superficial inguinal rings are superimposed so direct dissection of sac is possible.

In older children, the direct dissection is not possible. Inguinal canal is opened. External ring is not opened.

Q: **What are the indications of herniorrhaphy in children?**

A: • Ventriculoperitoneal shunt
• CAPD (Continuous Ambulatory Peritoneal Dialysis)
• Malnutrition
• Growth failure
• Connective tissue disorders
e.g. Marfan's syndrome and Ehler Danlos syndrome

Q: **What are the chances of developing contralateral hernia in children?**

A: 20%.

Q: **What are the main differences between umbilical hernia and exomphalos?**

A: • A umbilical hernia is herniation through weak umbilical cicatrix which fails to close after birth. It is covered with skin.
• Exomphalos occurs through umbilicus. It is due to failure of return of midnut into peritoneal cavity completely. It is covered by transparent membrane and not by skin.

Q: **What are the ususal contents of paraumbilical hernia?**

A: Commonly it contains greater omentum.
Less commonly it contains:
• Small intestine
• Transverse colon
• Urinary bladder

Q: **Why paraumbilical hernia is more common in females?**

A: It is due to:
• Obesity
• Repeated pregnancies

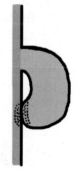

Q: **What is intertrigo?**

A: A superficial dermatitis occurring on apposing skin surfaces caused by moisture, friction, warmth etc. Obese patients with large paraumbilical hernia may have intertrigo.
Ulceration in skin between redundant skin folds occurs (Fig. 31.6).

Fig. 31.6. Intertrigo in large paraumbilical hernia.

Q: **When normal activities can be started after hernia operation?[2]**

A: Patient can return to normal activities as soon as pain and discomfort subside. Recurrence depends more upon the technique of operation than activities.

Q: **What is false epigastric hernia?**

A: Epigastric hernia without a peritoneal sac, only protrusion of extraperitoneal fat occurs.

Q: **What are the usual contents of epigastric hernia?**

A: An empty peritoneal hernia sac or only omentum.

Q: **What is the cause of pain in paraumbilical hernia?**

A: Usually it is asymptomatic, pain is due to traction on omentum or due to strangulation of omentum.

Q: **What structures are drained by Cloquet's lymph node?**

A: Clitoris in females and glans penis in males.

Q: **What is La Rocque's Maneuver?**

A: Sometimes it is required to return the herniated viscera inside abdomen by pulling the viscus from within abdominal cavity. In such a situation La Roque's maneuver is done. It is used specially for sliding hernia.

The incision of hernia is extended laterally and up in same line of incision.

The external oblique aponeurosis is incised further up. The internal oblique and the transversus abdominis muscles are split above the deep inguinal ring by an incision.

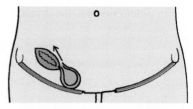

Fig. 31.7. La Rocque's maneuver.

The peritoneum is now opened from this incision and the viscus is pulled in from this incision.

Q: **What are the sites of recurrence of inguinal hernia?**

A: • At the pubic tubercle in direct inguinal hernia.
   • At deep inguinal ring in indirect inguinal hernia.

Q: **What is "Swiss - Cheese hernia"?**

A: It is a variety of ventral hernia, specially incisional hernia. When it is seen from inside, laparoscopically, lots of small and big defects are seen, like holes of Swiss-cheese.

Q: **Which organs can be found in sliding inguinal hernia[3]?**

A: • Colon
   • Caecum
   • Appendix
   • Ovary
   • Bladder
   • Fallopian tube
   • Uterus (rare)

Q: **What is "Howship Romberg's Sign"?**

A: It is the pain along the medial aspect of the thigh in obturator hernia. It is due to obturator nerve compression.

Q: **What is Gornall's test?**

A: It is to diagnose inguinal hernia in infant, when other methods fail. The child is held from his back by placing both hands on abdomen and lifting infant, this increases intra-abdominal pressure and hernia protrudes out.

Q: **Why incisional hernia is not common with transverse abdominal incisions?**

A : When intra-abdominal pressure increases on straining, the abdominal wall bulges more transversely and less longitudinally so longitudinal scar separates but not transverse scar.

Q: **Why incisional hernia is common in lower abdominal scar than upper abdominal scar?**

A: It is due to the following facts:
   • There is no posterior rectus sheath in lower abdomen. It makes this area weak.
   • In erect posture, there is more strain in lower abdomen than in upper adomen due to gravity.

Q: **Why midline scars are more prone to incisional hernia than lateral scars or paramedian scars?**

A: • In midline scars, there is no protection of muscles. In lateral scars, muscles support the scar.
   • When abdominal muscles contract, midline gap increases due to lateral contraction of abdominal muscles.

Q. What is ping-pong hernia?
A. It is a layman's term for ping-pong ball-sized umbilical hernia.
It is also sometimes used for bilateral inguinal hernia. Sometimes on coughing and straining hernia bulges on one side and sometimes on other side.

Q. What is the process of biologic response to a synthetic prosthetic mesh?
A. The following process happens after prosthetic mesh implantation
Prosthesis implantated → Protein coagulum → Platelet adherance → Release of Chemoattractants → Polymorphonucleocyts collection → Macrophages, Fibroblasts and Smooth muscle cell increase and collected → Collagen is secreted by all three cells → Connective tissue forms → Scar and connective tissue contraction (contraction of prosthetic mesh).[5]

Q. Why are groin hernias more common on right side?
A: Following reasons have been put forward:
- Processus vaginalis closes later on right side than left side and thus causes more hernias on right side.
- Right side is usually the dominant side of body, so hernias on right side are more common due to more strain on right side.
- Presence of sigmoid colon on left side gives support to left groin and thus presents hernias on left side. Sigmoid colon gives a tamponding effect to left femoral canal.

KEY POINT

Always examine groin for femoral hernia in an old lady with acute intestinal obstruction.

REFERENCES

1. **Harken AH, Moore EE.**, (2004). Abernathy's surgical secrets, 5th edition, pp. 199–205.
2. **Robert MY.**, (1993). The surgery book, pp. 282–285.
3. **Williams R,** *et al.*, (2004). Bailey and Love's short practice of surgery, 24th edition, pp. 1268–93.
4. **La Roque GP.**, (1919). *Surg. Gynaecol. Obstet.*, 29: 507.
5. **Earl DB.,** *et al.*, (2008). Prosthetic material. Inguinal hernia, repair: How do I choose., *Surg. Clin. N Am.*, 88, 185.

True or False

2

"Whoever is careless with truth in small matters cannot be trusted in important affairs."
— **Albert Einstine, April 1955, written about one week before his death**

Q: Black children are more likely to have umbilical hernia than white.
A: True.

Q: The risk of myxedema is higher in children with umbilical hernia.
A: True.

Q: Paraumbilical hernia always requires surgery.
A: True.

Q: Femoral hernia is common in nulliparous women.
A: False

Q: Males are 20 times more affected with inguinal hernia than females[1].
A: True.

Q: In males 35% inguinal hernias are direct and 12% are bilateral.
A: True.

Q: Laugier's femoral hernia occurs through Gimbernat's ligament.
A: True.

Q: In Cloquet's femoral hernia, sac lies under fascia of pectineus muscle.
A: True.

Q: Presence of Malgaigne's bulge is an absolute indication for hernioplasty.
A: True.

Q: If the caecum and appendix are the contents of hernia sac, it is not a sliding hernia.[2]
A: True.

Q: In females the most common hernia is inguinal hernia then incisional hernia and least common is femoral hernia
A: True.

Q: Direct hernia does not descend into scrotum as it pushes the posterior wall of inguinal canal.
A: True.

Q: Femoral hernia is never congenital.
A: True.

Q: Femoral hernia is more affected on right side due to dominant nature of right side of body.
A: True.

Q: Direct inguinal hernia is more common on left side.[3]
A: True.

Q: Sliding hernia is more common on left side and almost always occurs in males.
A: True.

Q: 90% of umbilical hernia in infants disappear by 2 years age.
A: True.
Q: In epigastric hernia the common finding is a tender nodule which is irreducible and without impulse on coughing.
A: True.
Q: Patient with Down's Syndrome and Prune Bully Syndrome are commonly affected with interstitial or interparietal hernia.
A: True.
Q: In scintigraphy, a radionuclide material is added to the ambulatory dialysis fluid and scanning is done to detect a patent processus vaginalis. It is used to detect an occult hernia.
A: True.
Q. Irreducibility is the first sign of strangulation in inguinal hernia.
A: False.
   Tenderness is the first sign.
Q. Parastomal hernia incidence is 30 to 50%.
A: True.[4]

Q: Most important step in repair of indirect inguinal hernia is herniotomy.
A: False.
   (Narrowing of the internal inguinal ring is the most important step.)

KEY POINT

Femoral hernia is more common in females but the commonest hernia in females is inguinal hernia.

REFERENCES

1. **Harken AH, Moor EE.**, (2000). Abernathy's surgical secrets, 4th edition, 5th edition, 2004.
2. **Dharmendra Sharma** *et al.,* (2004). *Surgery Buster.* pp. 118–122.
3. **Way WL and Doherty GM.**, (2003). Current surgical diagnosis and treatment. 11th edition.
4. **Israelsson LA.**, (2008). Parastomal hernias. *Surg. Clin. N. Am.*; 88, 113.

33 Multiple Choice Questions

"Good surgeons operate well; great surgeons know how to manage their own complications."
— **Moshe Schein**

"The wise man avoids crisis, by anticipating it"
— **P. Syrus**

1. **Which of the following is the first sign of strangulation of inguinal hernia:**
a) Tense
b) Tender
c) Irreducible
d) Redness

2. **In examination of the patient for a hernia, it is useful to realise that:**
a) An impulse is often much better seen than felt.
b) The internal abdominal ring lies 1.25 cm above the midpoint of Poupart's ligament.
c) The external abdominal ring lies 1.25 cm above and external to pubic symphysis.
d) None of the above

3. **Richter's hernia is commonly associated with:**
a) Direct inguinal hernia
b) Femoral hernia
c) Indirect inguinal hernia
d) Obturator hernia

4. **Richter's hernia contains:**
a) Portion of intestine
b) Bladder
c) Meckel's diverticulum
d) Sigmoid colon

5. **Preservation of ilioinguinal nerve is an important step during inguinal hernia operation while:**
a) Incising the subcutaneous tissue
b) Incising the external oblique aponeurosis
c) Incising the cremasteric fascia
d) Isolating the sac

6. **Inguinal canal is not bounded posteriorly by:**
a) Transversalis fascia
b) Internal oblique muscle
c) Conjoint tendon
d) Lacunar ligament

7. **The superficial inguinal ring is a defect in:**
a) Transversalis fascia
b) Internal oblique muscle
c) External oblique muscle
d) External oblique aponeurosis

8. **On an average, the distance between femoral ring and saphenous opening (length of femoral canal) is:**
a) 1.25 cm
b) 2.50 cm
c) 3.75 cm
d) 5.00 cm

9. **Most common hernia of abdominal wall is:**
a) Ventral
b) Inguinal
c) Umbilical
d) Femoral

10. **Which of the following are true regarding hernias?**
a) >90% are external abdominal hernias.
b) Femoral hernias are more likely to strangulate.
c) >50% of direct hernias are acquired.
d) Treatment of choice is surgery.
e) Indirect hernias are more common in adults.

11. **Most important step in the repair of an indirect inguinal hernia is:**
a) Herniotomy
b) Narrowing of the internal ring
c) Bassini's repair
d) Transfixation of the neck of the sac

12. **The treatment of choice for inguinal hernia in infants is:**
a) Herniotomy
b) Herniorrhaphy
c) Truss
d) Hernioplasty

13. While performing a hernia operation, a patient develops tingling sensation over the dorsal surface of penis and over the scrotum. The nerve implicated is:
a) Genitofemoral nerve
b) Ilioinguinal nerve
c) Hypogastric plexus
d) Pudendal nerve

14. **Which one of the following hernias is least likely to strangulate?**
a) Direct inguinal hernia
b) Indirect inguinal hernia
c) Femoral hernia
d) Umbilical hernia

15. The ideal treatment for congenital inguinal hernia is:
a) Herniotomy
b) Herniorrhaphy
c) Hernioplasty
d) Preperitoneal repair

16. All of the following are features of direct inguinal hernia except:
a) Rarely descends into the scrotum
b) Strangulation rarely occurs
c) Passes through the internal ring
d) Contents may be bladder

17. Strangulation is most common with which hernia:
a) Femoral
b) Inguinal
c) Obturator
d) Epigastric

18. Differential diagnosis of acute funiculitis with a small inguinal swelling is:
a) Undescended testes
b) Acute orchitis
c) Lymphadenitis
d) Small strangulated inguinal hernia

19. In strangulated hernia, the incision is given at:
a) Neck
b) Body
c) Fundus
d) Inguinal ring

20. During repair of indirect inguinal hernia, while releasing the constriction at the deep inguinal ring, the surgeon takes care not to damage which one of the following structures?
a) Falx inguinalis (conjoint tendon)
b) Interfoveolar ligament
c) Inferior epigastric artery
d) Spermatic cord

21. Which one of the following statements is NOT true about direct inguinal hernia?
a) The sac is medial to inferior epigastric artery.
b) The coverings of sac include cremasteric and internal spermatic fascia.
c) The sac is anterolateral to cord structures.
d) The direct hernias are rarely congenital.

22. A patient undergoing open inguinal hernia repair can have neuralgia due to the involvement of any of the following nerves except:
a) Ileoinguinal nerve
b) Ileohypogastric nerve
c) Lateral cutaneous nerve of thigh
d) Genitofemoral nerve

23. **Which one of the following is not the aetiology of strangulating hernia?**
a) Volvulus
b) Mesenteric vascular occlusion
c) Intussusception
d) Gallstone ulcers

24. **In hernia-en-glissade the most common content is:**
a) Omentum
b) Urinary bladder
c) Caecum
d) Sigmoid colon

25. **Amyand's hernia contains:**
a) Meckel's diverticulum
b) Appendix
c) Caecum
d) Ileum

26. **Strangulation is a frequent complication of:**
a) Paraumbilical hernia
b) Incisional hernia
c) Inguinal hernia
d) Femoral hernia

27. **A Littre's hernia contains:**
a) Meckel's diverticulum
b) Appendix
c) Fallopian tube
d) Sigmoid colon

28. **Truss cannot prevent progression of which of the following types of inguinal hernia?**
a) Sliding
b) Littre's
c) Indirect
d) Direct

29. **Femoral hernia is characteristically.... the pubic tubercle:**
a) Lateral and below
b) Medial and above
c) Lateral and above
d) Medial and below

30. **Femoral hernia and inguinal hernia are differentiated by landmark:**
a) Pubic tubercle
b) Inferior epigastric vessel
c) Inguinal ligament
d) None of the above

31. **Abnormal obturator artery creates a dangerous situation in the repair of**
a) Direct inguinal hernia
b) Indirect inguinal hernia
c) Femoral hernia
d) Obturator hernia

32. Exomphalos major should be operated at:
a) Birth
b) 3 months of age
c) 1 year
d) 3 years

33. Exomphalos is a disease involving:
a) Umbilicus
b) Cervix
c) Abdominal wall
d) Urinary bladder

34. The covering over an omphalocele is:
a) Skin
b) Amniotic membrane
c) Chorionic membrane
d) None of the above

35. Mayo's operation is done for:
a) Spigelian hernia
b) Femoral hernia
c) Richter's hernia
d) Umbilical hernia

36. Regarding gastroschisis and omphalocele, which one of the following is false
a) Umbilical cord is attached in normal position in gastroschisis.
b) Liver is the content of omphalocele.
c) Gastroschisis associated with multiple anomalies.
d) Intestinal obstruction is common in gastroschisis.

37. The hernia which often simulates a peptic ulcer is:
a) Umbilical hernia
b) Fatty hernia of the linea alba
c) Incisional hernia
d) Femoral hernia

38. Spigelian hernia is in:
a) Supraumbilical
b) Subumbilical
c) Paraumbilical
d) Lumbar

39. Which hernia occurs into pouch of Douglas?
a) Amyand's hernia
b) Beclard's hernia
c) Berger's hernia
d) Bladin's hernia

40. Ventral hernia is:
a) Inguinal hernia
b) Incisional hernia
c) Umbilical hernia
d) Femoral hernia

41. **Treatment of strangulated hernia is**
a) Observation
b) Immediate surgery
c) Manual reduction
d) Analgesia

42. **Cause of recurrent hernia:**
a) Infection
b) Absorbable sutures
c) Sliding hernia
d) Missed sac

43. **Richter's hernia is commonly associated with:**
a) Direct inguinal hernia
b) Femoral hernia
c) Indirect inguinal hernia
d) Obturator hernia

44. **Most common type of hernia in female is:**
a) Femoral
b) Inguinal
c) Ventral
d) Epigastric

45. **Which of the following does not differentiate between direct and indirect hernias:**
a) Direct inguinal hernia appears itself whenever the patient stands up.
b) Impulse on coughing is quite strong in direct inguinal hernia.
c) Direct inguinal hernia is prevented from appearance by pressing upon internal ring.
d) Direct inguinal hernia does not get strangulated commonly.

46. **Which of the following is of least importance as far as diagnosis of inguinal hernia is concerned?**
a) Impulse on coughing.
b) Herniation of abdominal viscera into scrotal sac.
c) The size of external inguinal ring.
d) All of the above.

47. **Which one of the following is incorrect about strangulated hernia:**
a) Sudden onset of pain in pre-existing hernia.
b) Forceful vomiting.
c) Tense and tender feeling of hernia.
d) Loss of expansile impulse on coughing.
e) History of recent regression in the size of hernia.

48. **Usually the inguinal hernia gets constricted due to:**
a) External abdominal ring.
b) Adhesions within the hernia sac.
c) Neck of the sac.
d) Narrowing of the inguinal canal.

49. During herniorrhaphy, the relation of the sac to the cord following mobilization is:

a)   Sac is anteromedial to the cord.

b)   Sac is posteromedial to the cord.

c)   Sac is anterolateral to the cord.

d)   Sac is posteolateral to the cord.

50. A patient is advised to avoid strenuous activity following herniorrhaphy for a period of:

a)   One day

b)   One week

c)   Six weeks

d)   Six months

e)   Three weeks

51. A hernia incarcerating only a portion of the lumen of intestine is known as:

a)   Obturator

b)   Richter

c)   Littre

d)   Hiatus

52. Which of the following is not true regarding inguinal canal?

a)   Its anterior wall is formed by external oblique muscle.

b)   Ileo-inguinal nerve passes through it.

c)   Internal oblique forms the outer 1/3rd of anterior wall.

d)   Conjoint tendon forms the inner 1/3rd of anterior wall.

53. Impulse on coughing is not present in which of the following:

a)   Uncomplicated femoral hernia.

b)   Varicocele of pampiniform plexus.

c)   Lipoma of the spermatic cord.

d)   Irreducible inguinal hernia.

54. Which of the following is true regarding hernias?

a)   Obstruction is more frequent in inguinal than femoral hernia.

b)   Pain in abdomen offers clue to diagnosis of obstructed hernia.

c)   Some inguinal hernias of infancy are cured spontaneously.

d)   Protrusion of viscus is through a weak area.

55. The common cause of strangulation of femoral hernia is:

a)   Sharp and crescent-shaped upper border of fossa ovalis.

b)   Many changes in the direction during its course.

c)   Tight neck formed by fascia transversalis.

d)   All of the above.

e)   None of the above.

56. The neck of a femoral hernia is situated:

a)   Above the inguinal ligament and lateral to pubic tubercle.

b)   Below the inguinal ligament and lateral to pubic tubercle.

c)   Above the inguinal ligament and medial to pubic tubercle.

d)   Below the inguinal ligament and medial to pubic tubercle.

e)   At mid-inguinal canal.

57. In an adult, major predisposing factor of hernia is:
a) Muscular weakness.
b) Neurological weakness.
c) Increased intra-abdominal pressure.
d) None of the above.

58. Obesity is the predisposing factor for:
a) Inguinal hernia.
b) Femoral hernia.
c) Paraumbilical hernia.
d) Obturator hernia.

59. Neuritic pain following herniorrhaphy is usually due to injury to:
a) Genito-femoral nerve.
b) Ilio-inguinal nerve.
c) Ilio-hypogastric nerve.
d) Any of the above.

60. Predisposing factors for incisional hernia is/are:
a) Old age
b) Obesity
c) Midline incision
d) Infection in operation wound
e) All of the above.

61. An umbilical hernia should preferably be operated:
a) Soon after birth.
b) At the age of two months.
c) At the age of two years.
d) After gaining adulthood.

62. Pregnancy is a causative factor of:
a) Epigastric hernia.
b) Inguinal hernia.
c) Femoral hernia.
d) Obturator hernia.

63. Ideal treatment for epigastric hernia is:
a) Use of abdominal belt.
b) Reduction in body weight.
c) Surgical repair.
d) None of the above.

64. Appearance of right direct inguinal hernia after appendicectomy is usually due to:
a) Post-operative weakness of abdominal muscles.
b) Gaping due to wound infection.
c) Injury to ileo-hypogastric and or ilio-inguinal nerve.
d) None of the above.

65. Which of the following is true about pantaloon hernia?
a) Bilateral direct inguinal hernia.
b) Bilateral indirect inguinal hernia.
c) Direct inguinal hernia on one side and indirect on the other side.
d) Both direct and indirect hernia on the same side.

66. The two limbs of a pantaloon sac are separated by:
a) Spermatic cord.
b) Superficial external pudendal vessels.
c) Obturator artery and vein.
d) Inferior epigastric vessels.

67. Regarding the use of truss in inguinal hernia, the pad of truss should press upon:
a) The external inguinal ring.
b) The internal inguinal ring.
c) The canal itself.
d) Any of the above.

68. During reduction of a devitalised bowel in strangulated inguinal hernia, the danger is that of:
 a) Rupture of bowel at fundus.
b) Rupture of sac at fundus.
c) Rupture of bowl at neck of sac.
d) None of the above.

69. Which of the following is not true regarding femoral hernia?
a) Posterior wall of femoral sheath is a continuation of fascia iliaca.
b) Anterior wall of femoral sheath is downward.
c) Posterior to the femoral ring is the horizontal pubic ramus.
d) It appears more frequently in males than females.

70. During operative reduction of strangulated inguinal hernia, the neck of sac should be divided in:
a) Upward and lateral directions.
b) Medial direction.
c) Lateral direction.
d) Upward and medial directions.

71. The complications of a hernia include:
a) Irreducibility.
b) Strangulation.
c) Inflammation.
d) All of the above.

72. Which of the following is contraindicated as a treatment for femoral hernia?
a) Operative reduction.
b) Conservative treatment.
c) Laparoscopic repair.
d) Tension-free repair.

73. Ventral hernia is also known as:
a) Inguinal hernia.
b) Femoral hernia.
c) Incisional hernia.
d) Obturator hernia.

74. An epigastric hernia is:
a) A fatty hernia of linea alba.
b) Divarication of abdominal muscles.
c) Same as umbilical hernia.
d) None of the above.

75. A paraumbilical hernia is:
a) Congenital.
b) Seen more commonly in women.
c) May get strangulated.
d) Seen more commonly in men.

76. The contents of an inguinal hernia sac may include:
a) Omentum.
b) Appendix.
c) Ovary
d) Meckel's diverticulum.
e) All of the above.
f) None of the above.

77. In a case of strangulated Richter's hernia:
a) A portion of the circumference of intestine is involved.
b) Vomiting is pathognomonic.
c) Absolute constipation is pathognomonic.
d) Severe pain is pathognomonic.

78. While operating upon a case of indirect inguinal hernia one should:
a) Use general anaesthesia.
b) Strengthen the internal inguinal ring in adults.
c) Do not operate if the patient is having chronic bronchitis.
d) Always use spinal anaesthesia.

79. A strangulated hernia is:
a) Tense.
b) Tender.
c) Irreducible.
d) To be operated immediately
e) All of the above.
f) None of the above.

80. Which of the following is not true regarding boundaries of inguinal canal?
a) Anteriorly – Fascia transversalis.
b) Posteriorly – Conjoined tendon.
c) Superiorly – Internal oblique.
d) Inferiorly – Inguinal ligament.

81. An obstructed hernia:
a) Is strangulated.
b) Can be caused by a truss.
c) Is irreducible.
d) Needs immediate operation
e) Both (b) and (c) are correct.

82. An inguinal hernia in female should be differentiated from:
a) Bartholin cyst.
b) Vaginal hydrocele.
c) Femoral hernia.
d) None of the above.

83. In strangulation of inguinal hernia:
a) Irreducibility of hernia is pathognomonic.
b) Reduction of herniated mass improved the situation.
c) The large intestine may be involved.
d) Omentum may be strangulated.
e) Urgent operation is required.

84. Which of the following is not true regarding paraumbilical hernia?
a) It is seen unusually in females.
b) Omentum in the sac is usually adherent.
c) It is often troubled by intertrigo.
d) It is unlikely to be strangulated.

85. An epigastric hernia:
a) Has a sac containing small intestine.
b) Is through linea semilunaris.
c) Requires Mayo's operation.
d) Commences as an extrusion of extraperitoneal fat.

85. What is parastomal hernia?[7]
a) Paravertebral hernia.
b) Paraumbilical hernia.
c) An incisional hernia related to abdominal wall stoma.
d) Pararectal hernia.

ANSWERS

1B	2B	3B	4A	5B	6D	7D	8A	9B	10B,E	11B
12A	13D	14A	15A	16C	17A	18D	19C	20C	21B	22C
23D	24A	25B	26D	27A	28A	29A	30A	31C	32A	33C
34B	35D	36A	37B	38B	39B	40B	41B	42B	43B	44B
45C	46C	47E	48B	49C	50C	51B	52A	53D	54D	55C
56B	57C	58C	59D	60E	61C	62D	63D	64C	65D	66D
67D	68D	69D	70B	71D	72B	73C	74A	75B	76E	77A
78B	79E	80A	81D	82C	83E	84C	85D	86C		

KEY POINT

"Surgeon like the captain of the ship or a pilot of an aircraft, is responsible for everything that happened."

-Francis D. Moore, (1913-2001)

REFERENCES

1. **Townsend CM,** *et al.,* (2005). Sabiston's textbook of surgery, 17th edition.
2. **Kirk RM.,** (2000). General Surgical operations, 4th edition.
3. **Doherty GM** *et al.,* (2002). The Washington manual of surgery, 3rd edition.
4. **Eric S.,** (2002). Wilson's surgery, A current clinical strategies medical book.
5. **Ghosal SR.,** (2005). Practical and viva in surgery, Elsevier.
6. **Brown P.,** (2005). Core topics in general and emergency surgery, 3rd edition.
7. **Israelsson LA.,** (2008). Parastomal hernias. *Surg. Clin. N. Am.*; 88, 113.

34 Epilogue

"Once you start studying medicine, you never get through with it."
— **Charles H. Mayo, 1865-1939**

WHAT IS THE FUTURE OF HERNIA?

The process of origin of human life on planet earth is studied by either of the following methods:
• Study of fossils
• Comparative study of anatomy and genetics in humans

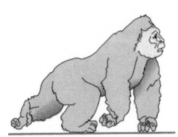

Fig. 34.1. Thousands of years back probably quadripedal species, used to have thick abdominal fascia to avoid abdominal wall hernias.

These studies have shown that human body has undergone a series of transformations and developments due to environmental threats and need to survive under those threats. According to Darwin's theory of evolution,[1] principle of survival of the fittest and "the show must go on" (genesis must not stop), body is forced to change itself to survive in the presence of threats and keep itself in optimum condition of reproduction.

Bipedal gait came with various changes in shape, size, strength and orientation of pelvis and groin areas which helped man to sustain bipedal posture, but also made him hernia prone (In Chapter 5: Aetiology of hernia, see hypothesis of aetiology of inguinal hernia, and hypothesis of aetiology of femoral hernia). The endoabdominal fascia must have been very thick and strong under anterior abdominal wall when humans had quadripedal posture. But it remained thin at groin as it was not required to be thick and strong in those days, as the groin was not affected by intra-abdominal pressure.

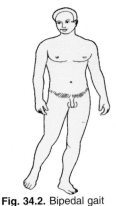

Fig. 34.2. Bipedal gait and erect posture will make groin tissues and fascia transversalis stronger in due course of time to avoid abdominal wall hernias.

Now the bipedal gait, upright posture, lifting of weight, running and the effects of gravity are putting strain on groin and making the groin susceptible to develop hernia.

Evolutionary changes like forward growth of iliac crests and thinning of origin of oblique muscles, make groin areas hernia susceptible, as these changes weaken the sphincteric action of inguinal canal.

Evolutionary changes will definitely make transversalis fascia and other layers in groin tougher and stronger in future.

To completely avoid hernia just wait for a few more million years.

> **KEY POINT**
>
> *Evolutionary changes will alter the future of hernia and its treatment.*

REFERENCE

Darwin CR., (1859). On the origin of species by means of natural selection.

Resources and Further Reading

"Reach what you can, my child......... Reach What you cannot"
— **Nikos Kazantzakis**

1. A concise text book of surgery, 3rd Edition, 2001, Das S.
2. A manual on Clinical Surgery, 6th edition, Das S, 2004, Das S.
3. A practical guide to operative surgery, 4th, Das S, 1999, Das S.
4. A textbook on Surgical Short Cases 2nd edition, Das S, 2000, Das S.
5. Abdominal Wall Hernias: Principles and Management, Bendavid R, 2001, New York: Springer.
6. Abernathy's Surgical Secrets, 4th edition, Harken AH, and Moore EE, 2000, Hanley and Belfus.
7. Abernathy's Surgical Secrets, 5th edition, Harken AH, and Moore EE, 2005. Hanley and Belfus.
8. An introduction to the Symptoms & Signs of Surgical Disease, 3rd edition, Browse NL, 1997, Arnold.
9. Atlas of Anatomy, Eagle editions, 2002.
10. Atlas of Hernia Surgery, Wantz GE, 1991, New York Raven Press.
11. Atlas of Human Anatomy, 3rd edition, Netter Frank H, 2003, ICON Learning System.
12. Bailey & Love's Short Practice of Surgery, 15th edition. Rains JH, Capper WM, 1971, HK Lewis & Co. Ltd.
13. Clinical and Operative Surgery, 3rd edition, Charry AY, 2007, Paras Publications.
14. Common Sense Emergency Abdominal Surgery, 2nd edition, Schein M, Rogers PN, 2005, Springer.
15. Comprehensive Laparoscopic Surgery, 1st edition, Kriplani A, Bhatia P, Prasad A, Govil D, Garg HP, 2007 IAGES.
16. Core Topics in General and Emergency Surgery, 3rd edition, Simon Paterson–Brown, 2005, Elsevier.
17. Current Review of Minimally Invasive surgery, Brooks DC, 1998, Springer.
18. Current Surgical Diagnosis & Treatment, 11th edition, Way LW, Doherty GM, 2003. McGraw Hill.
19. Endoscopic Repair of Abdominal Wall Hernias, 1st edition, Chowbey, Pradeep, 2004, Word Viva Publishers Pvt. Ltd.
20. Essential Anatomy, 11th edition, Snell RS, 2004, Churchill Livingstone.
21. Essential Surgery, 3rd edition, Burkitt HG, Quick CRG, 2001, Churchill Livingstone.
22. Essential Surgical Practice,4th edition, Cuschieri A, Steele RJC, Moossa AR, 2002, Arnold.
23. General Surgical Operations, 4th edition, Kirk RM, (2000), Churchill Livingstone.
24. Gray's anatomy for students Companion Workbook, 1st edition, Dark RL, Vogl W, Mitchell AWM, 2005, Elsevier.
25. Gray's Anatomy, 37th edition, Williams PL, Warwick R, Dyson M, Bannister LH, 1989, Churchill Livingstone.
26. Gray's Anatomy: the anatomical basis of clinical practice, 39th edition, Standring S, 2005, Edinburgh: Elsevier Churchill Livingstone.
27. Hernia repair; Open Vs Laparoscopic approaches, Maddern GJ, Hiatt JR, Philips EH, 1997, New York, Churchill Livingstone.
28. Hernias and Surgery of the abdominal wall, Chevrel JP, 1998, Berlin: Springer.
29. Human Anatomy, 4th edition, Chaurasia BD, 2004, CBS Publishers & Distributors.
30. Incisional Hernia, Schumpelick V, Kingsnorth AN, 1999, Berlin Heidelberg, Springer.
31. Inguinal Hernias: Advances and Controversies? Arregui M, Nagan R, 1994, Oxford Radcliffe Medical Press.

32. Laparoscopic Hernia Repair, A Step by Step approach, 1st edition, Bhatia P, John SJ, 2003, Global digital services.
33. Lee McGergor's Synopsis of surgical anatomy, 12th edition, Decker GAG, du Plessis DJ, 1986, John Wright & Sons Ltd.
34. Lee's Synopsis of anaesthesia, 13th edition, Davies NJH, Cashman JN, 2006, Elsevier.
35. Maingot's Abdominal Operations, 11th edition, Zinner MJ, Ashley SW, 2007, McGraw Hill.
36. Manipal Manual of Surgery, 2nd edition, Shenoy KR, 2005, CBS Publishers & Distributors.
37. Master of surgery, 4th edition, Baker RJ, Fischer JE, 2002, Philadelphia; Lippincott Williams & Wilkins.
38. Mastery of Surgery, 5th edition, Fischer JE, Bland KI, 2007, Lippincott Williams & Wilkins.
39. Medical Quotations 1st edition, Singh M, 2003, Sagar.
40. Modern Hernia Repair, Skandalakis L, Gadacz T, Mansberger A, 1996, New York: Perthenon.
41. New Procedures in open Hernia Surgery, Corcione Francesco, 2004, Springer.
42. Nyhus and Condon's Hernia, 5th edition, Fitzgibbons RJ, Jr. Greenburg AG, 2003, Philadelphia JB, Lippincott Co.
43. Princples of Laparoscopic Surgery: Basic and Advanced Techniques, Arregui ME, Fitzgibbons RJ, Katkhouda N, 1995, New York: Springer–Verlag.
44. Problems in General Surgery. Philadelphia: 1995, Lippincott-Raven Publications.
45. Prosthesis and Abdominal Wall Hernia, 1st edition, Austin, TX, 1994, RG Landes.
46. Prosthesis and Abdominal Wall hernias, Bendavid R, 1994, Austin (TX): RG Landes.
47. Sabiston textbook of Surgery, 24th edition, Townsend Jr. CM, Beauchamp RD, Evers BM, Mattox KL, 2004, Arnold.
48. Schwartz's Principles of Surgery, 8th edition, Brunicardi FC, Andersen DK, Billar, Dunn DL, Hunter JG, Pollock RE, 2005, McGraw Hill.
49. Skandalakis' Surgical Anatomy: The Embryologic and Anatomic Basis of Modern Surgery, Skandalakis JE, Colborn GL, Weidman TA, *et al.*, 2004, Athens, Greece: Paschalidis Medical Publication.
50. SRB's Manual of Surgery, 2nd edition, Bhat SR, 2007, JP.
51. Surgery Buster, Sharma D, & Sharma R, 2004, Jaypee.
52. Surgical Anatomy and Techniques-A Pocket Manual, 2nd edition, Skandalakis JE, Skandalakis PN, Skandalakis LJ, 2000, Springer.
53. Surgical Clinics of North America, 83, 2003.
54. Surgical Management of Abdominal Wall Hernias, Kurzer M, Kark AE, Wantz GE, 1998, London: Martin Dunitz.
55. The Association of the Surgeons of India Textbook of Surgery, 15th edition, Hai AH, Srivastava RB, 2003, Tata McGraw Hill Publication Company Ltd.
56. The New Airds Companion in Surgical Studies, 3rd edition, Burnand KG, Young AE, Lucas J, Rowlands BJ, & Scholefield J, 2005, Elsivier.
57. The SAGES Manual, 2nd edition, Scott-Conner CEH, 2006, Springer.
58. The Surgical Anatomy of the inguinal area, Skandalakis JE, Colborn GL, Gray SW, *et al.*, 1991, Contemp Surg.
59. The Washington Manual of Surgery, 4th edition, Klingensmith ME *et al.*, 2005, Lippincott Williams & Wilkins.
60. The Washington Manual of Surgery, 3rd edition, Doherty GM, *et al.*, 2002, Lippincott Williams & Wilkins.
61. Tips and Techniques in Laparoscopic Surgery, Jean Louis Dulucq, 2005, Springer.
62. Ultrapro Pamphlet by Ethicon.
63. Zollinger's Atlas of Surgical Operations, 8th edition, Zollinger Jr, Robert M, Zollinger Sr, Robert M, 2006, McGraw Hill.

Index